The Women's Health DATA BOOK

A Profile of Women's Health in the United States

Dawn Misra, Editor

Third Edition

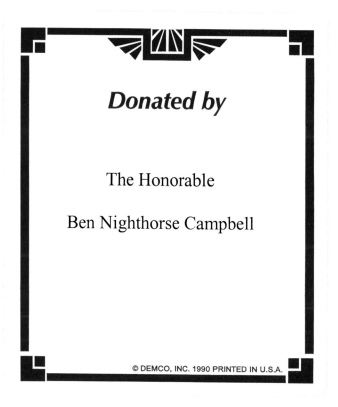

Donated by

The Honorable

Ben Nighthorse Campbell

Preface

As the field of women's health has evolved and grown, the breadth of information needed to understand its many dimensions is greater than ever. We live in the information age—a time of unprecedented access to data and information—yet we may lack the time to navigate through the many available sources of information or the expertise to judge which sources are the most reliable. With this new edition, the *Women's Health Data Book: A Profile of Women's Health in the United States* continues to offer readers current information gleaned from a host of sources on a variety of women's health issues ranging from contraceptive use to heart disease, from intimate partner violence to managed care.

Since the preparation of the first edition of the *Women's Health Data Book,* there have been many important accomplishments in the field of women's health. We now accept that women and men have different patterns of illness and care-seeking behavior, and can have different physiologic responses to health conditions and to medical treatments. Practically all federal agencies that oversee health care research and services now have staff dedicated to assuring attention to women's health issues. National data collection efforts have also improved, particularly with respect to domestic violence and adolescent health, and greater detail is now available from national surveys on health and health behaviors by gender, age, and race.

There are several new and exciting aspects to the third edition of the *Women's Health Data Book,* among them a new partnership between the Jacobs Institute of Women's Health and the Henry J. Kaiser Family Foundation. This collaboration permitted us to broaden the scope of the book, to improve the layout and presentation of data, and to make the information presented even more accessible to the reader. As in earlier editions, the goal of the third edition of the *Women's Health Data Book* is to provide readers with a current, comprehensive, and reliable compilation of data and trends on women's health in the United States.

New and notable in this edition is an introductory chapter on social factors that firmly establishes the link between women's health and the broader context of women's lives. Social roles as mothers and caregivers and membership in groups defined by race and ethnicity, age, income, education, employment, and marital status have profound effects on women's health status and access to and use of health services. Subsequent chapters use this lens to offer detailed information on how these factors relate to specific health indicators.

With more women living longer and with improved therapies for life-threatening or debilitating diseases, access to health care services and individual health behaviors play an increasingly important role in determining women's quality of life. We have expanded the focus of chapter 6 on health behaviors to include data on diet and exercise, and broadened the scope of chapter 8 on access, utilization, and quality of health care. New topics include preventive health services, physician counseling, and a discussion of quality measurement.

New material in chapter 2 on reproductive health includes information on chronic but non-life-threatening conditions such as endometriosis and uterine fibroids. Although, these conditions affect large numbers of women with serious implications for their quality of life, data are scarce. Chapter 5 on mental health has been revised and updated with new analyses of studies on mental health problems among women. Unfortunately, no new nationally representative prevalence studies on mental health have been conducted for more than 20 years, a serious gap in the information available on a topic vital to women and society.

Major gaps also remain in our understanding of differences in health conditions and access to care among subgroups of women. Unfortunately, there is frequently a significant lag time in publication of data and details on minority groups such as Native Americans and Asian/Pacific Islanders are often lacking. While disparities are widely acknowledged, progress documenting and addressing them has been painfully slow.

Although the authors have attempted to be inclusive, not every women's health topic could be addressed. Data and space limitations necessitated difficult choices. Nevertheless, we hope that health care providers, policymakers, researchers, writers, teachers, and students will find this volume a useful resource in their work and one they consult frequently. As always, we welcome readers' suggestions for future editions of this book.

We would like to extend a special thank you to some of the many individuals who made this *Women's Health Data Book* a reality. First and foremost, we would like to express our heartfelt appreciation to the new principal author, Dawn Misra, Ph.D., who stepped into the giant shoes of her predecessor and editor of the first two editions, Jacqueline Horton, Sc.D., and ably filled them. She is to be commended for thoughtfully building on the structure of the two previous editions, while expanding into new areas to take into account new data and emerging issues in women's health. We would also like to extend a special thank you to Zoë Beckerman of the Kaiser Family Foundation for her critical role though the entire review and publication process.

Martha C. Romans
Executive Director
Jacobs Institute of Women's Health

Alina Salganicoff, Ph.D.
Vice President and Director
Women's Health Policy
Henry J. Kaiser Family Foundation

Editor's Acknowledgments

This book represents the contributions of many people who served as coauthors, researchers, reviewers, and editors. I would like to extend a special thank you to my collaborators on each of the chapters who are listed on page vi. I would also like to express my appreciation to the reviewers who generously gave their time and effort to provide external reviews of the materials in each chapter. Specifically, I would like to thank Bill Andrews, Douglas Ball, Fred Brancati, Carol Bruce, Charlyn Cassady, Willard Cates, Laura Caufield, Gary Chase, Louis Floyd, Francis Giardiello, Mary Goodwin, Juliette Kendrick, Karen McDonnell, Roberta Ness, Patricia O'Campo, Robert Park, Melissa Perry, Mary Rogers, Jonathan Samet, Ulonda Shamwell, Cheryl Warner, Carol Weisman, Lynn Wilcox, and Sara Wilcox for their efforts to assure the material included was as accurate as possible.

I would like to acknowledge the individuals who provided much needed data and other relevant information: Linda Bartlett, Trude Bennett, Cynthia Berg, Kate Brett, Ronald Brookmeyer, Holly Grason, Jennifer Madans, and Carol Weisman. Many colleagues at Johns Hopkins, too numerous to name, also provided support and advice throughout the writing of this book.

My graduate research assistants, Patti Ephraim, Ruby Nguyen, and Anjel Vahratian, made invalu-able contributions to this project, assisting me with the collection and synthesis of data and the writing of the text. Amy Jacobs, a research assistant at the Jacobs Institute, carefully reviewed all references and tracked down needed data and sources in the final stages of editing. I also thank my administrative assistant, Elizabeth Curry, for her many careful readings of the book and excellent work in preparing figures and tables throughout the book. I was also fortunate to have the able assistance of Melissa Hawkins in the final stages of work on this book. I thank her for her dedication to completing this project. I would also like to express my appreciation to Jane Stein and her staff at The Stein Group for their editorial assistance and management of the production process.

Finally, I thank Martha Romans at the Jacobs Institute of Women's Health and Alina Salganicoff and Zoë Beckerman at the Henry J. Kaiser Family Foundation for providing me with this opportunity and for their support and guidance throughout the process. This was an extremely gratifying project in many respects because of the pleasure of working with these individuals.

Dawn Misra, Ph.D., Editor

The Women's Health Data Book:
A Profile of Women's Health in the United States
Third Edition

Contributors

(in Alphabetical Order)

Chapter 1:
Impact of Social and Economic Factors on Women's Health

Holly Grason, Cynthia Minkovitz, Dawn Misra, Donna Strobino

Chapter 2:
Perinatal and Reproductive Health

Patty Ephraim, Melissa Hawkins, Dawn Misra, Ruby Nguyen, Kendra Rothert, Donna Strobino, Anjel Vahratian

Chapter 3:
Infections

Ruby Nguyen, Dawn Misra, Anjel Vahratian

Chapter 4:
Chronic Conditions

Patty Ephraim, Dawn Misra, Ruby Nguyen, Anjel Vahratian

Chapter 5:
Mental Health

Courtney Denning Johnson, Dawn Misra

Chapter 6:
Health Behaviors

Patty Ephraim, Dawn Misra, Donna Strobino, Anjel Vahratian

Chapter 7:
Violence Against Women

Nancy Berglas, Dawn Misra

Chapter 8:
Access, Utilization and Quality of Health Care

Zoë Beckerman, Melissa Hawkins, Dawn Misra, Alina Salganicoff, Roberta Wyn

Contents

Figures

Tables

Chapter 5 Mental Health (no tables)

Chapter 6 Health Behaviors

Chapter 7 Violence Against Women

Chapter 8 Access, Utilization, and Quality of Health Care

The Women's Health

DATA BOOK

A Profile of Women's Health in the United States

Third Edition

Chapter 1

Impact of Social and Economic Factors on Women's Health

Contents

Introduction

This chapter explores the social context of women's health in the United States. Within the arena of public health, various frameworks have been used to understand women's health. The dominant model has been biomedical with a focus on the prevention, detection, and treatment of disease. The emphasis frequently has been on individual responsibility for personal health behaviors (e.g., smoking, diet) and medical care (e.g., annual Pap smear, prenatal care). Biomedical models have helped improve public health but have neglected the influence of the social context of women's lives.

Recently, however, there have been efforts to broaden the biomedical framework by considering social factors. Some have called for a fundamental shift to a framework that models the underlying social dynamics of what actually produces health for different groups of women.[1] The third edition of *The Women's Health Data Book* does just that: It provides an expanded model that builds upon the most up-to-date *biomedical and social data*. This expanded biomedical model relies upon data on individual-level factors, such as education attainment, and on group-level or social factors, such as the male-female income gap. Subsequent chapters consider social factors as they relate to specific health conditions and causes of death.

Social Context of Women's Health

The social context of women's health covered in this section includes several interrelated factors: age, race/ethnicity, women's status, social class, and family and household.

Age

Currently, nearly 140 million girls and women live in the United States. Figure 1-1 shows the distribution of U.S. adult women (103.8 million) by age

Figure 1-1

U.S. women by age, 1998

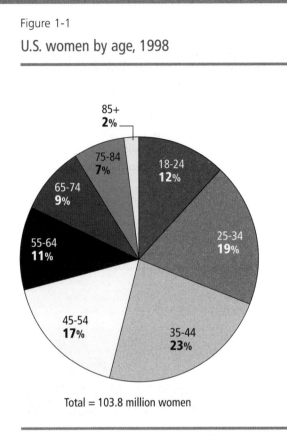

Total = 103.8 million women

Source: Henry J. Kaiser Family Foundation estimates based on Urban Institute analyses of the March 1999 Current Population Survey, U.S. Bureau of the Census. Includes women aged 18 years and older.

Figure 1-2

U.S. women by race/ethnicity, 1998

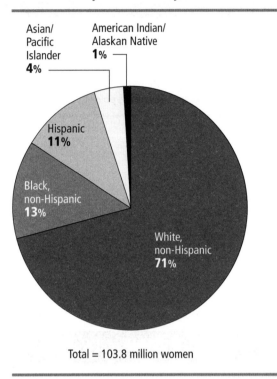

Total = 103.8 million women

Source: Henry J. Kaiser Family Foundation estimates based on Urban Institute analyses of the March 1999 Current Population Survey, U.S. Bureau of the Census. Includes women aged 18 years and older.

for 1998. The majority of U.S. women are between 15 and 44 years old, considered to be of reproductive age. Over the next 50 years, however, this distribution will shift toward an increasingly older U.S. female population. Since 1950, the number of women aged 65 or older has tripled from 6.5 million in 1950 to more than 20 million in 1998. By July 2020, the U.S. Bureau of the Census estimates that this number will exceed 29 million and represent close to one-fifth of the total female population, and, by 2050, there will be more than 42 million women aged 65 years or older, accounting for 21% of the total female population.[2] The rise is due in part to an increase in life expectancy for women (see chapter 4), but it primarily results from the aging of the baby boom population born between 1946 and 1964. The aging of the female population is likely to result in increasing numbers

of women living longer but with more chronic illnesses and functional disabilities.

Race/Ethnicity

The U.S. female population is also ethnically diverse (Figure 1-2). Although the population growth rate is greatest for Asians, the growth in absolute numbers is greatest for Hispanic women because the Hispanic population is considerably larger than the Asian population in the United States. Hispanic women currently constitute about 11% of the female population, but estimates indicate that they will make up 16% by 2020 and 24% by 2050.[2] They will constitute a greater proportion of women of childbearing ages (see chapter 2) because the Hispanic population is younger than other ethnic groups. The Asian female population is expected to rise from 4% of the total population

Table 1-1

U.S. population aged 18 years and older by gender and poverty level, 1998

Income as a proportion of federal poverty level	Female (Total=103.8 million)		Male (Total=95.1 million)	
	Number (x1 million)	Percent	Number (x1 million)	Percent
Poor (<100% FPL*)	13.8	13	8.2	9
Near-poor (100-199% FPL)	19.1	18	14.6	15
Non-poor (≥200% FPL)	70.9	68	72.4	76

Note: Details may not add to totals due to rounding.
*FPL is the federal poverty level, which was $16,660 for a family of four in 1998.
Source: Henry J. Kaiser Family Foundation estimates based on Urban Institute analyses of the March 1999 Current Population Survey, U.S. Bureau of the Census.

Table 1-2

U.S. women aged 18 years and older by race/ethnicity and poverty level, 1998

Race/ethnicity	Total	Poor (<100% FPL*)		Near-poor (100-199% FPL)		Non-poor (≥200% FPL)	
	Number (x1 million)	Number (x1 million)	Percent	Number (x1 million)	Percent	Number (x1 million)	Percent
White, non-Hispanic	76.1	7.1	9	12.3	16	56.7	75
Black, non-Hispanic	12.7	3.4	27	3.1	24	6.2	49
Hispanic	10.3	2.7	26	2.9	28	4.7	46
Asian/Pacific Islander	4.0	0.5	13	0.6	15	2.8	71
American Indian/ Alaskan Native	0.7	0.1	21	0.1	19	0.4	60

Note: Details may not add to totals due to rounding.
*FPL is the federal poverty level, which was $16,660 for a family of four in 1998.
Source: Henry J. Kaiser Family Foundation estimates based on Urban Institute analyses of the March 1999 Current Population Survey, U.S. Bureau of the Census.

in 1996 to 6% in 2020 and close to 9% in 2050. It is estimated that non-Hispanic white women, who currently account for more than 70% of the female population, will make up 60% of the population in 2030 and only 35% in 2050.[2]

Figure 1-3

U.S. women's participation in the labor force, 1950–1998

Percent participating

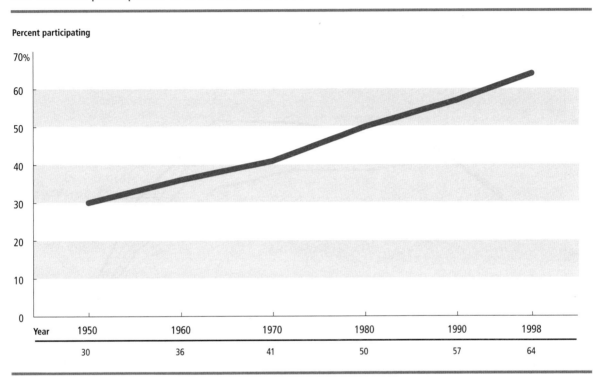

Year	1950	1960	1970	1980	1990	1998
	30	36	41	50	57	64

Source: Wagener D, Walstedt J, Jenkins L, Burnett C, Lalich N, Fingerhut M. Women: Work and health. Vital Health Stat 1997;3(31). U.S. Bureau of the Census. Work experience of the population (annual): Current Population Survey. Washington: U.S. Department of Labor; 1999.

Women's Status

Social factors related to gender may influence a woman's health. In 1998, the Institute for Women's Policy Research compiled data for each U.S. state on indicators of women's status in four areas: political participation and representation; employment and earnings; economic autonomy; and reproductive rights.[3,4,5,6,7] For each area, a composite index was derived from a set of component indicators. For example, the employment and earnings composite index was based on four indicators of women's economic status: women's earnings, the female/male income ratio, women's representation in managerial and professional jobs, and women's participation in the labor force. Generally, the four indices were highly correlated.[8] Stated another way, women tended either to fare well across all four areas or to fare poorly across all four areas, depending upon which state was examined.

Seeking to uncover the societal-level determinants of women's health, researchers have used data from the composite indices to examine the effect of women's status on women's overall and cause-specific mortality and on activity limitations.[8] As income distribution and poverty rates also are valid predictors of mortality and morbidity, analyses were adjusted to control for these factors. The political participation and economic autonomy composite indices were both inversely correlated with total female mortality, that is, there were fewer deaths among women as they participated politically and had greater economic autonomy. Higher scores on the political participation, economic autonomy, and employment and earnings composite indices were also significantly related with fewer self-reported days of activity limitation among women.[8]

Figure 1-4

Women's labor force participation rates by age, 1960–1996 and projected 2000 and 2005*

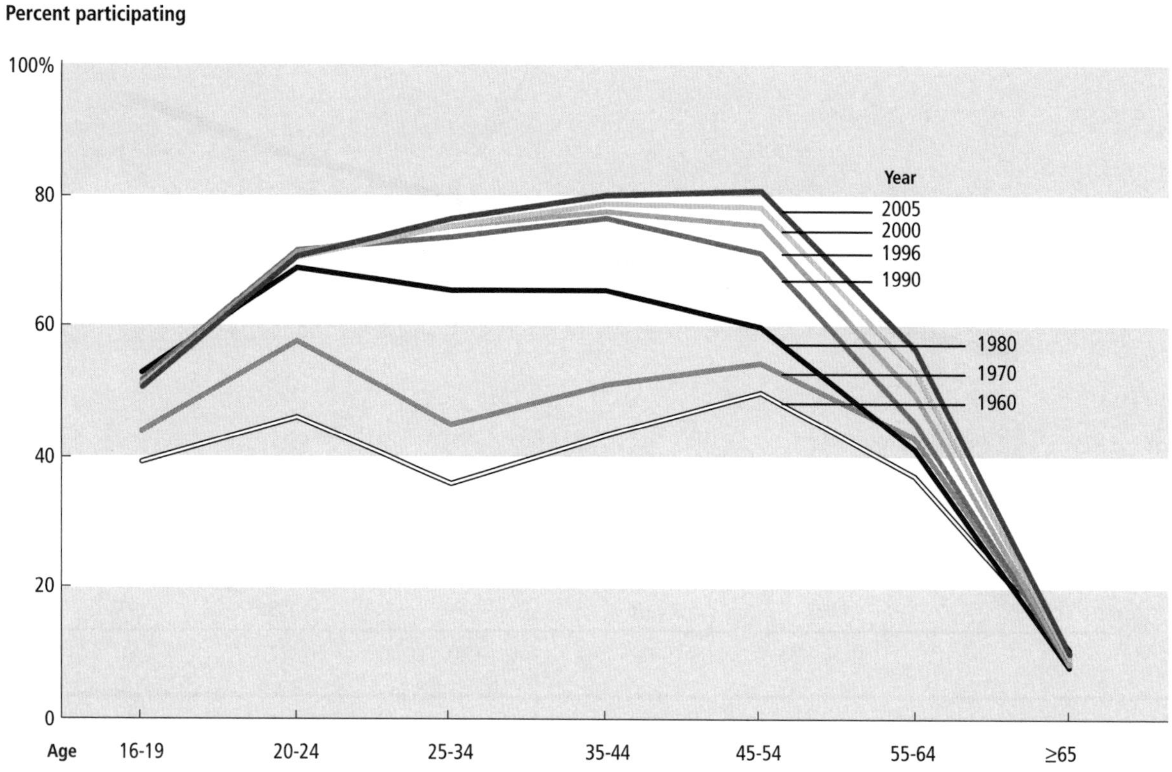

Percent participating

Age	16-19	20-24	25-34	35-44	45-54	55-64	≥65
1960	39.3	46.1	36.0	43.4	49.9	37.2	10.8
1970	44.0	57.7	45.0	51.1	54.4	43.0	9.7
1980	52.9	68.9	65.5	65.5	59.9	41.3	8.1
1990	51.8	71.6	73.6	76.5	71.2	45.3	8.7
1996	51.3	71.3	75.2	77.5	75.4	49.6	8.6
2000	51.2	70.5	75.3	78.7	78.2	53.4	9.5
2005	50.7	70.7	76.4	80.0	80.7	56.6	10.2

* Civilian women aged 16 years and older. Labor force participants as a percentage of all women in age group.

Source: Bureau of Labor Statistics. Handbook of labor statistics. Table 5. Washington: U.S. Department of Labor; 1989. Bureau of Labor Statistics. Labor force projections: the baby boom moves on. Table 3. Mon Labor Rev 1991 Nov. Bureau of Labor Statistics. The 2005 labor force: growing but slowly. Table 10. Mon Labor Rev 1995 Nov. Bureau of Labor Statistics. Employment and earnings, January 1997. Tables 2 and 3. Bureau of Labor Statistics; February 29, 1997. Available from: URL: http://stats.bls.gov.

Social Class

Social class has profound effects on health and is certainly influenced by gender. Employment, education, and income represent different dimensions of social class. Across racial/ethnic groups, women are more likely than men to live

Figure 1-5

Mothers in U.S. labor force by age of children, 1975–1997

Percent of mothers in labor force

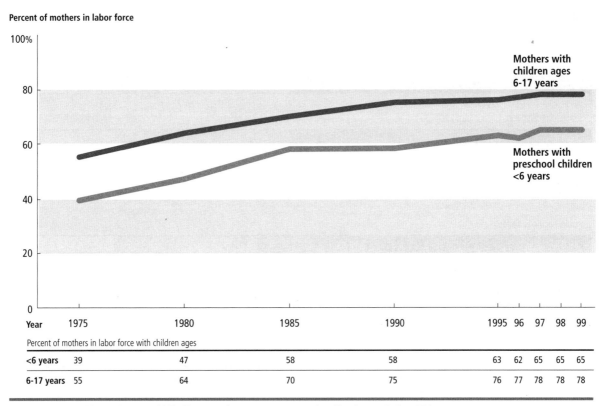

Year	1975	1980	1985	1990	1995	96	97	98	99
Percent of mothers in labor force with children ages									
<6 years	39	47	58	58	63	62	65	65	65
6-17 years	55	64	70	75	76	77	78	78	78

Source: Maternal and Child Health Bureau. Child health USA. Washington: U.S. Department of Health and Human Services; 1998

in poverty (Table 1-1). Table 1-2 describes the number and percentage of U.S. adult women living in poverty by race/ethnicity. Black (non-Hispanic) and Hispanic women are the most likely to be poor (approximately 25%) but most women living in poverty are white (approximately 7 million women).

In the last half of the twentieth century, there was a dramatic rise in the formal labor force participation by women of all ages in the United States, but the trend is strongest among young women. The percentage of women aged 16 or older participating in the formal labor force nearly doubled from 30% in 1950 to 57% in 1990 (Figure 1-3); it reached 64% in 1998, representing approximately 63 million employed

women.[9] The rate of labor force participation more than doubled for women aged 25–34 from 1960 to 2000 (Figure 1-4).[3,4,5,6,7] In addition, although in 1960, rates of labor force participation were lowest among women in their twenties and early thirties, when women were caring for young children in their homes, this pattern had largely disappeared by 1980.[3,4,5,6,7] In 1999, 65% of women with children under 6 years of age and 78% of women with children 6–17 years of age worked in the formal labor force (Figure 1-5).[10]

Although the labor force participation rate has increased among all women since 1980, the increase has been greater for whites than for blacks or Hispanics. From 1990 to 1994, the employment rate continued to climb for white

Figure 1-6

Educational attainment of women aged 25 years or older by race/ethnicity, 1998

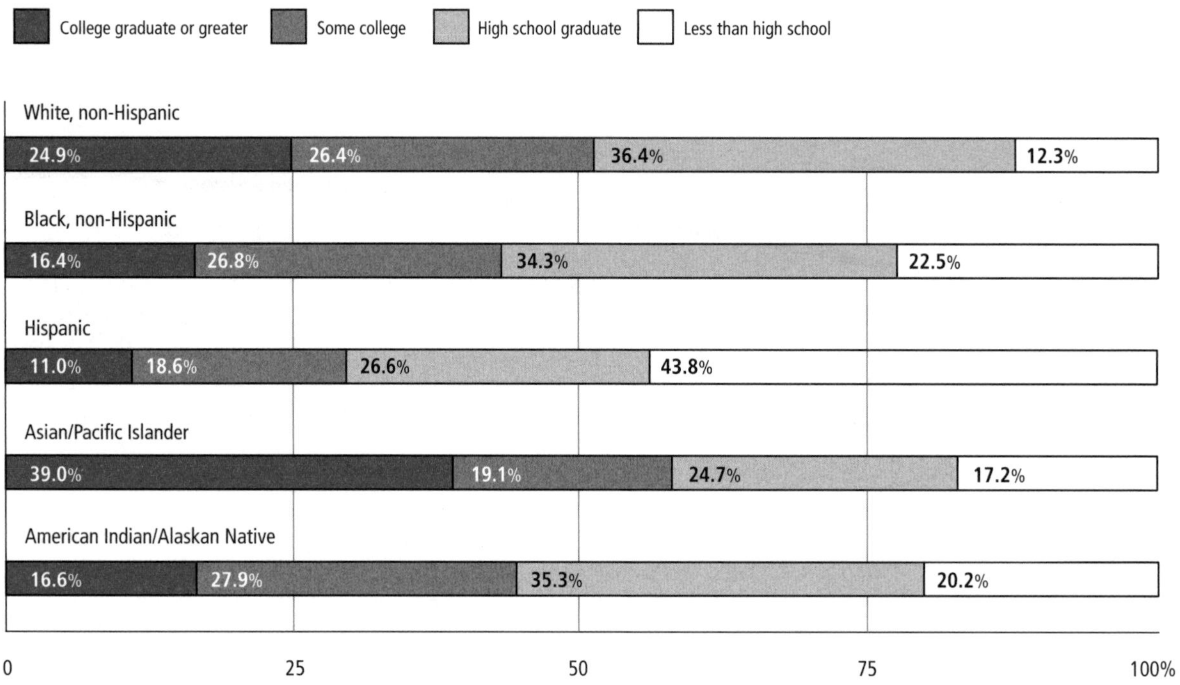

■ College graduate or greater   ■ Some college   ■ High school graduate   □ Less than high school

White, non-Hispanic

| 24.9% | 26.4% | 36.4% | 12.3% |

Black, non-Hispanic

| 16.4% | 26.8% | 34.3% | 22.5% |

Hispanic

| 11.0% | 18.6% | 26.6% | 43.8% |

Asian/Pacific Islander

| 39.0% | 19.1% | 24.7% | 17.2% |

American Indian/Alaskan Native

| 16.6% | 27.9% | 35.3% | 20.2% |

0   25   50   75   100%

Source: Henry J. Kaiser Family Foundation estimates based on Urban Institute analyses of the March 1999 Current Population Survey, U.S. Bureau of the Census.

and black women but it stabilized for Hispanic women and dropped for Asian American women. Employment rates in 1994 were similar across racial and ethnic categories, but slightly lower proportions of Asian American (56.3%) and Hispanic (52.9%) women were employed in the formal labor force.[9]

The industries where women work have also changed dramatically since 1950. Women are more likely now to work in finance (4.8% in 1950 versus 8.5% in 1994), business (1.0% versus 4.7%), and professional industries (17.1% versus 35.3%) and are less likely to work in manufacturing (23.1% versus 11.4%) and personal services (14.6% versus 5.3%).[9] With these changes also come potential increases in exposures to hazardous job conditions. Twenty-three

percent of currently employed women indicate that they have been exposed to substances at work that were, in their opinion, potentially harmful. Many employed women also have jobs with high physical demands that may stress the body. In 1988, more than one-third of women reported spending more than 4 hours per day in activities involving bending or twisting of the hands or wrists. More than 40% of women reported some time spent in repeated bending, twisting, or reaching activities in the workplace.[9]

As labor force participation has risen among American women, so have their educational levels. Moreover, the gap between black and white women with regard to completion of secondary education is closing. Figure 1-6 describes the educational attainment in 1998 for women 25 years and older by race/ethnicity. Although black women historically have had lower educational achievement than white women, 88% of white women and 77% of black women aged 25 years or older in 1998 had completed a high school education. Hispanic women lagged behind all other groups of women; only 56% aged 25 years or older had completed high school in 1998.[11]

A gender gap in education has historically favored men, but this trend actually reversed in recent years, and women are now slightly more likely to complete college than men (Figure 1-7). In 1997, women were 10% more likely to have earned a bachelor's degree than men, whereas in 1970 they were only about two-thirds as likely to have attained one.[11] Education also has implications for health behaviors. As will be seen in

Figure 1-7

Attainment of bachelor's degree, U.S. women and men aged 25–29 years, 1970 and 1998

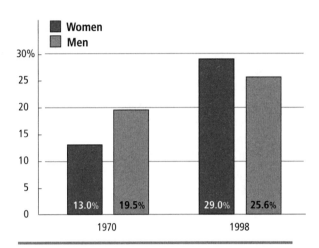

Source: Day J, Curry A. Educational attainment in the United States: March 1998. Washington: U.S. Bureau of the Census; 1998.

Figure 1-8

Income gap for U.S. women and men by age, 1996

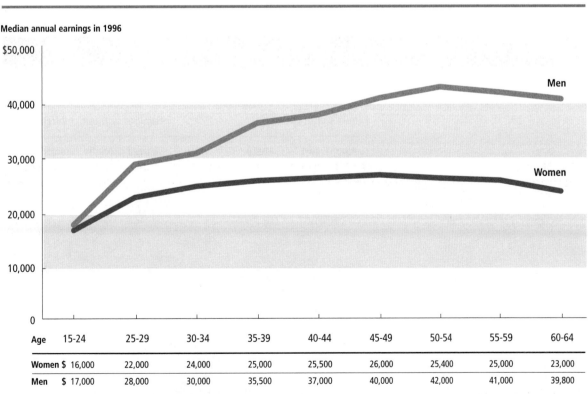

Age	15-24	25-29	30-34	35-39	40-44	45-49	50-54	55-59	60-64
Women $	16,000	22,000	24,000	25,000	25,500	26,000	25,400	25,000	23,000
Men $	17,000	28,000	30,000	35,500	37,000	40,000	42,000	41,000	39,800

Source: Bureau of Labor Statistics. Highlights of women's earnings in 1998, Report 928. Washington: U.S. Department of Labor; 1999. Available from: URL: http://stats.bls.gov/cpswom98.htm.

chapter 6, women who have less education are less likely to engage in health promoting behaviors and more likely to engage in unhealthy behaviors such as smoking.

Despite the advances in education for women and their increased participation in the labor force, women still earn less than men, although the gap in wages has narrowed slightly. Women earned only 76% of men's median earnings in 1998, when earnings are adjusted for education. This represents a narrowing of the wage gap by 11.9% between 1979 and 1997. Unfortunately, this change has been attributed to a decline in men's wages rather than a real rise in women's wages. The gap in women's earnings relative to men's increases with age (Figure 1-8).[12] A gap in earnings is also evident for black women relative to white women at all educational levels, although differences are greatest for women with the lowest levels of education.[11]

Family and Household

Women in the United States are marrying later in life, and the average age of women having their first child has risen from 21.3 years in 1969 to 24.4 years in 1994 (see chapter 2). These changes have been accompanied by a rise in single parent households, the majority of which are headed by women.[13] Table 1-3 describes the distribution of family structure and of adult women by race/ethnicity. Among women with children, Hispanic and Asian/Pacific Islander women are the most likely to report being in a two-parent household and whites and blacks are the least likely to report this arrangement. Black women with children, however, are the most likely to report living in multigenerational/other household structure. High divorce rates are a primary reason for the rise in female-headed households, with an increase in childbearing outside of marriage only of secondary importance.[13] Women-headed households have

Table 1-3

U.S. women aged 18 years and older by household type and race/ethnicity, 1998

| | | Percent | | | | | |
| | | Families with children | | | Families without children | | |
Race/Ethnicity	Total	Single parent	Two parents	Multi-generational/other	Married couple	Adults alone	Adults living together
Total	103.8 million	9	28	5	31	15	12
White, non-Hispanic	76.1 million	6	28	3	35	16	11
Black, non-Hispanic	12.7 million	21	18	12	16	16	16
Hispanic	10.3 million	14	38	9	20	7	13
Asian/Pacific Islander	4.0 million	5	40	4	30	8	13
American Indian/ Alaskan Native	0.7 million	14	27	7	24	10	17

Note: Rows may not total 100% due to rounding.

Source: Henry J. Kaiser Family Foundation estimates based on Urban Institute analyses of the March 1999 Current Population Survey, U.S. Bureau of the Census.

Table 1-4

U.S. median family income by household type, 1997

Type of household	Median family income
Female-headed	$23,040
Male-headed	$36,634
Married couple	$51,681

Source: U.S. Bureau of the Census. Money income in the United States, 1997 (with separate data on valuation of noncash benefits). Washington: U.S. Bureau of the Census; 1998.

a distinct economic disadvantage relative to households headed by men or married couple households (Table 1-4).[14]

Mothers not employed in the formal labor force ("stay-at-home" mothers) likely shoulder the bulk of the responsibility for child care in their households, particularly in women-headed households without another adult. Nevertheless, the majority of women with children, even young children, are employed. This trend towards employment of mothers does not necessarily imply that women are no longer the primary caregiver for their children. Mothers who work may still provide and be responsible for care of children even in two-parent households.

As with the care of young children, the responsibility of caregiving for a sick or disabled family member (e.g., child, spouse, or parent) more often falls to women than men. Based on data from the 1998 Commonwealth Fund Survey of Women's Health, 9% of women as compared to 4% of men in the United States provide care for a sick or disabled relative.[15] This gender gap exists although most working-age women are employed outside the home. The proportion of

women providing care is likely to rise in future years as the U.S. population ages and as life expectancy continues to increase. Women between 45 and 64 years of age are the most likely to provide caregiving.[15] Women who are married are more likely (11%) than single (8%) or divorced, separated, or widowed women (7%) to be caregivers.[15] Approximately equal proportions of women above (9%) and below (11%) the national median income ($35,000 per year) are caregivers.

Nevertheless, there are large differences by income for more intensive involvement in caregiving (Table 1-5). Among women caregivers, more than half of those with incomes at or below the median provide more than 20 hours of care per week as compared with less than one-third of women caregivers with incomes

Table 1-5

Women caring for sick or disabled family member, 1998

	Percent		
	All women	Income $35,000 or less	Income above $35,000
Percent of women who are currently caregivers	9	11	9
Percent of women caregivers who:			
Provide more than 20 hours of care per week	43	52	29
Provide care to a relative living with them	51	62	36
Have some paid home health care or assistance	24	18	35

Source: Collins K, Schoen C, Joseph S, Duchon L, Simantov E, Yellowitz M. Health concerns across a woman's lifespan: The Commonwealth Fund 1998 Survey of Women's Health. New York: The Commonwealth Fund; 1999.

above the median. Fewer than one in five women caregivers in the lower income group have some paid assistance as compared with one in three of the women caregivers in the higher income group.[15] Caregiving may have important detrimental effects on a woman's health. Those with caregiving responsibilities are less likely to practice preventive health behaviors.[16] In recent studies, those who provide caregiving also had lower levels of immunity[17] and greater cardiovascular reactivity.[18] Caregiving may even increase a woman's risk of death. In the caregiver health effects study, a substudy of a population-based study of the elderly, caregivers who were experiencing mental or emotional strain related to their role had a 63% increase in mortality during the 4-year follow-up period. In contrast, however, there was no increased risk among caregivers who were not experiencing strain or among spouses who had a disabled spouse for whom they did not provide care.[19]

In addition to caregiving roles, women often carry the primary burden of household maintenance. The juggling and interaction of women's multiple roles (work outside of the home, work at home, child rearing, family and marital relationships) may have significant implications for women's health—both positive and negative. Health scientists and policy makers are currently examining this topic.[20,21]

Conclusion

The social context of women's lives in the United States has changed enormously over the past half-century. Women are more likely than ever to complete high school and college and to work outside the home. Paralleling these trends, women are marrying later and delaying their first births. Despite these gains, some inequalities persist: the male-female wage gap and the disproportionate responsibility of women for caregiving, for example. Finally, demographic trends toward an increasingly aged and ethnically diverse population of U.S. women are likely to continue into this new century. These changes will likely affect women's health and influence the way that women's health needs are addressed. Furthermore, the social context of women's lives is an important influence and determinant of women's health and should be incorporated into biomedical models.

References

1. Ruzek, SB, Clarke AE, Olesen, VL. Social, biomedical, and feminist models of women's health. In: Ruzek, SB, Olesen, VL, Clarke, AE, editors. Women's health: complexities and differences. Ohio: Ohio State University Press; 1997.

2. National Center for Health Statistics. Health, United States, 1998. Hyattsville (MD): U.S. Department of Health and Human Services; 1998.

3. Bureau of Labor Statistics. Handbook of labor statistics, 1989. Table 5. Washington: U.S. Department of Labor; 1989.

4. Bureau of Labor Statistics. Labor force projections: the baby boom moves on. Table 3. Mon Labor Rev 1991 Nov.

5. Bureau of Labor Statistics. The 2005 labor force: growing but slowly. Table 10. Mon Labor Rev 1995 Nov.

6. Bureau of Labor Statistics. Employment and earnings. Tables 2 and 3. 1997 Jan. Available from: URL: http://stats.bls.gov.

7. Bureau of Labor Statistics. Bureau Website. 1997 Feb. Available from: URL: http://stats.bls.gov.

8. Kawachi I, Kennedy B, Gupta V, Prothrow-Stith D. Women's status and the health of women and men: a view from the states. In: Kawachi I, Kennedy B, Wilkinson R, editors. The society and population health reader: income inequality and health. New York: The New Press; 1999:474–491.

9. Wagener D, Walstedt J, Jenkins L, Burnett C, Lalich N, Fingerhut M. Women: work and health. Vital Health Stat 3 1997;3:1–16.

10. Maternal and Child Health Bureau. Child health USA, 1996–1997. Rockville (MD): U.S. Department of Health and Human Services; 1998.

11. Day J, Curry A. Educational attainment in the United States: March 1997. Number P20–505. Washington: U.S. Bureau of the Census; 1998.

12. Bureau of Labor Statistics. Highlights of women's earnings in 1998. Washington: U.S. Department of Labor; 1999.

13. Saluter A. Marital status and living arrangements. Number P20–496. Washington: U.S. Bureau of the Census; 1998.

14. U.S. Bureau of the Census. Money income in the United States: 1997 (with separate data on valuation of noncash benefits). Washington: The Bureau; 1998.

15. Collins K, Schoen C, Joseph S, Duchon L, Simantov E, Yellowitz M. Health concerns across a woman's lifespan: The Commonwealth Fund 1998 survey of women's health. New York: The Commonwealth Fund; 1999.

16. Schulz R, Newsom J, Mittelmark M, Burton L, Hirsch C, Jackson S. Health effects of caregiving: the Caregiver Health Effects Study: an ancillary study of the Cardiovascular Health Study. Ann Behav Med 1997;19:110–116.

17. Kiecolt-Glaser J, Glaser R, Gravenstein S, Malarkey W, Sheridan J. Chronic stress alters the immune response to influenza virus vaccine in older adults. Proc Natl Acad Sci USA 1996; 93:3043–3047.

18. King AC, Oka RK, Young DR. Ambulatory blood pressure and heart rate responses to the stress of work and caregiving in older women. J Gerontol 1994;94:M239–245.

19. Schulz R, Beach SR. Caregiving as a risk factor for mortality: the Caregiver Health Effects Study. JAMA 1999;282:2215–2219.

20. Waldron I, Weiss CC, Hughes ME. Interacting effects of multiple roles on women's health. J Health Soc Behav 1998;39:216–236.

21. Ross CE, Mirowsky J. Does employment affect health? J Health Soc Behav 1995;36:230–243.

Chapter 2

Perinatal and Reproductive Health

Contents

Introduction

Women's health has been expanded in recent years beyond the traditional emphasis on reproductive health to include other health and lifestyle issues relevant to women. Notwithstanding, reproductive health plays a critical role in women's overall physical, social, and psychological well-being. Decisions regarding pregnancy and childbearing, in particular, have both a personal and larger social impact ranging from the demographic characteristics of the population to policy makers' health care decisions. This chapter reviews and describes perinatal and reproductive trends in the United States in the last several decades.

Natality

Women of Childbearing Age

Between 1988 and 2000, the overall number of women of childbearing age (15–44 years) increased 3.8% to 60.1 million women (Table 2-1). The number of teenagers remained relatively stable at approximately 9.5 million, while the number of those between 20 and 34 years of age decreased by approximately 7%, from 30 million to 27 million. At the same time, the number of women between the ages of 35 and 44 increased 28%, from nearly 18 million to more than 22 million.[1,2] These changes may be attributed to the baby boomers, the group of women born after World War II. As we move into the new millennium, the women of the baby boom generation will be moving out of their reproductive years. In 1988, this group of women made up 50% of the childbearing population, but in 1997, this proportion dropped to less than 18%.

Among racial and ethnic sub-populations, the Hispanic subpopulation is the fastest growing, with an increase of 65% between 1988 and 1998, from approximately 4.4 million women of childbearing age to almost 7.3 million.[3] In contrast, the number of non-Hispanic white women has

Table 2-1

U.S. women of childbearing age by age and race/ethnicity, 1988 and 2000

Characteristic	1988		2000	
	Number (x1,000)	Percent	Number (x1,000)	Percent
Age (years)				
15-44	57,900	100%	60,127	100%
15-19	9,179	16	9,658	16
20-24	9,413	16	9,033	14
25-29	10,796	19	8,977	16
30-34	10,930	19	9,874	17
35-39	9,583	17	11,205	19
40-44	7,999	13	11,380	18
Race/ethnicity				
White, non-Hispanic*	42,882	79	100,320	74
Black, non-Hispanic	6,824	13	17,596	14
Hispanic	4,393	8	16,093	12

*Includes Asians and others who are not black or Hispanic.

Source: U.S. Bureau of the Census. Resident population estimates of U.S. by age, sex and origin. Washington: The Bureau; 2000.

increased only 4%, from 42.9 million women of childbearing age to 44.7 million, and the number of non-Hispanic black women has increased 20%, from 6.8 million women of childbearing age to 8.2 million during that same time period.

Pregnancy Rates

Birth and fertility data represent easily measured endpoints of pregnancy because all live births in the United States are registered and reported by state health departments to the National Center for Health Statistics (NCHS). These data, while informative, do not provide a complete picture of pregnancy as not all pregnancies end in a live birth. There is no registration of pregnancies in the United States, precluding direct estimation of the number and rate of pregnancies. Pregnancy data can be indirectly assembled by combining data on all endpoints of pregnancy: live births, induced abortions, and fetal losses (spontaneous abortions and stillbirths). The national vital registration system does not collect data on induced abortions and all fetal losses, but other sources of data on these endpoints can be used. The number and rate of pregnancies in the United States have been estimated by using live birth data collected by NCHS; from induced abortion data collected by the Alan Guttmacher Institute and the National Center for Chronic Disease Prevention and Health Promotion within the Centers for Disease Control and Prevention (CDC); and fetal loss data from the National Survey of Family Growth (NSFG).[4] These data sources are of high quality, but it is likely that some degree of selection bias exists compared to the live birth data collected through a vital registration system with nearly universal coverage.

Figure 2-1

U.S. pregnancy rates by maternal age, 1976–1996

Pregnancy rate per 1,000 women

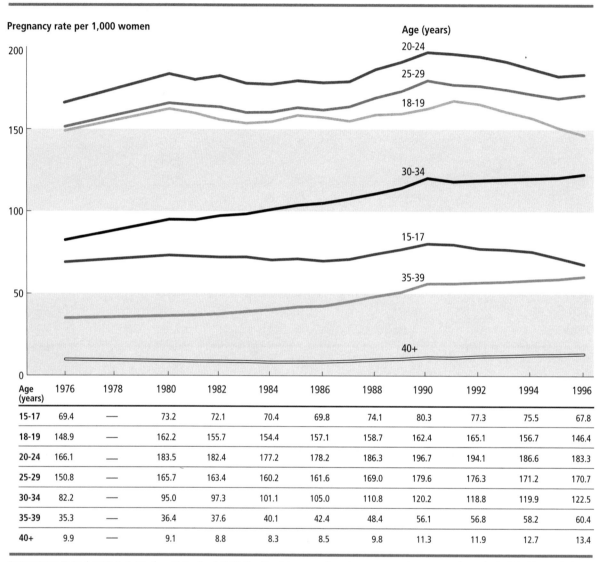

Age (years)	1976	1978	1980	1982	1984	1986	1988	1990	1992	1994	1996
15-17	69.4	—	73.2	72.1	70.4	69.8	74.1	80.3	77.3	75.5	67.8
18-19	148.9	—	162.2	155.7	154.4	157.1	158.7	162.4	165.1	156.7	146.4
20-24	166.1	—	183.5	182.4	177.2	178.2	186.3	196.7	194.1	186.6	183.3
25-29	150.8	—	165.7	163.4	160.2	161.6	169.0	179.6	176.3	171.2	170.7
30-34	82.2	—	95.0	97.3	101.1	105.0	110.8	120.2	118.8	119.9	122.5
35-39	35.3	—	36.4	37.6	40.1	42.4	48.4	56.1	56.8	58.2	60.4
40+	9.9	—	9.1	8.8	8.3	8.5	9.8	11.3	11.9	12.7	13.4

Source: Ventura SJ, Mosher WD, Curtin SC, Abma JC, Henshaw S. Highlights of trends in pregnancies and pregnancy rates by outcome: estimates for the United States, 1976–96. Natl Vital Stat Rep 1999;47(29):1–12.

This bias may lead to inaccuracies in estimates of pregnancy numbers and rates.

Using this method, there were an estimated 6.24 million pregnancies in the United States in 1996,[4] a decline from the peak of 6.78 million in 1990. Nearly two thirds (62%) ended in a live birth. The remainder ended in either induced abortion (22%) or fetal loss (16%). In 1996, the pregnancy rate was an estimated 104.7 pregnancies per 1,000 women aged 15–44 years. This represents the lowest rate in two decades. In general, there has been a steady downward trend in the overall pregnancy rate that mirrors the trend in the overall live birth rate. Similar to live birth rates, women in their early twenties have the highest pregnancy rate (an estimated 183 per 1,000 in

Figure 2-2

U.S. live births, 1930–1998

Number of births in millions

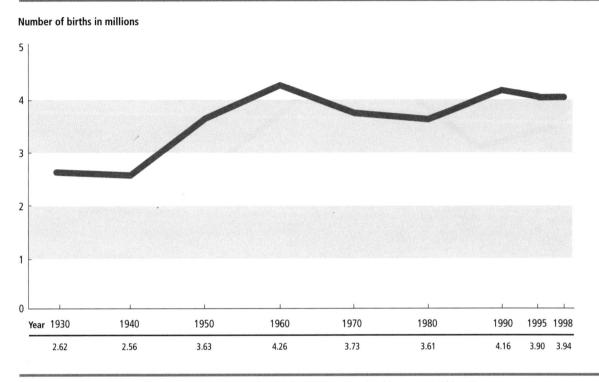

Year	1930	1940	1950	1960	1970	1980	1990	1995	1998
	2.62	2.56	3.63	4.26	3.73	3.61	4.16	3.90	3.94

Source: Ventura SJ, Martin JA, Curtin SC, Matthews TJ, Park MM. Births: final data for 1998. Figure 1. Natl Vital Stat Rep 2000;48(3):1–100.

1996 Figure 2-1). Pregnancy rates among women in their thirties run counter to the overall trend; the pregnancy rates for these women have been increasing in the 1990s, similar to the birth rate trends in this group.

Births

Between 1990 and 1998, there was a slight decline in the annual number of births in the United States. This decline has been attributed to the stable or declining birth rates in women under 30 years of age.[1] In 1998, there was a reversal in this trend with an increase in the number of births in the United States to 3,941,553 (Figure 2-2). Although this is 7% less than 1990 and the lowest number since 1987, it represents a 2% increase since 1997.[1]

The crude birth rate—the number of births by the total population—also increased in 1998 to 14.6

births per 1,000 total population, 1% higher than the 1997 rate, yet 13% lower than in 1990. Likewise, the fertility rate, the number of births by the number of women of childbearing age (15–44 years), increased in 1998 to 65.6 births per 1,000 women of childbearing age (Figure 2-3). The latest estimates of birth and fertility rates and trends in the rates related to maternal age and race/ethnicity are discussed in the following sections.

Maternal Age. In 1998, births to women in their twenties and early thirties accounted for 75% of all births. The remaining one-quarter of births, in approximately equal proportions, were to older women (35–44 years, 13% of births) and younger women (15–19 years, 12% of births).

The most recent birth and fertility rates by maternal age are described in Table 2-2. Birth rates for women in their twenties were relatively

Figure 2-3

U.S. fertility rates, 1930–1998

Number of live births per 1,000 women aged 15–44 years

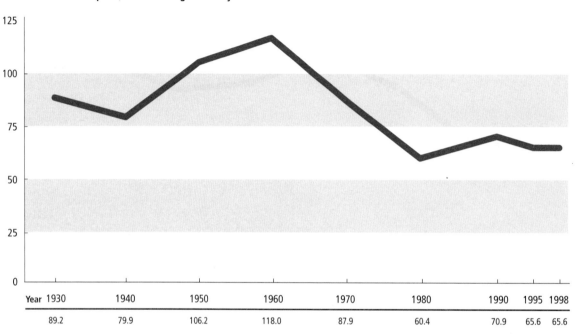

Year	1930	1940	1950	1960	1970	1980	1990	1995	1998
	89.2	79.9	106.2	118.0	87.9	60.4	70.9	65.6	65.6

Source: Ventura SJ, Martin JA, Curtin SC, Matthews TJ, Park MM. Births: final data for 1998. Figure 1. Natl Vital Stat Rep 2000;48(3):1–100.

Table 2-2

U.S. birth rates* by age of mother, 1960–1998

Year	Mother's age (years)							
	15–19	15–17	18–19	20–24	25–29	30–34	35–39	40–44
1960	89.1	43.9	166.7	258.1	197.4	112.7	56.2	15.5
1965	70.5	36.6	124.5	195.3	161.6	94.4	46.2	12.8
1970	68.3	38.8	114.7	167.8	145.1	73.3	31.7	8.1
1975	55.6	36.1	85.0	113.0	108.2	52.3	19.5	4.6
1980	53.0	32.5	82.1	115.1	112.9	61.9	19.8	3.9
1985	51.0	31.0	79.6	108.3	111.0	69.1	24.0	4.0
1990	59.9	37.5	88.6	116.5	120.2	80.8	31.7	5.5
1995	56.8	36.0	89.1	109.8	112.2	82.5	34.3	6.6
1998	51.1	30.4	82.0	111.2	115.9	87.4	37.4	7.3

*Live births per 1,000 women.

Source: Ventura SJ, Martin JA, Curtin SC, Matthews TJ, Park MM. Births: final data for 1998. Figure 2. Natl Vital Stat Rep 2000;48(3):1–100.

Figure 2-4

U.S. birth rates for teenagers aged 15–19 years and proportion of births to unmarried teenagers aged 15–19 years, 1950–1998

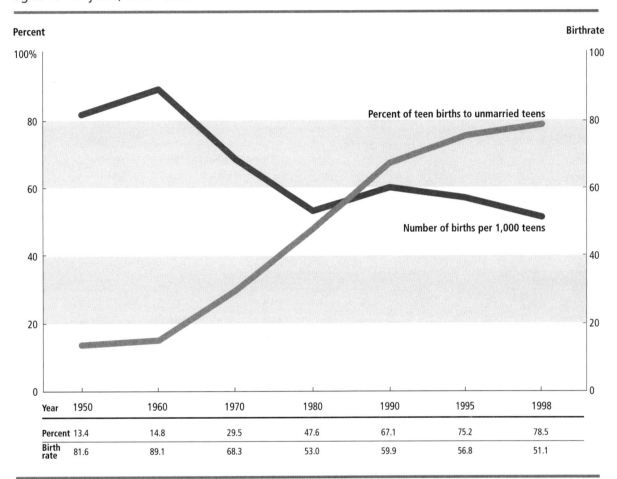

Year	1950	1960	1970	1980	1990	1995	1998
Percent	13.4	14.8	29.5	47.6	67.1	75.2	78.5
Birth rate	81.6	89.1	68.3	53.0	59.9	56.8	51.1

Source: Ventura SJ, Curtin SC, Mathews TJ. Variations in teenage birth rates, 1991–98: national and state trends. Figure 3 and Table B. Natl Vital Stat Rep 2000;48(6).

stable in the 1980s and this trend continued in the 1990s. In contrast, birth rates for women in their thirties increased between 1975 and 1990 by 54% for women aged 30–34 years and 63% for women aged 34–39 years. During the 1990s, the rate of increase slowed, especially for women aged 30–34 years. Birth rates for women in their forties have increased 33% in the 1990s. In 1998, the birth rate for women aged 40–44 years increased to 7.3 per 1,000. This is a substantial increase, but the rates for this age group remain much lower than even the rates for women aged 30–34 years (87.4 per 1,000) or 35–39 years (37.4 per 1,000).

Paralleling the increase in the birth rate among women over 30 years old is the increasing mean age at first birth. The average age at first birth edged upwards from 21.3 years in 1969 to 24.4 years in 1994.[5] The proportion of women over 30 years old who are first-time mothers has accordingly risen from 4.1% in 1969 to 21.2% in 1994.[5] This shift, however, was not uniformly distributed and was concentrated among women with 12 or more years of education, with nearly half of women with a college education having their first birth after age 30.[5]

Table 2-3

U.S. birth and fertility rates by age and race/ethnicity, 1998

Race/ ethnicity	Birth rate*	Fertility rate**	Birth rate by maternal age***							
			10–14	15–19	20–24	25–29	30–34	35–39	40–44	45–49
Total[†]	14.6	65.6	1.0	51.1	115.9	115.9	87.4	37.4	7.3	0.4
Hispanic										
Total	24.3	101.1	2.1	93.6	178.4	160.2	98.9	44.9	10.8	0.6
Mexican	26.4	112.1	2.2	102.7	197.6	173.5	103.7	48.4	10.9	0.6
Puerto Rican	19.0	75.5	1.9	81.2	164.2	104.4	67.6	26.7	7.2	0.4
Cuban	10.0	50.1	0.8	24.2	85.6	95.2	64.5	34.2	7.1	—
Other Hispanic[††]	23.2	90.2	1.9	80.0	137.4	157.2	106.9	46.9	12.9	0.6
Non-Hispanic[†††]										
Total	13.2	60.7	0.9	44.3	99.9	109.3	83.5	36.5	7.0	0.4
White	12.1	57.7	0.3	35.2	90.7	109.7	85.2	36.4	6.7	0.4
Black	18.1	73.0	3.0	88.2	146.4	104.6	65.8	31.2	6.8	0.3
American Indian	17.1	70.7	1.6	72.1	139.3	102.2	64.2	30.2	6.4	—
Asian/Pacific Islander	16.4	64.0	0.4	23.1	68.8	110.4	110.3	52.8	12.0	0.9

*Rate per 1,000 total population.

**Rate per 1,000 women aged 15–44 years.

*** Rate per 1,000 women in specified age group.

[†]Includes origin not stated.

[††]Includes Central and South American and other Hispanics of unknown origin.

[†††]Includes races other than white and black.

— Figures do not meet standards of reliability or precision based on fewer than 20 births in numerator.

Source: Ventura SJ, Martin JA, Curtin SC, Matthews TJ, Park MM. Births: final data for 1998. Tables 1 and 6. Natl Vital Stat Rep 2000;48(3):1–100.

The teenage birth rate has continued to fall in the 1990s (Figure 2-4), as reflected in concurrent declines in birth and abortion rates.[1] The declining teenage birth rate has been attributed to both reduced sexual activity and increased use of contraception among those teens who are sexually active.[6] In 1998, the birth rate for teenagers aged 15–19 years fell 2%, to 51.1 births per 1,000 women. The rate for young teenagers, aged 15–17 years, declined 6% to 30.4 per 1,000; the rate for older teenagers, 18–19 years old, declined 2% to 82.0 per 1,000.

Maternal Race/Ethnicity. Fertility rates for non-Hispanic white and black women declined 9% and 19%, respectively, between 1990 and 1997. In 1998, fertility rates for non-Hispanic black and non-Hispanic white women increased less than 1% from the previous year, indicating a reversal in this downward trend.

Between 1990 and 1997, there was a 5% decline in the fertility rate of Hispanic women. Among subgroups of Hispanic women, fertility rates during that same period declined 2% for Mexican

Table 2-4

U.S. birth rates for unmarried women* by maternal age and race/ethnicity, 1980, 1990, and 1998

	Total	Maternal age (years)							
	15–44	15–17	18–19	20–24	25–29	30–34	35–39	40–44**
Year	**All races***								
1980[†,††]	29.4	20.6	39.0	40.9	34.0	21.1	9.7	2.6
1990[†]	43.8	29.6	60.7	65.1	56.0	37.8	17.3	3.6
1998[†]	44.3	27.0	64.5	72.3	58.4	39.1	19.0	4.6
	White								
1980[†,††]	18.1	12.0	24.1	25.1	21.5	14.1	7.1	1.8
1990[†]	32.9	20.4	44.9	48.2	43.0	29.9	14.5	3.2
1998[†]	37.5	21.8	53.5	60.5	50.9	34.9	17.0	4.0
	Black								
1980[†,††]	81.1	68.8	118.2	112.3	81.4	46.7	19.0	5.5
1990[†]	90.5	78.8	143.7	144.8	105.3	61.5	25.5	5.1
1998[†]	73.3	56.5	123.5	131.0	90.3	51.7	24.7	6.1
	Hispanic[†††]								
1990[†]	89.6	45.9	98.9	129.8	131.7	88.1	50.8	13.7
1998[†]	90.1	53.0	107.8	135.0	136.0	85.4	40.1	12.0

*Rates per 1,000 unmarried women computed by relating total number of births to unmarried mothers (regardless of age of mother) to number of unmarried women aged 15–44 years.

**Rates computed by relating numbers of births to unmarried mothers aged 40 years and older to number of unmarried women aged 40–44 years.

***Includes races other than white and black.

[†]Data for states in which marital status was not reported have been inferred and included with data from the remaining states.

[††]Based on 100% of births in sampled states and 50% of births in all other states.

[†††]Includes all persons of Hispanic origin of any race.

Source: Ventura SJ, Martin JA, Curtin SC, Matthews TJ, Park MM. Births: final data for 1998. Natl Vital Stat Rep 2000;48(3):1–100.

women, 16% for Puerto Rican women, and 17% for other Hispanic women which includes all births to Central and South American and Hispanic women of unknown origin. An exception to this downward trend was a 9% increase in the fertility rate among Cuban women. The fertility rate for Hispanic women overall in 1998 was 101.1 per 1,000 women aged 15–44 years, the lowest reported since 1989 (104.9 per 1,000) when data collection for all Hispanic births in the United States first became available.[1] Fertility rates for each Hispanic subgroup are reported in Table 2-3; Mexican women have the highest rate among Hispanics whereas Cubans have the lowest.

Figure 2-5

U.S. births to unmarried women, 1980–1998

Percent of all births

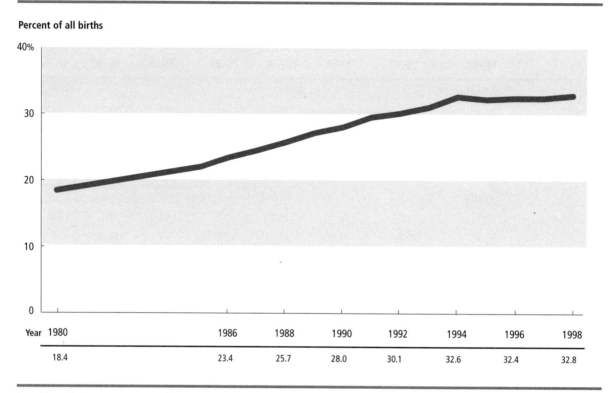

Year	1980		1986	1988	1990	1992	1994	1996	1998
	18.4		23.4	25.7	28.0	30.1	32.6	32.4	32.8

Source: Ventura SJ, Martin JA, Curtin SC, Matthews TJ, Park MM. Births: final data for 1998. Table 17. Natl Vital Stat Rep 2000;48(3):1–100.

Among teenagers, the largest decline from 1991 to 1998 occurred among non-Hispanic black teenagers aged 15–19 years for whom the overall birth rate fell 35% to the lowest rate ever recorded for that subpopulation—88.2 births per 1,000. Likewise, the birth rate for Puerto Rican teenagers dropped 26%. Despite these declines, birth rates for non-Hispanic black and Hispanic teenagers continue to be two to three times higher than those of non-Hispanic whites.

Maternal Marital Status. Overall, the proportion of births to unmarried women has increased since 1980. Much of the increase occurred between 1980 and 1990 (Figure 2-5), with 32.8% of all births in 1998 to unmarried women. The birth rate for unmarried women aged 15–44 years in 1998 was 44.3 births per 1,000 unmarried women, less than 1% higher than in 1997 yet 6%

lower than the highest level, 46.9, in 1994. The overall decline in the rate and number of births to unmarried women has occurred in conjunction with a decline in the number of total births.[3]

Over the past three decades, birth rates for unmarried women have been highest for women aged 18–19 and 20–24 years, followed closely by birth rates for women aged 25–29 years. Rates for younger teenagers and women aged 30 years and above are considerably lower. In addition, the proportion of births to unmarried women varies by maternal age. Although the proportion of births to unmarried women overall has declined, it has risen steeply over the past two decades among teenagers. This reflects primarily a decrease in the proportion of teenagers who marry rather than an increased birth rate among teenagers.[3]

The proportions of births to unmarried black women (69%) and unmarried Hispanic women

(42%) have changed little between 1991 and 1998. Over the past decade, birth rates for unmarried women have declined 23% for black women and 4% for Hispanic women. In contrast, birth rates for unmarried, non-Hispanic white women have increased 11%. Despite these opposing trends, birth rates for unmarried black and Hispanic women remain three times those of non-Hispanic white women. Table 2-4 describes birth rates for unmarried women by race/ethnicity and maternal age.

Infertility

In 1995, as estimated from the most recent NSFG, only 8.9% of married U.S. women who were childless did not expect to have a child. Eighty-seven percent of these women were voluntarily sterile; that is, they were fecund but sterile because of contraceptive intervention. Thirteen percent were involuntarily sterile as defined by impaired fecundity or sterile for noncontraceptive reasons.[7] In examining infertility rates from

Figure 2-6

U.S. infertility rates, 1965–1995

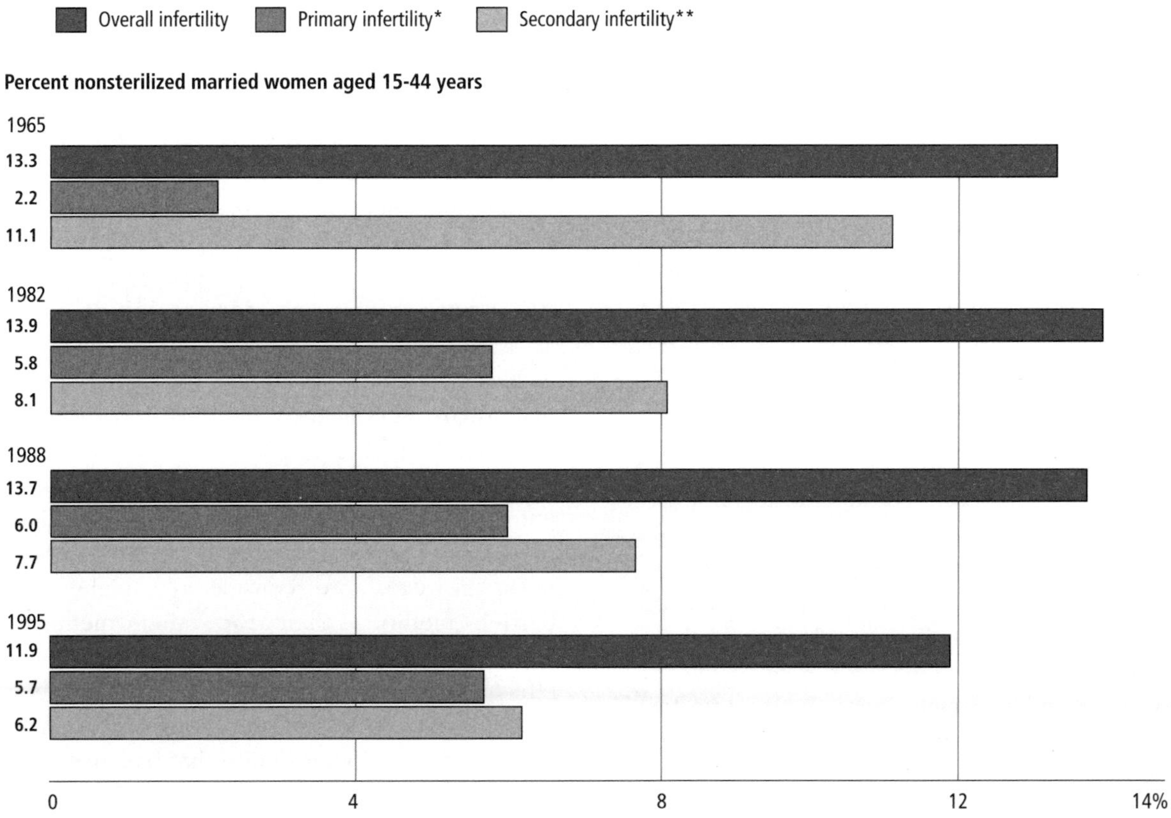

■ Overall infertility   ■ Primary infertility*   ■ Secondary infertility**

Percent nonsterilized married women aged 15-44 years

1965	
13.3	
2.2	
11.1	

1982	
13.9	
5.8	
8.1	

1988	
13.7	
6.0	
7.7	

1995	
11.9	
5.7	
6.2	

0   4   8   12   14%

*No prior pregnancy
**At least one prior pregnancy achieved

Source: Abma JC, Chandra A, Mosher WD, Peterson LS, Piccinino LJ. Fertility, family planning, and women's health: new data from the 1995 National Survey of Family Growth. Vital Health Stat 1997;23(19):1–114.

the NSFG data, it is important to remove women who are voluntarily sterile from the group of women at risk for infertility. Based on data from the NSFG and taking this factor into account, the rate of involuntary infertility overall in U.S. married women of childbearing age has not changed substantially over the past 40 years (Figure 2-6) although there was a small decline from 1988 (13.7%) to 1995 (11.9%). However, the rate of primary infertility (no prior pregnancy) has increased (to 5.7% in 1995), whereas the rate of secondary infertility (at least one prior pregnancy achieved) has decreased (to 6.2% in 1995).

The immediate causes of infertility in women are ovulation defects, luteal phase defects, cervical factors, endometriosis, and tubal obstruction.[8] Differences in infertility rates by social class or race/ethnicity have not been widely reported. Risk of infertility and time to conception both increase with maternal age.[9,10] Women with a history of pelvic inflammatory disease and/or sexually transmitted infections are at increased risk for tubal obstruction, a major cause of infertility.[9,11] Smoking[12] and high doses of caffeine[13] have also been associated with infertility and/or conception delay. It is important to note that fertile partners of infertile men have not been included in the above descriptions.

A wide range of treatment options, usually referred to as assisted reproductive technologies (ART), are available for infertile couples. These include "low-tech" therapies (e.g., drugs to stimulate the ovaries to produce more than one egg, intrauterine insemination) and "high-tech" therapies (e.g., in vitro fertilization, zygote intrafallopian transfer, gamete intrafallopian transfer). The federal government now collects data on the outcomes of high-tech therapies. The overall rate of pregnancies per cycle of ART was 27 per 100 in 1997 with a live birth rate of 22.6 per 100.[14] The risk of multiple gestations is high; 26.3% of all pregnancies achieved by ART in 1996 resulted in twins and 5.8% resulted in triplets or greater. Not all ART pregnancies result in a live birth of either a singleton or multiple; 15.6% end in ectopic pregnancy, induced abor-

tion (possibly the result of selective termination or congenital malformations), spontaneous abortion, or stillbirth.[14]

Contraception

The availability of safe and reliable methods of contraception has been a primary factor in demographic changes in birth rates and the ability of women to make decisions about childbearing.

The oral pill is the most popular contraceptive method and has been widely used since the 1960s. Oral contraceptives have been studied extensively and, in addition to pregnancy prevention, they provide health benefits including regular menses and protection against ectopic pregnancy and ovarian and endometrial cancers. The data on relationships between long-term oral contraceptive use and breast cancer are conflicting. Other hormonal methods include implants (e.g., Norplant) and injectables (e.g., depomedroxyprogesterone). There has been renewed interest in the intrauterine device (IUD) since studies have documented its safety as a contraceptive method. Barrier methods include the male condom, female condom, diaphragm, spermicide, and the cervical cap. The main benefits of these methods include ease in accessibility and availability, affordability, immediate effectiveness, and protection against sexually transmitted diseases (STDs). Failure rates, however, are considerably higher for barrier methods than for other methods. Furthermore, although barrier methods are most effective in preventing the spread of STDs, they are less effective in preventing pregnancy. Sterilization is another option that has increased in recent decades; it is highly effective in preventing pregnancy, but this method does not offer protection from the spread of STDs.

The 1995 NSFG reported that 64% of reproductive-aged women were using some method of contraception (Table 2-5). Among the women who reported not using any method of contraception, most (85%) were reportedly not at risk

Table 2-5

Current reproductive status of U.S. women aged 15–44 years, 1982, 1988, and 1995			
	1982	**1988**	**1995**
All women (x1,000)	54,099	57,900	60,201
Percent			
Using a method	55.7	60.3	64.2
Contraceptive sterilization	19.0	23.6	24.8
Nonsurgical methods	36.7	36.7	39.4
Not using a method	44.3	39.7	35.8
Pregnant, postpartum, or seeking pregnancy	9.2	8.6	8.6
Infertile	8.2	6.1	4.3
Never had intercourse	13.6	11.5	10.9
Had not had intercourse in last 3 months	5.9	6.9	6.2
Had intercourse in last 3 months	7.4	6.7	5.2

Source: National Survey of Family Growth, 1982 and 1988. Adapted from Mosher, WD. Contraceptive practice in the United States, 1982–1988. Fam Plann Perspect 1990;22:199. Abma JC, Chandra A, Mosher WD, Peterson LS, Piccinino LJ. Fertility, family planning, and women's health: new data from the 1995 National Survey of Family Growth. Vital Health Stat 1997;23(19):1–114.

of unintended pregnancy. This group includes women who had been surgically sterilized for noncontraceptive reasons, were knowingly sterile, were pregnant, had delivered within the last 2 months, were attempting pregnancy, or had not had sexual intercourse within the 3 months before the interview.

Trends in Contraceptive Use

In 1995, 93% of women who were at risk of unintended pregnancy reported use of some type of contraception, primarily female sterilization (10.7 million), oral contraceptives (10.4 million), male

condoms (7.9 million), and male sterilization (4.2 million).[7] Descriptions of the contraceptive methods of choice for U.S. women of childbearing age in 1995 are described in Table 2-6.[7]

Comparing data from the 1988 and 1995 NSFG indicates an increase in condom use by the male partner across all age groups, but the largest increases were among women aged 20–24 and 25–29 years. It is postulated that this is primarily because of increased awareness of sexually transmitted diseases, particularly human immunodeficiency virus (HIV), and the desire to prevent their transmission. There was a modest decline from 1988 to 1995 in oral contraceptive use among women less than 30 years old. Closer examination of the data reveals that there were substantial decreases in oral contraceptive use among women 15–19 and 20–24 years of age. Interestingly, among these same young women, there was a concomitant increase in injectable and implanted progestin-only contraceptives.[7] Diaphragm use declined among women in all age groups with the largest decline among women aged 30–34 years.[7] The choice of sterilization by married couples has increased dramatically in the past 20 years, with more than a third of couples choosing male or female sterilization.[7]

Failure, Discontinuation, and Resumption of Contraception

Discontinuation of a contraceptive method is an important factor to consider when estimating the failure rates of various methods. The failure rate may differ for women who use a method for 3 months as compared to experienced users who continue for 1 or more years. Yet, only one failure rate is usually cited. This issue can be ignored if only a few women discontinue the selected method or change (resume with a new method). In fact, many women discontinue using their method within a few months of starting it. Furthermore, those who resume contraception often choose a different method. Overall, 31% of women discontinue use within the first 6 months, and 44% do so in the first 12 months.[15] Sixty-eight

Table 2-6

Contraceptive method of choice of U.S. women aged 15–44 years by age, 1995						
	Age					
	15–19	**20–24**	**25–29**	**30–34**	**35–39**	**40–44**
All women (x1,000)	8,961	9,041	9,693	11,065	11,211	10,230
Percent						
Any method of contraception	29.8	63.4	69.3	72.7	72.9	71.5
Female sterilization	0.1	2.5	11.8	21.4	29.8	35.6
Male sterilization	0.0	0.7	3.1	7.6	13.6	14.5
Pill	13.0	33.1	27.0	20.7	8.1	4.2
Condom	10.9	16.7	16.8	13.4	12.3	8.8
Injectable	2.9	3.9	2.9	1.3	0.8	0.2
Withdrawal	1.2	2.1	2.6	2.1	2.3	1.4
Implant	0.8	2.4	1.4	0.5	0.2	0.1
Diaphragm	<0.05	0.4	0.6	1.7	2.2	1.9
Periodic abstinence	0.4	0.6	1.2	2.3	2.1	1.8
Natural family planning	0.0	0.1	0.2	0.3	0.4	0.2
Other methods*	0.3	0.9	1.2	1.3	0.9	1.8
Female condom	0.0	0.1	0.0	0.0	0.0	0.0

*Includes morning-after pill, foam, cervical cap, Today spermicidal sponge, suppository, jelly or cream (without diaphragm), and other methods not shown separately.

Source: Abma JC, Chandra A, Mosher WD, Peterson LS, Piccinino LJ. Fertility, family planning, and women's health: new data from the 1995 National Survey of Family Growth. Vital Health Stat 1997;23(19):1–114.

percent of couples report that they resume contraception with a different method within 1 month, while 76% resume within 3 months.[15]

Contraceptive failure and discontinuation was the subject of a study based upon NSFG data.[15] Overall, 9% of women experienced a pregnancy during 12 months of typical use of a reversible contraceptive, and 17% became pregnant during 24 months of typical use. Excluding the residual category of other methods, the probability of becoming pregnant during a typical first year of using a method ranged from a low of 2% for implants (e.g., Norplant) to a high of 20% for

periodic abstinence. Women who discontinue use of oral contraceptives are more likely to switch to the male condom, regardless of length of time since they switched. Women whose partners initially used male condoms are more likely to resume using this method rather than changing to oral contraceptives.

Consequences of Contraceptive Failure

Approximately 47% of all pregnancies in the United States are unintended.[16] Of these, half occur to women who reported practicing contraception in the month that they conceived, and others occur when couples stop contraceptive use because their method of contraception is too difficult or inconvenient to use properly.[15] Because methods such as oral contraceptives do not offer protection against STDs, other methods are relied upon to prevent transmission (e.g., condoms). Therefore, ineffective barrier methods and/or ineffective use of barrier methods can not only lead to pregnancy but also to infections with STDs because of compromised protection against disease (see chapter 3).

Emergency contraceptive pills (i.e., "morning-after pills"), which are usually a higher, concentrated dose of birth control pills, can prevent pregnancy after unprotected intercourse or after a contraceptive failure. Scant data are available on the use of this method by women. Lack of knowledge on the part of both health care providers and consumers suggest low levels of utilization.[17] In a recent national survey, most women (72%) did not know that this method was available in the United States, and only 1% had ever used it.[17]

Unintended Pregnancy

Unintended pregnancies fall into two categories: mistimed and unwanted. A mistimed pregnancy is one that occurs when the woman expected to become pregnant but the pregnancy occurred earlier than anticipated. An unwanted pregnancy is one that occurs if the woman does not anticipate pregnancy at that time or any time in the future.[18] Whether unwanted or mistimed, unintended pregnancies have a substantial effect on women, reproductive outcomes, and the family structure within society. Goals of contraceptive programs are primarily targeted to reduce chances of unintended pregnancy and subsequent adverse outcomes.[18] Based on data from the 1995 NSFG, it is estimated that 31% of births are unintended at the time of conception.[7]

The proportion of births that are unintended clearly varies with maternal age. Using 1995 NSFG

data, it is estimated that 66% of births to women aged 15–19 were unintended as compared with 39% of births to women aged 20–24. The Pregnancy Risk Assessment Monitoring System (PRAMS) provides estimates that are consistent with the NSFG estimates. According to PRAMS data, approximately 65% to 78% of live births were unintended among women aged 15–19 years, compared with 48% to 60% among women aged 20–24 years. Other demographic factors are also related to the risk of unintended pregnancy, with higher rates for women who are unmarried, low income, black, or Hispanic.[19]

In a recent study that examined this problem in eight states, several sociodemographic factors influenced the likelihood of giving birth as a result of an unintended pregnancy. Black women, unmarried women, those between the ages of 15 and 24, women who have had a previous child, and women who received aid under the Women, Infants, and Children (WIC) program were more likely to continue with a pregnancy that was unintended at conception.[20]

This problem can also be examined from the perspective of the impact of unintended pregnancy on women rather than its impact on births. Using data collected in 1994 from several sources on a cohort of women, one study found that 48% of women aged 15–44 years had had at least one unplanned pregnancy at some time in their life. Among these women, approximately 28% had given birth to at least one baby who was not planned, and 30% had one or more induced abortions. Approximately 11% of the women had not only given birth to a child as the result of an unintended pregnancy, but they also had a history of induced abortion.[19]

Abortion

The rate of induced abortions is another measure of the problem of unintended pregnancy. Data on induced abortions have been collected systematically over the past two decades by The Alan Guttmacher Institute and by the National

Figure 2-7

U.S. induced abortion rates by age, 1976–1996

Abortion rate per 1,000 women

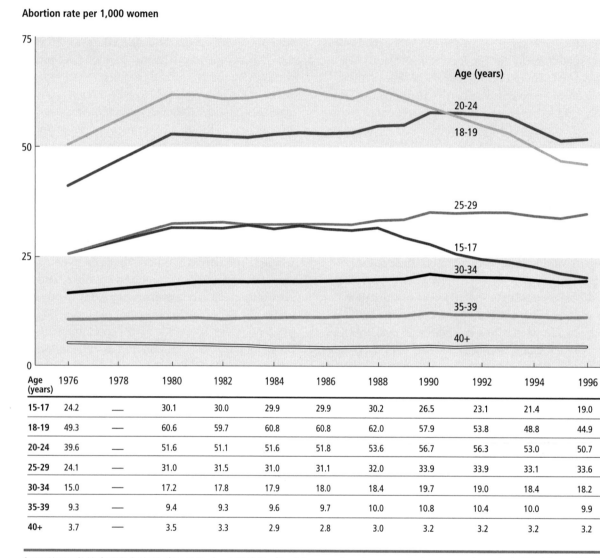

Age (years)	1976	1978	1980	1982	1984	1986	1988	1990	1992	1994	1996
15-17	24.2	—	30.1	30.0	29.9	29.9	30.2	26.5	23.1	21.4	19.0
18-19	49.3	—	60.6	59.7	60.8	60.8	62.0	57.9	53.8	48.8	44.9
20-24	39.6	—	51.6	51.1	51.6	51.8	53.6	56.7	56.3	53.0	50.7
25-29	24.1	—	31.0	31.5	31.0	31.1	32.0	33.9	33.9	33.1	33.6
30-34	15.0	—	17.2	17.8	17.9	18.0	18.4	19.7	19.0	18.4	18.2
35-39	9.3	—	9.4	9.3	9.6	9.7	10.0	10.8	10.4	10.0	9.9
40+	3.7	—	3.5	3.3	2.9	2.8	3.0	3.2	3.2	3.2	3.2

Source: Ventura SJ, Mosher WD, Curtin SC, Abma JC, Henshaw S. Highlights of trends in pregnancies and pregnancy rates by outcome: estimates for the United States, 1976–96. Table 2. Natl Vital Stat Rep 1999;47(29):1–12.

Center for Chronic Disease Prevention and Health Promotion of the CDC. Starting from 1976, the rate of abortion peaked in 1980 at 29.4 per 1,000 women aged 15–44 years and has declined steadily since that time (Table 2-7). Abortion rates have fallen for most age groups of women (Figure 2-7). Abortion rates have generally been much lower for white women as compared with women of other racial/ethnic backgrounds; in 1995, the rate for whites was 17 as compared to 48.1 per 1,000 for women of other racial/ethnic groups. Data were not available by race/ethnicity for 1996. In 1996, the overall induced abortion rate was 22.9 per 1,000 women aged 15–44 years. In 1998, it was estimated that by age 45 (the end of the childbearing years) 43% of women will have had an abortion.[21]

Table 2-7

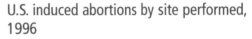

Year	Rate per 1,000 women aged 15–44 years		
	1980	**1990**	**1995**
Total	29	27	23
Race			
White	24	22	17
Other	57	55	48
Marital Status			
Married	12	11	8
Unmarried	52	48	39

Source: Ventura SJ, Mosher WD, Curtin SC, Abma JC, Henshaw S. Trends in pregnancies and pregnancy rates by outcome: estimates for the United States, 1976–96. Vital Health Stat 2000;21(56):1–47.

Based on the 1995 NSFG data, 49% of unintended (at conception) pregnancies ended in induced abortion.[19] The true proportion may be even higher given that induced abortion is known to be substantially underreported in population surveys. The respondents of the 1995 NSFG have been estimated to have underreported induced abortions by at least 40%.[16]

There are two primary types of abortions: medical (induced by a drug combination) and surgical. To date, most abortions in the United States (99%) have been performed surgically.[22] Abortion is one of the safest and most frequently performed surgical procedures in the country.[23,24] It is also one of the most regulated and restricted procedures. Legal surgical abortion carries a risk of death estimated to be 0.3 per 100,000 and a risk of major complications estimated at less than 1%.[25] In September 2000, the U.S. Food and Drug Administration approved mifepristone (RU486) for use in medical abortions.

Approximately 88% of abortions in the United States occur within the first trimester of pregnancy, with more than half (approximately 54%)

before 9 weeks of gestation.[22] More than 90% are performed in clinics, with 7% performed in hospitals and 3% in physicians' offices (Figure 2-8). In 1996, the number of abortion providers fell 14% to 2,042 providers; of these, 42% were abortion or other clinics, 34% were hospitals, and 23% were physicians' offices.[21]

Pregnancy and Childbirth

Pregnancy and childbirth are critical experiences in the lives of women. They shape a woman's relationship with her partner and family. They affect her role in the workforce. They can also have a major impact on her health. Maternal morbidity and mortality can result from problems throughout pregnancy, labor and delivery, and

Figure 2-8

U.S. induced abortions by site performed, 1996

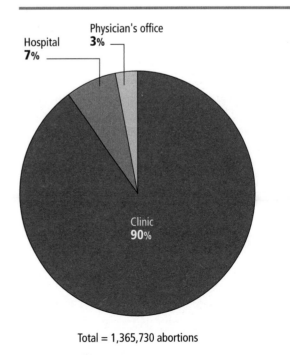

Total = 1,365,730 abortions

Source: Henshaw SK. Abortion incidence and services in the U.S., 1995–1996. Fam Plann Perspect 1998;30:263–270, 287.

postpartum. Defining and measuring maternal mortality and morbidity are complex tasks. The following sections discuss maternal mortality and the broader topic of maternal health related to the antenatal (during pregnancy), intrapartum (labor and delivery), and postpartum (after delivery) periods.

Maternal Mortality

Maternal mortality rates reflect a nation's health status. In the United States, there has been a steady downward trend in maternal deaths from causes related to pregnancy since the early 1900s. In 1930, the maternal mortality ratio was 670 deaths per 100,000 live births; this ratio declined during the 1940s and has continued to decline substantially over the years.[26] This is due in large part to the determination that the majority of maternal deaths were preventable.[27] Additional factors that have contributed to the decrease in maternal mortality include the introduction of antibiotics, increased use of blood transfusions for treating hemorrhage, and overall improvements in social and economic conditions.

Only deaths classified as a complication of pregnancy, childbirth, or the postpartum period are counted as maternal deaths in vital statistics compiled by NCHS. Recent figures for maternal deaths based on the standard classification of deaths using vital statistics indicate that the ratios fluctuated between 7.0 and 8.0 per 100,000 live births during the period from 1982 to 1996.[28] The actual magnitude of maternal mortality in the United States is estimated to be 1.3 to 3.0 times higher than that reported in vital statistics data.[28] Pregnancy-related deaths may be missed unless the death certificate includes a checkbox inquiring about pregnancy during the past year or if the data are manually coded; many states currently do not include a checkbox about pregnancy on death certificates. More complete counts can also be achieved by linking deaths to women aged 10–50 years with live births and fetal deaths in the previous year.[29,30] Based on data from the Pregnancy-Related Mortality Surveillance System

(PRMSS) of the CDC, the average maternal mortality ratio was 9.1 deaths per 100,000 live births for the period from 1987 to 1990, rising from 7.2 in 1987 to 10.0 in 1990. This increase may be due in part to improved surveillance.[29]

According to PRMSS data, pregnancy-induced hypertension, infection, and ectopic pregnancy accounted for most maternal deaths (59%). Women who give birth by cesarean delivery are also at greater risk than women who give birth vaginally; their ratio is estimated to exceed that for women with vaginal births by two- to eleven-fold.[29] This increased risk is due in part to the greater likelihood of a cesarean delivery for women with severe complications rather than cesarean delivery itself causing the death. Additional research suggests that unmarried women, women with low levels of education, women with inadequate prenatal care, and women with higher numbers of previous pregnancies and births are also at increased risk of maternal death.[29]

Data from the PRMSS also indicate that although the maternal mortality rate rose for all racial groups from 1987 to 1990, the rate of increase was greatest for black women. Their maternal mortality rates are higher than those of other racial/ethnic groups (Table 2-8) and are more than three times higher than the rate for white women in 1998 (17.1 versus 5.1 deaths per 100,000 live births, respectively). Differences in the rates between black women and other groups increase as age increases, with the divergence being especially great for women aged 35 years and older.[29] This disparity is apparent in every U.S. state for which maternal mortality can be reliably calculated.[31]

Antenatal Maternal Health

Two proxy measures of morbidity during pregnancy are antenatal hospitalization (hospitalization not related to delivery) and emergency department visits. Both represent the need for medical intervention and, as such, are indirect measures of the occurrence of significant

Table 2-8

U.S. maternal mortality rates by age and race/ethnicity, 1998

Age (years)	Deaths per 100,000 live births
All races	
All ages	7.1
< 20	5.7
20–24	5.0
25–29	6.7
30–34	7.5
35+	14.5
White	
All ages	5.1
< 20	—
20–24	3.1
25–29	4.7
30–34	4.9
35+	11.0
Black	
All ages	17.1
< 20	—
20–24	12.7
25–29	17.2
30–34	27.7
35+	37.2

— Based on fewer than 20 deaths.

Source: National Center for Health Statistics. Health, United States, 2000 with adolescent health chartbook. Table 44. Hyattsville (MD): U.S. Department of Health and Human Services; 2000.

complications during pregnancy. Hospitalizations, however, represent only the most severe complications. Therefore, trends in hospitalizations may reflect changes in outpatient management rather than changes in the occurrence of complications.[32]

Among the 4 million or so women who give birth annually, between 12% and 27% are hospitalized during pregnancy.[32,33,34,35,36] The most common reason is preterm labor, representing about one-third of antenatal hospitalizations.[33,35] Other common reasons are genitourinary infection, pregnancy-induced hypertension, placental bleeding/placenta previa, vomiting, and diabetes.[33,35] In a recent analysis of National Hospital Discharge Survey (NHDS) data, an estimated 18.0 pregnancy-associated hospitalizations were reported per 100 deliveries (including all hospitalizations in which the woman was pregnant) in 1991–1992.

A history of medical or obstetrical problems is strongly associated with an increased risk of hospitalization, as is a lack of prenatal care.[34,35,37] Ensuring increased prenatal care will not necessarily alter the reasons for hospitalization, but improved management of some conditions in the course of prenatal care may prevent some hospitalizations.[37] The evidence is mixed regarding an effect of race/ethnicity on antenatal hospitalization; some studies found higher rates of hospitalization for black women,[32,35] and others found no difference.[36,37]

There are no routinely collected data from which the frequency of emergency department visits during pregnancy can be estimated. If such a statistic were available, it would be an important indicator of morbidity that would capture more than hospitalization statistics alone.

Chronic Disease. Women with chronic diseases who become pregnant may be more likely to experience adverse maternal outcomes because pregnancy may exacerbate the disease. No single chronic disease is common among women of childbearing age, but, taken as a group, chronic diseases affect substantial numbers of women (see chapter 4). Furthermore, low-income[38,39,40] and minority women[39,41,42] are at increased risk for chronic conditions. In a study of low-income African American women of childbearing age, more than 25% of the women reported a chronic illness (i.e., diabetes, hypertension, asthma, or other conditions requiring regular medication).[43]

Complications of Pregnancy. Currently, birth certificates are the only available source of annual data on medical complications of pregnancy for the entire population of women who give birth to live-born infants. In 1989, improvements were made in the reporting of data on medical complications by introducing a checklist of 16 complications of pregnancy on the standard birth certificate. Although the completeness of reporting has improved since the introduction of this checklist, the prevalence of complications is still underreported.[44] The prevalence of both pregnancy-induced hypertension (PIH) and chronic hypertension appear to be underreported in birth certificate data compared to clinical studies of pregnant women.[45] Table 2-9 describes the prevalence of the most common complications of pregnancy for which accurate and meaningful data are available from the birth certificate. The prevalence of PIH has been rising across all age, race, and ethnic groups since 1990, which may be due to improved reporting on birth certificates.

Ectopic pregnancy is an infrequent complication that is very dangerous for the mother. The ectopic pregnancy rate has been climbing steadily since 1970. The most recent estimate of the ectopic pregnancy rate is based on aggregate inpatient and outpatient data for 1992[46] when the estimated rate of ectopic pregnancy was 19.7 per 1,000 reported pregnancies (108,800 ectopic pregnancies). This represents approximately 2% of reported pregnancies.[46] More recent estimates of the incidence rate are not available because the shift to outpatient medical and surgical management of this condition has made it more difficult to track. Nevertheless, it remains the leading cause of maternal death in the first trimester for U.S. women,[47] representing 9% of all pregnancy-related deaths.[48] Pelvic inflammatory disease[11,49,50] and prior infection with chlamydia[51,52,53,54,55] are strongly associated with an increased risk of ectopic pregnancy. Among women who experience an ectopic pregnancy, 20% to 40% are unable to conceive again.[56,57]

Table 2-9

Prevalence of complications of pregnancy from U.S. birth certificates, 1997

Complication of pregnancy	Percent of births
Pregnancy-induced hypertension	3.68
Chronic hypertension	0.69
Diabetes*	2.64
Anemia	2.02

*Birth certificate checklists do not differentiate gestational diabetes from pre-existing diabetes, and, therefore, interpretation of these data is problematic.

Source: Ventura, SJ, Martin, JA, Curtin, SC, Mathews, TJ, Park MM. Births: final data for 1997. Natl Vital Stat Rep 1999;47(18):10.

Intrapartum Maternal Health

Several factors contribute to a woman's health status during the intrapartum period. Among them are cesarean delivery, the use of other obstetric interventions during labor and delivery, the place of birth, and birth attendants.

Cesarean Delivery. Historically, cesarean delivery has been performed for maternal complications (i.e., obstructed labor, maternal diabetes, severe hemorrhage, toxemia). Recently, however, the procedure has been performed more frequently for fetal indications (i.e., fetal distress, breech presentation).[58] Cesarean deliveries (cesarean section) in the United States have increased fivefold since 1970, but a downward trend had been observed from 1989–1996 (Figure 2-9).[59] The decline in cesarean section rates appears to have ended in 1996, and the rate rose from 20.7% in 1997 to 21.2% in 1998.[1] The increase is the result of both more primary cesarean sections (first cesarean for the mother) as well as a tendency to rely upon cesarean births rather than vaginal births for subsequent deliveries.[1] Cesarean delivery is more costly than vaginal delivery both in terms of dollars and its effects for the mother.[60]

Figure 2-9

U.S. cesarean delivery rates, 1970–1998

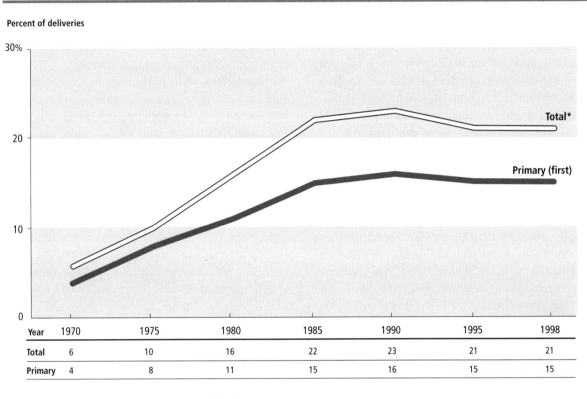

Percent of deliveries

Year	1970	1975	1980	1985	1990	1995	1998
Total	6	10	16	22	23	21	21
Primary	4	8	11	15	16	15	15

*Total includes all primary and repeat cesarean deliveries.

Source: Centers for Disease Control and Prevention. Rates of cesarean delivery, United States, 1991. MMWR Morb Mortal Wkly Rpt 1993;42:286. Ventura SJ, Martin JA, Curtin SC, Matthews TJ, Park MM. Births: final data for 1998. Natl Vital Stat Rep 2000;48(3):1–100.

Recently, controversy has arisen about how low the rate of cesarean deliveries can go without compromising quality of care.[61]

The risk factors for cesarean delivery include clinical and nonclinical factors. Older women are more likely to deliver via cesarean section possibly, but not necessarily, because of increased risks of complications of pregnancy.[62] Women giving birth for the first time and women who have had more than five births are at increased risk of cesarean delivery.[63,64,65] Women with a high body mass index[66,67] or who experience greater weight gain during pregnancy are also at increased risk for giving birth via cesarean section.[66] Both pre- and post-term fetuses are at higher risk of being delivered abdominally.[65] Malpresented fetuses (e.g., breech) are almost exclusively delivered by cesarean.[60,65] Finally, despite guidelines advocating a trial of labor and the established safety of vaginal birth after cesarean delivery, more than 30% of cesareans are repeat cesareans.[68]

Clinical risk factors alone cannot account for the variation in cesarean delivery rates among groups of women, nor can risk factors explain rising rates over the past 20 years. Findings consistently show that white,[69] married,[65] and higher income/more educated[69] women are more likely to deliver by cesarean. In general, obstetricians have higher cesarean rates than do family practitioners and nurse-midwives, even among low-risk women.[70,71,72] Older, more experienced providers are less likely to perform a cesarean.[73] Women with private insurance are most likely to have a cesarean delivery, whereas uninsured women are the least likely.[74] Findings also reveal higher rates of cesarean deliveries during daytime and weekday hours.[75,76,77] Cesarean deliveries are more common in hospitals that are large,[78] privately owned,[58] and affiliated with a medical school.[78] Fear of malpractice actions has also been linked to the practice of defensive medicine, including increased use of cesarean delivery.[78,79,80] Some work suggests that technology, such as electronic fetal monitoring, is used more than is medically warranted and that any obstetric intervention can lead to reliance upon more technology during labor and delivery, ultimately resulting in cesarean delivery.[81,82] Finally, the cesarean delivery rate varies by geographic region, with the highest rates occurring in the southern and northeastern states, possibly because of differences in professional training, core shared values, or underlying population risk.[79,80,83]

Obstetric Interventions in Labor and Delivery. Trends in the use of obstetric interventions between 1989 and 1997 have been examined using birth certificate data.[84] In 1997, approximately 18% of deliveries were induced by medical or surgical means; this figure represents a doubling of the rate of 9% in 1989. Stimulation of labor with dilute oxytocin to normalize irregular or ineffective contractions occurred in 11% of deliveries in 1989, a rate that nearly doubled to 17% of deliveries in 1997. In approximately 34% of deliveries in 1997, women had their labor induced or stimulated or both (2%).[84]

This review of obstetric procedures did not examine trends in episiotomy rates. Episiotomy is understood to be sometimes necessary, but controversy remains regarding liberal or prophylactic use of episiotomy. Systematic reviews of randomized studies conclude that there is no evidence that such use is beneficial.[85] Episiotomy is the most frequent surgical procedure performed on women of childbearing age in the United States; approximately 1,295,000 episiotomies were performed in 1996, resulting in a rate of 108.6 episiotomies per 10,000 women of childbearing age (15–44 years). There are no published data on the proportion of vaginal births for which an episiotomy is performed in the United States, but this number can be estimated by using the number of vaginal births in 1996 computed by subtracting births delivered by cesarean (20.7%, or 805,539) from the total live births (3,891,494).[84] Based on this estimate of vaginal births (3,085,954), an episiotomy was performed for approximately 42% of births. This represents a continuation of a downward trend; the proportion of vaginal births accompanied by episiotomy declined from 64% in 1981[86] to 50.4% in 1993.[87]

Place of Delivery and Birth Attendants. Nearly 99% of births in 1998 occurred in hospitals, a rate that has remained relatively constant since 1975. The majority of nonhospital setting births took place at home (63%), and 29% were in freestanding birth centers in 1998.[1]

In 1998, 91.9% of births were attended by a physician in a hospital; this represents, however, an overall decline in physician-attended births from 92.3% in 1997 and 98.4% in 1975.[1] The percentage of births attended by a midwife was 7.4 in 1998, and this percentage has increased sharply in the past 30 years (1.0% in 1975). Approximately 95% of midwife-attended births were by certified nurse midwives. Hispanic women were more likely to have midwife-attended births (9%) compared to white (6%) or black women (7%). Doctors of medicine (MDs) attended the majority of births (95.7%) in 1998.[1]

Postpartum period

Among the factors that affect a woman's health and well-being during the postpartum period are the length of hospitalization and breast-feeding.

Length of Postpartum Hospitalization.

Length of hospitalization does not directly reflect women's postpartum health because it is determined by a diverse set of factors. It is, nevertheless, an important part of any discussion of postpartum health. Clearly, medical care for the mother following childbirth is a goal of postpartum hospitalization, but this stay has also been used to educate families about the care of the newborn and to establish feeding practices. To reduce health care costs, early discharge has become a common practice. Briefer stays certainly reduce costs, but many argue that the health of women (and their newborns) may be compromised. For a number of reasons, research in this area has been difficult and an evidence-based optimal length of stay has not yet been determined. Guidelines published by the American Academy of Pediatrics and the American College of Obstetricians and Gynecologists recommend an average of 48 hours for uncomplicated vaginal births and 96 hours for uncomplicated cesarean births.[88]

Using NHDS data, average length of stay and trends in the length of stay have been examined. For women delivering vaginally, the average length of stay decreased from 3.9 days in 1970 to 2.1 days in 1992. For women delivering by cesarean, the average length of stay decreased from 7.8 in 1970 to 4.0 days in 1992. These numbers and trends appear to be independent of mother's age, race, hospital location, and hospital size.[89] In 1996, federal legislation was enacted that banned "drive-through deliveries" or very short hospitalizations required by insurance companies. The legislation mandated that insurers cover a minimum stay of 48 hours following a vaginal birth and 96 hours following a cesarean birth. This legislation was enacted in response to consumer and professional concerns about the trend towards brief postpartum stays. A recent analysis examined the length of stay in New Jersey hospitals before and after a state law similar to the federal one was passed. The average length of stay for both vaginal and cesarean deliveries rose after the passage of the law.[90]

Breast-feeding.

In addition to the benefits to the newborn, breast-feeding is associated with improved health outcomes in both the short and long term for the mother, including more rapid return to prepregnancy weight and reduced risk for obesity, ovarian cancer, premenopausal breast cancer, and osteoporosis.[91] Breast-feeding initiation rates have fluctuated over the past three decades (Table 2-10).[92,93] During the 1970s and early 1980s, there was an increase in the percentage of women who initiated breast-feeding, both overall and in each racial/ethnic group. This was followed by a decline in the late 1980s and early 1990s. Most recently, in the mid- to late 1990s, there has been an upswing in the proportion of women who initiated breast-feeding. This has been especially dramatic for women of color with increases of 80% for black women and 33% for white women from 1990 to 1997. In 1997, approximately 62.4% of all mothers initiated breast-feeding,[93] including 41% of black mothers, 64% of Hispanic mothers, and 56% of American Indian/Alaskan Native mothers.[92]

Related Reproductive Health Conditions

Pregnancy and childbirth profoundly affect the health of a woman, but reproductive health encompasses more than childbearing. Reproductive health encompasses all health concerns of women that relate to the well-defined anatomical differences between men and women. Reproductive health, although an important dimension, is only part of women's

Table 2-10

U.S. breast-feeding rates for mothers aged 15–44 years by race/ethnicity and education, 1972–1994

Characteristic of mother	Percent of babies breastfed							
	1972–74	1975–77	1978–80	1981–83	1984–86	1987–89	1990–92	1993–94
All mothers	30.1	36.7	47.5	58.1	54.5	52.3	54.2	58.1
Race								
White, non-Hispanic	32.5	38.9	53.2	64.3	59.7	58.3	59.1	61.2
Black, non-Hispanic	12.5	16.8	19.6	26.0	22.9	21.0	22.9	27.5
Hispanic	33.1	42.9	46.3	52.8	58.9	51.3	58.8	67.4
Education*								
No high school diploma or GED**	14.0	19.4	27.6	31.4	36.8	30.0	38.6	43.0
High school diploma or GED	25.0	33.6	40.2	54.3	46.7	46.6	46.0	51.2
Some college, no bachelor's degree	35.2	43.5	63.2	66.7	66.1	57.8	60.7	65.9
Bachelor's degree or more	65.5	66.9	71.3	83.2	75.3	79.2	80.8	80.6

*For women aged 22–44 years. Education is as of year of the interview.

**General equivalence diploma.

Source: National Center for Health Statistics. National Survey of Family Growth, cycle 4 1988, cycle 5 1995. Hyattsville (MD): U.S. Department of Health and Human Services; 1988 and 1995.

health. A woman's reproductive health profile certainly changes over her lifespan, but most adverse conditions occur after the onset of menarche. Disorders of the reproductive system represent a wide spectrum of conditions, ranging from those that are easily treatable (e.g., bacterial vaginosis) to others that are life threatening (e.g., breast cancer). Some conditions are of an acute nature (e.g., chlamydia infection), whereas others are of a more chronic nature (e.g., endometriosis, genital herpes infection). Reproductive tract infections are discussed in chapter 3. Cancers of the reproductive organs (e.g., breast, cervical, ovarian, and endometrial) are discussed with other cancers in the chapter on chronic conditions (chapter 4). The following sections address what are usually referred to as benign uterine and ovarian conditions as contrasted with malignant (i.e., cancerous) conditions. For the women who experience these problems, however, the word *benign* may be a misnomer. The effect of these reproductive health problems on women's overall health can be enormous; the sequelae can affect physical and mental health as a whole although no data are readily available to document such effects.

Endometriosis

A disorder of the reproductive system that can cause painful menstrual periods and, in some instances, lead to infertility, endometriosis is the third leading cause of gynecologic hospitalizations in the United States and one of the most common indications for hysterectomy.[94] Symptoms include painful menstrual cramps, pain during intercourse, fatigue, pain during bowel movements or urination, pain from surgical adhesions, abdominal bloating, heavy or irregular periods, and an inability to get pregnant.[95,96] Moreover, the severity of symptoms does not always correlate with the severity of the disease. Women with less severe disease may experience more debilitating symptoms than those who have more advanced disease. Furthermore, many of these symptoms are nonspecific. Women may dismiss the pain as a component of their regular menstrual cycle and not distinguish it as a symptom of something potentially more serious.[98]

There is no clear, standard case definition for endometriosis, making it difficult to estimate accurate incidence or prevalence rates for the general population. It is conservatively estimated that between 3% and 10% of all women of reproductive age have endometriosis.[98,99] Other, more liberal estimates assert that endometriosis affects 10% to 20% of women of reproductive age in the United States.[100] Only three studies have tried to estimate the prevalence of endometriosis in the general population. However, each of these studies was limited by the absence of an effective, noninvasive, diagnostic tool for the disease.[101] At present, the diagnosis must be confirmed by laparoscopic examination. Other ways to diagnose endometriosis are being investigated, including laboratory tests for surrogate markers, which may prove more reliable in diagnosis. One of the most promising is CA-125, an antigenic determinant.[95] Imaging studies, such as ultrasonography and magnetic resonance imaging (MRI) have also been useful in identifying patients with endometriosis.[95] Their reliability depends in part on the extent of endometrial lesions.

A woman's age is the only sociodemographic factor that has been consistently and positively associated with endometriosis.[101] Endometriosis is most common in women aged 25–40 years. Although the disease frequently begins in a woman's twenties, clinical symptoms may not develop until her thirties. Endometriosis typically subsides after the cessation of menstruation at menopause.[102] This association with a woman's menstrual cycle suggests a positive relationship exists between estrogen levels and endometriosis, but further research is needed.[101] In addition, a family history of endometriosis is associated with a six- to eightfold increased risk.[103,104] The worldwide OXEGENE study is currently trying to identify the genetic component of this disease.[105,106,107] Environmental toxins, such as dioxin and polychlorinated biphenyls (PCBs), disrupt hormone levels and may contribute to the development of endometriosis. Recent research indicates that animals exposed to various environmental toxins develop endometriosis.[108]

The primary goal of endometriosis treatment is to alleviate symptoms (including pain and infertility) and prevent progression of the disease.[109] If a woman's symptoms are mild, medical therapy is commonly recommended. Surgical treatment may be recommended in more severe cases. Surgical treatment can also often be combined with the diagnostic laparoscopic procedure.[100] Endometriosis is one of the two leading indicators for hysterectomy for women under age 50.[110] Recent research suggests that medical therapy along with surgical treatment may be the most efficacious management of endometriosis and may reduce the incidence of hysterectomies for this population.[111]

Much work remains to be done in the study of this disease. Noninvasive diagnostic techniques and a universal case definition are sorely needed. Without such developments, estimates of the prevalence of this disorder, identification of its causes, and prevention of the disease will continue to be elusive.

Uterine Fibroids

One in five women of reproductive age has uterine fibroids, although it is estimated that 40% to 50% of women with fibroids have no symptoms.[112] Other women experience a variety of symptoms that may include excessive menstrual bleeding, anemia, menstrual pain, and aching or sharp pain in the abdomen or lower back, and infertility.[112,113] Fibroids can often be detected through internal pelvic examination and diagnosed or monitored by ultrasound or MRI. Uterine fibroids are one of the most frequent reasons for performing a hysterectomy in the United States. During 1988–1993, this diagnosis was the primary indication for hysterectomy among 62% of the African American women, 29% of the white women, and 45% of the women of other races undergoing hysterectomy.[110]

In the Nurses' Health Study, a cohort of premenopausal nurses ages 25–44 with no history of uterine fibroids was followed to estimate the incidence of uterine fibroids and to identify risk factors for incident fibroids. The incidence increased with age, reaching a peak at 40–44 years (the oldest group in the study cohort). Standardized for age, 8.0 new cases per 1,000 woman-years were identified over a 4-year period. The investigators estimated 30.6 new cases per 1,000 woman-years among African American women, 11.0 new cases per 1,000 woman-years among Hispanic women, and 8.9 new cases per 1,000 woman-years among white women.[115]

Beyond race and ethnicity, the only definite risk factor associated with the development of uterine fibroids is being a female of reproductive age.[113] It is postulated that uterine fibroids are a hormone-dependent condition and that women receiving estrogen-only hormone replacement may be at increased risk of developing fibroids.[114] However, studies examining other factors that affect a woman's hormone levels, such as obesity[114], smoking, or oral contraceptive use,[116]

have yet to definitively establish a link to an increased risk of developing uterine fibroids.[117] A recent study showed that a diet high in red meat and low in green vegetables and fruits might increase the risk of developing fibroids.[117] The effect of diet on estrogen levels may explain these findings, but further study is needed.

Medical (nonsurgical) therapies can reduce the size of the fibroids and symptoms. These treatments have some serious side effects and may fail to permanently shrink the tumor.[113] Surgical management includes abdominal hysterectomy, vaginal hysterectomy, myomectomy, and uterine artery embolization (an experimental treatment).[113,118]

Hysterectomy

As the second most frequently performed surgical procedure among women of reproductive age, hysterectomy rates are a significant public health concern of women. Approximately 600,000 hysterectomies are performed each year in the United States; rates vary by disease, age, and race.[119] Hysterectomy rarely leads to serious complications, but the removal of the uterus and possibly other reproductive organs (e.g., ovaries) may adversely affect a woman's physical and mental health. Therefore, alternative procedures, which may decrease morbidity and ensure reproductive capacity for those who desire it, are emerging. Endometrial ablation and myomectomy are less invasive alternatives that can preserve a woman's fertility. Less is known about the epidemiology and practice of these procedures, but their use is increasing. Less invasive methods of hysterectomy have also been developed (e.g., vaginal hysterectomy).

Data on hysterectomies are collected as part of the ongoing NHDS conducted by NCHS. The rates of hysterectomies declined somewhat over the period from 1980–1987, beginning at 7.1 per 1,000 and declining to 6.6 by 1987. This downward trend appeared to level off after

Table 2-11

U.S. hysterectomy rates* by age and primary discharge diagnosis, 1988–1993**

Age (years)	Rate per 1,000 women						
	Total	Cancer	Endometrial hyperplasia	Endometriosis	Uterine leiomyoma	Uterine prolapse	Other
Total	5.5	0.6	0.3	1.0	1.8	0.9	0.9
15–24	0.4	—	—	0.1***	—	0.1***	0.2
25–29	3.5	0.3	—	1.0	0.3	0.5	1.3
30–34	6.0	0.4	0.2***	1.8	1.1	0.9	1.6
35–39	9.9	0.7	0.3	2.6	3.3	1.3	1.7
40–44	12.9	0.6	0.4	2.7	6.3	1.3	1.6
45–54	9.9	0.6	0.8	1.4	5.2	1.1	0.8
≥55	3.3	0.9	0.3	0.1	0.4	1.2	0.4

*Per 1,000 female civilian residents in each age category. Rates were calculated by applying population weights to the sum of the number of hysterectomies obtained each year and then dividing this value by the sum of the population estimates for each year. Population estimates were obtained from the U.S. Department of Commerce, Bureau of the Census.

**Standard error data are available in source.

***Based on 30–59 women in the sample; figure is unreliable.

— Fewer than 30 women in the sample; numbers were too small for meaningful analysis.

Source: Centers for Disease Control. Hysterectomy surveillance: United States, 1980–1993. Mor Mortal Wkly Rep CDC Surveill Summ 1997 Aug 8.

1987; the average annual rate from 1988 through 1993 was 5.5 and remained relatively stable over this time period.[110]

The highest rates of hysterectomy were for women 40–44 years of age (Table 2-11). Rates were similar for blacks and whites (Table 2-12). Indicators for hysterectomy, however, differed by race. The rate of hysterectomy associated with uterine leiomyoma (i.e., fibroids) was higher for African Americans, and rates associated with endometriosis and uterine prolapse were higher for whites. Geographic region was related to rate of hysterectomy, with rates lowest in the Northeast and highest in the South.

Women in the Northeast were older when they underwent hysterectomy (average age 47.7 years) and women in the South were younger (average age 41.6 years), as compared with women from the other regions.[111]

Limitations of the NHDS should be considered when interpreting these findings. First, the survey was redesigned in 1988, a factor which may affect the comparability of data prior to 1988. Second, data on important clinical variables, such as parity, are not collected and cannot be examined. Third, race/ethnicity is missing for a substantial proportion of the discharge data, and this affects the validity of

Table 2-12

U.S. hysterectomy rates* by race and primary discharge diagnosis, 1988–1993

Diagnosis	Rate per 1,000 women			
	All races	White	Black	Other**
Total	5.5	5.5	5.9	4.8
Cancer	0.6	0.6	0.4	0.8
Endometrial hyperplasia	0.3	0.3	0.1	—
Endometriosis	1.0	1.1	0.5	0.6
Uterine leiomyoma	1.8	1.6	3.6	2.2
Uterine prolapse	0.9	1.0	0.3	0.6
Other	0.9	0.9	0.9	0.5

*Per 1,000 female civilian residents in each age and race category. Rates by race were adjusted by redistributing the number of women for whom race was unknown according to the known distribution of race in the NHDS. Rates were calculated by applying population weights to the sum of the numbers of hysterectomies obtained each year and then dividing this value by the sum of the population estimates for each year. Population estimates were obtained from the U.S. Department of Commerce, Bureau of the Census.

**Included Asian/Pacific Islander, American Indian, Alaskan Native, and other races.

— Fewer than 30 women in the sample; numbers too small for meaningful analysis.

Source: Centers for Disease Control. Hysterectomy surveillance: United States, 1980–1993. Mor Mortal Wkly Rep CDC Surveill Summ 1997 Aug 8.

the finding of racial differences in rates and indicators.[110]

Hysterectomy rates alone do not tell the complete story. The prevalence of hysterectomy for the older age groups would also be informative, but such national estimates are not readily available.

Lower levels of education are associated with an increased likelihood of hysterectomy.[120,121] Early age at first birth also increases the risk of hysterectomy.[120,121] Correlates of hysterectomy among African American women were examined as part of the Black Women's Health Study. As in the analysis of the NHDS, geographic region emerged as a predictor. Less education and early age at first birth were also predictors of hysterectomy risk.[122]

References

1. Ventura SJ, Martin JA, Curtin SC, Matthews TJ, Park MM. Births: final data for 1998. Natl Vital Stat Rep 2000;48(3):1–100.

2. Forrest J, Singh S. The sexual and reproductive behavior of American women, 1982–1988. Fam Plann Perspect 1990;22:26–214.

3. Mathews TJ, Ventura SJ, Curtin SC, Martin JA. Births of Hispanic origin, 1989–95. Mon Vital Stat Rep 1998;46 Suppl 6:1–28.

4. Ventura SJ, Mosher WD, Curtin SC, Abma JC, Henshaw S. Highlights of trends in pregnancies and pregnancy rates by outcome: estimates for the United States, 1976–96. Natl Vital Stat Rep 1999;47(29):1–12.

5. Heck KE, Schoendorf KC, Ventura SJ, Kiely JL. Delayed childbearing by education level in the United States, 1969–1994. Matern Child Health J 1997;1:81–88.

6. Piccinino LJ, Mosher WD. Trends in contraceptive use in the United States: 1982–1995. Fam Plann Perspect 1998;30:4–10,46.

7. Abma JC, Chandra A, Mosher WD, Peterson LS, Piccinino LJ. Fertility, family planning, and women's health: new data from the 1995 National Survey of Family Growth. Vital Health Stat 1997;23(19):1–114.

8. Gondos B, Riddick D. Pathology of infertility. New York: Thieme Medical Publishers; 1987:388.

9. Menken J, Trussel J, Larsen U. Age and infertility. Science 1986;233:1389–1394.

10. Stein ZA. A woman's age: childbearing and childrearing. Am J Epidemiol 1985;121:327–342.

11. Westrom L, Joesoef R, Reynolds G, Hadgu A, Thompson SE. Pelvic inflammatory disease and fertility: a cohort study of 1,844 women with laparoscopically verified disease and 657 control women with normal laparoscopic results. Sex Trans Dis 1992;19(4):185–192.

12. Baird DD, Wilcox AJ. Cigarette smoking associated with delayed conception. JAMA 1985;253:2979–2983.

13. Hatch EE, Bracken MB. Association of delayed conception with caffeine consumption. Am J Epidemiol 1993;138:1082–1092.

14. Centers for Disease Control and Prevention. 1996 assisted reproductive technology success rates. Atlanta: Centers for Disease Control and Prevention, National Center for Chronic Disease Prevention and Health Promotion; 1998.

15. Trussell J, Vaughan B. Contraceptive failure, method-related discontinuation and resumption of use: results from the 1995 National Survey of Family Growth. Fam Plann Perspect 1999;31:64–72, 93.

16. Fu H, Darroch JE, Haas T, Ranjit N. Contraceptive failure rates: new estimates from the 1995 National Survey of Family Growth. Fam Plann Perspect 1999;31:56–63.

17. DelBanco SF, Mauldon J, Smith MD. Little knowledge and limited practice: emergency contraceptive pills, the public, and the obstetrician-gynecologist. Obstet Gynecol 1997;89:1006–1011.

18. Institute of Medicine Committee on Unintended Pregnancy. The best intentions: unintended pregnancy and the well-being of children and families. In: Brown S, Eisenberg L, editors. Washington: National Academy Press; 1995.

19. Henshaw SK. Unintended pregnancy in the United States. Fam Plann Perspect 1998;30:24–29,46.

20. Dietz PM, Adams MM, Spitz AM, Morris L, Johnson CH. Live births resulting from unintended pregnancies: is there variation among states? The PRAMS Working Group. Fam Plann Perspect 1999;31:132–136.

21. Henshaw SK. Abortion incidence and services in the U.S., 1995–1996. Fam Plann Perspect 1998;30:263–270, 287.

22. Koonin LM, Smith JC, Ramick M, Strauss LJ. Abortion surveillance: United States, 1995. Mor Mortal Wkly Rep CDC Surveill Summ 1998;47:31–40.

23. Cates W. Legal abortion: the public health record. Science 1982;215:1586–1590.

24. Centers for Disease Control and Prevention. CDC abortion surveillance. MMWR Morb Mortal Wkly Rep 1998:47(SS2).

25. Hatcher R. Contraceptive technology. 17th ed. New York: Ardent Media; 1998:688–694.

26. Linder FE, Grove RD. Vital statistics ratios in the United States, 1900–1940. Washington: U.S. Department of Commerce, Bureau of the Census; 1998.

27. Gold E. Maternal mortality and reproductive mortality. MCH Practices. 4th ed. Oakland (CA): Third Party Publishing Company; 1994:214–220.

28. Centers for Disease Control and Prevention. Maternal mortality: United States 1982–1996. MMWR Morb Mortal Wkly Rep 1998;47:705–707.

29. Koonin LM, MacKay AP, Berg CJ, Atrash HK, Smith JC. Pregnancy-related mortality surveillance: United States 1987–1990. Mor Mortal Wkly Rep CDC Surveill Summ 1997;46:17–36.

30. Atrash HK, Alexander S, Berg CJ. Maternal mortality in developed countries: not just a concern of the past. Obstet Gynecol 1995;86(4 Pt 2):700–705.

31. Centers for Disease Control and Prevention. State-specific maternal mortality among black and white women: United States 1987–1996. MMWR Morb Mortal Wkly Rep 1999;48:492–496.

32. Bennett TA, Kotelchuck M, Cox CE, Tucker MJ, Nadeau DA. Pregnancy-associated hospitalizations in the United States in 1991 and 1992: a comprehensive view of maternal morbidity. Am J Obstet Gynecol 1998;178:346–354.

33. Scott CL, Chavez GF, Atrash HK, Taylor DJ, Shah RS, Rowley D. Hospitalizations for severe complications of pregnancy, 1987–1992. Obstet Gynecol 1997;90:225–229.

34. Phillippe M, Frigoletto FD, VonOeyen P, Acker D, Koremiller JL. High risk antenatal hospitalization. Int J Gynaecol Obstet 1982;20:475–480.

35. Franks A, Kendrick J, Olson D, Atrash H, Saftlas AF, Maren M. Hospitalization for pregnancy complications, United States, 1986 and 1987. Am J Obstet Gynecol 1992;166:1339–1344.

36. Adams MM, Harlass FE, Sarno AP, Read JS. Antenatal hospitalization among enlisted servicewomen, 1987–1990. Obstet Gynecol 1994;84:35–39.

37. Haas JS, Berman S, Goldberg AB, Lee LW, Cook EF. Prenatal hospitalization and compliance with guidelines for prenatal care. Am J Public Health 1996;86:815–819.

38. Turkeltaub PC, Gergen PJ. Prevalence of upper and lower respiratory conditions in the U.S. population by social and environmental factors: data from the second National Health and Nutrition Examination Survey, 1976 to 1980 (NHANES II). Ann Allergy 1991;67:147–154.

39. Fraser GE. Preventive cardiology. New York: Oxford University Press; 1986.

40. Tyroler HA. Socioeconomic status in the epidemiology and treatment of hypertension. Hypertension 1989;13(5 Suppl):I94–I97.

41. Geronimus AT, Anderson HF, Bound J. Differences in hypertension prevalence among U.S. black and white women of childbearing age. Public Health Rep 1991;106:393–399.

42. Ries P. Health of black and white Americans, 1985–1987. Vital Health Stat 10 1990;171:1–114.

43. Kelley MA, Perloff JD, Morris NM, Liu W. Primary care arrangements and access to care among African American women in three Chicago communities. Women Health 1992;18:91–106.

44. Buescher PA, Taylor KP, Davis MH, Bowling JM. The quality of the new birth certificate data: a validation study in North Carolina. Am J Public Health 1993;83:1163–1165.

45. Misra DP. The effect of pregnancy-induced hypertension on fetal growth: a review of the literature. Paediatr Perinat Epidemiol 1996;10:244–263.

46. Centers for Disease Control and Prevention. Ectopic pregnancy: United States 1990–1992. MMWR Morb Mortal Wkly Rep 1995;44:46–48.

47. Berg CJ, Atrash HK, Koonin LM, Tucker M. Pregnancy-related mortality in the United States 1987–1990. Obstet Gynecol 1996; 88:161–167.

48. Kochanek KD, Hudson BL. Advanced report of final mortality statistics, 1992. Mon Vital Stat Rep 1995 Mar 22;43.

49. Brunham RC, Binns B, Guijon F, Danforth D, Kosseim ML, Rand F, et al. Etiology and outcome of acute pelvic inflammatory disease. J Infect Dis 1988;158:510–517.

50. Coste J, Job-Spira N, Fernandez H, Papierni KE, Spira A. Risk factors for ectopic pregnancy: a case-control study in France, with special focus on infectious factors. Am J Epidemiol 1991;133:839–849.

51. Cates W, Wasserheit JN. Genital chlamydial infections: epidemiology and reproductive sequelae. Am J Obstet Gynecol 1991;164:1771–1781.

52. Brunham RC, Binns B, McDowell J. Chlamydia trachomatis infection in women with ectopic pregnancy. Obstet Gynecol 1986; 67:722–726.

53. Chow JM, Yonekura ML, Richwald GA. The association between Chlamydia trachomatis and ectopic pregnancy. A matched-pair, case-control study. JAMA 1990;263:3164–3167.

54. Chrysostomou M, Karafyllidi P, Papdimitriou V, Bassiotou V, Mayakos G. Serum antibodies to Chlamydia trachomatis in women with ectopic pregnancy, normal pregnancy, or salpingitis. Eur J Obstet Gynecol Reprod Biol 1992;44:101–115.

55. Phillips RS, Tuomala RE, Feldblum PJ, Schachter J, Rosenberg MJ, Aronson MD. The effect of cigarette smoking, chlamydia trachomatis infection, and vaginal douching on ectopic pregnancy. Obstet Gynecol 1992;79:85–90.

56. Chow WH, Daling JR, Cates W, Greenberg RS. Epidemiology of ectopic pregnancy. Epidemiol Rev 1987;9:70–94.

57. Mueller BA, Daling JR, Weiss NR, Moore DC, Spadoni LR, Soderstrom RM. Tubal pregnancy and the risk of subsequent infertility. Obstet Gynecol 1987;69:722–725.

58. Taffel SM, Placek PJ, Moien M, Kosary CL. 1989 U.S. cesarean section rate studies: VBAC rate rises to nearly one in five. Birth 1991;18:73–77.

59. Curtin SC. Rates of cesarean birth and vaginal birth after previous cesarean, 1991–95. Mon Vital Stat Rep 1997 Jul 16;45.

60. Petitti DB. Maternal mortality and morbidity in cesarean section. Clin Obstet Gynaecol 1985;28:763–769.

61. Sachs B, Kobelin C, Castro M, Frigoletto F. The risks of lowering the cesarean delivery rate. N Engl J Med 1999;340:54–57.

62. Peipert JF, Bracken MB. Maternal age: an independent risk factor for cesarean delivery. Obstet Gynecol 1993;81:200–205.

63. Baruffi G, Strobino DM, Paine LL. Investigation of institutional differences in primary cesarean birth rates. J Nurse Midwifery 1990;35:274–281.

64. Myers SA, Gleicher N. A successful program to lower cesarean-section rates. N Engl J Med 1988;319:1511–1516.

65. Sokol RJ, Rosen MG, Bottoms SF, Chik L. Risks preceding increased primary cesarean birth rates. Obstet Gynecol 1982;59:340–346.

66. Witter FR, Caulfield LE, Stoltzfus RJ. Influence of maternal anthropometric status and birth weight on the risk of cesarean delivery. Obstet Gynecol 1995;85:947–951.

67. Thomson M, Hanley J. Factors predisposing to difficult labor in primiparas. Am J Obstet Gynecol 1988;158:1074–1078.

68. Eskew PN, Saywell RM Jr, Zollinger TW, Erner BK, Oser TL. Trends in the frequency of cesarean delivery. A 21-year experience, 1970–1990. J Reprod Med 1994;39:809–817.

69. Gould JB, Davey B, Stafford RS. Socioeconomic differences in rates of cesarean section. N Engl J Med 1989;321:233–239.

70. Butler J, Abrams B, Parker J, Roberts JM, Laros JK. Supportive nurse-midwife care is associated with a reduced incidence of cesarean section. Am J Obstet Gynecol 1993;168:1407–1413.

71. Rosenblatt RA, Dobie SA, Hart LG, Schneeweiss R, Gould D, Raine TR, et al. Interspecialty differences in the obstetric care of low-risk women. Am J Public Health 1997;87:344–351.

72. Ruderman J, Carroll JC, Reid AJ, Murray MA. Are physicians changing the way they practise obstetrics? CMAJ 1993;148:409–415.

73. Berkowitz GS, Fiarman GS, Mojica MA, Bauman J, de Regt RH. Effect of physician characteristics on the cesarean birth rate. Am J Obstet Gynecol 1989;161:146–149.

74. Gleicher N. Cesarean section rates in the United States: The short-term failure of the National Consensus Development Conference in 1980. JAMA 1984;252:3273–3276.

75. Burns LR, Geller SE, Wholey DR. The effect of physician factors on the cesarean decision. Med Care 1995;33:365–382.

76. Evans MI, Richardson DA, Sholl JS, Johnson BA. Cesarean section: assessment of the convenience factor. J Reprod Med 1984;29:670–676.

77. Fraser W, Usher RH, McLean FH, Bossenberry C, Thomson ME, Kramer MS, et al. Temporal variation in rates of cesarean section for dystocia: does "convenience" play a role? Am J Obstet Gynecol 1987;156:300–304.

78. Placek P, Taffel S, Moien M. Cesarean section delivery rates: United States, 1981. Am J Public Health 1983;73:861–862.

79. Localio AR, Lawthers AG, Bengston JM, Hebert LE, Weaver SL, Brennan TA, et al. Relationship between malpractice claims and cesarean delivery. JAMA 1993;269:366–373.

80. Tussing AD, Wojtowycz MA. The cesarean decision in New York State, 1986. Economic and noneconomic aspects. Med Care 1992;30:529–540.

81. Wertz R, Wertz DL. Lying-In: a history of childbirth in America. New York: The Free Press-MacMillan Publishing Company; 1997.

82. Davis-Floyd RE. Birth as an American rite of passage. Berkeley, CA: University of California Press; 1992.

83. Clarke SC, Taffel S. Changes in cesarean delivery in the United States, 1988 and 1993. Birth 1995;22:63–67.

84. Curtin SC, Park MM. Trends in the attendant, place, and timing of births, and in the use of obstetric interventions: United States, 1989–1997. Nat Vital Stat Rep 1999;47(27):1–12.

85. Sleep J, Roberts J, Chalmers I. Chapter 32. In: Chalmers I, Enkin M, Keirse M, editors. Effective care in pregnancy and childbirth. New York: Oxford University Press; 1989.

86. Kosak LJ. Surgical and nonsurgical procedures associated with hospital delivery in the United States: 1980–1987. Birth 1989;16:209–213.

87. Graham ID, Graham DF. Episiotomy counts: trends and prevalence in Canada, 1981/1982 to 1993/1994. Birth 1997;24:141–147.

88. Hauth J. In: Guidelines for perinatal care. 4th ed. Elk Grove Village (IL): American Academy of Pediatrics and American College of Obstetricians and Gynecologists; 1997.

89. Centers for Disease Control and Prevention. Trends in length of stay for hospital deliveries: United States 1970–1992. MMWR Morb Mortal Wkly Rep 1995;44:335–337.

90. Centers for Disease Control and Prevention. Average postpartum length of stay for uncomplicated deliveries: New Jersey, 1995. MMWR Morb Mortal Wkly Rep 1996;45:700–704.

91. Lawrence R. A review of the medical benefits and contraindications to breastfeeding in the United States (Maternal and Child Health Technical Information Bulletin). Arlington (VA): National Center for Education in Maternal and Child Health; 1997.

92. Maternal and Child Health Bureau, Health Resources and Services Administration. Child health USA 1999. Rockville (MD): U.S. Department of Health and Human Services; 1999.

93. National Center for Health Statistics. Healthy people 2000 review, 1998–1999. (PHS)99–1256. Hyattsville (MD): U.S. Department of Health and Human Services; 1999.

94. Velebil P, Wingo PA, Xia Z, Wilcox L, Peterson HB. Rate of hospitalization for gynecologic disorders among reproductive-age women in the United States. Obstet Gynecol 1995;86:764–769.

95. Duleba AJ. Diagnosis of endometriosis. Obstet Gynecol Clin North Amer 1997;24:331–346.

96. Mayo Foundation for Medical Education and Research. Mayo Clinic Health Oasis. Endometriosis: a common, sometimes painful disease. 1996 [cited 1999 Sep 15]. Available from: URL: www.mayohealth.org/mayo/9608/htm/endometr.htm.

97. Farley D. Endometriosis: painful, but treatable. Rockville (MD): U.S. Food and Drug Administration; 1997:53–55.

98. Gambone JC, DeCherney AH. Surgical treatment of minimal endometriosis. N Engl J Med 1997;337:269–270.

99. Endometriosis Association. Background information on endometriosis. ENDOnline [cited 1999 Sept 15]. Available from: URL: www.endometriosisassn.org.

100. National Institute of Child Health and Human Development. Facts about endometriosis. Washington: U.S. Department of Health and Human Services; 1999.

101. Eskenazi B, Warner ML. Epidemiology of endometriosis. Obstet Gynecol Clin North Amer 1997;24:235–258.

102. Moore J. Endometriosis and adenomyosis. In: Moore HA, editor. Essentials of obstetrics and gynecology. Philadelphia: WB Saunders Company; 1998.

103. Simpson J, Elias S, Malinak L, Buttram VC Jr. Heritable aspects of endometriosis. J Genetic Studies 1980;137:327–331.

104. Moen MH, Magnus P. The familial risk of endometriosis. Acta Obstet Gynecol Scand 1993;72:560–564.

105. Perloe M. Endometriosis update. Atlanta Reproductive Health Centre; 1999. Available from: URL: www.irf.com/endomp.html.

106. Witz CA. Current concepts in the pathogenesis of endometriosis. Clin Obstet Gynecol 1999;42:566–585.

107. Kennedy S. The genetics of endometriosis. J Reprod Med 1998; 43:263–268.

108. Guarnaccia M, Olive DL. The structure and future of endometriosis research. Obstet Gynecol Clin North Amer 1997;24:455–465.

109. Kettel LM, Hummel WP. Modern medical management of endometriosis. Obstet Gynecol Clin North Amer 1997;24:361–373.

110. Lepine L, Hillis S, Marchbanks P, Koonin LM, Morrow B, Kieke BA, et al. Hysterectomy surveillance: United States 1980–1993. Atlanta: National Center for Chronic Disease Prevention and Health Promotion, Centers for Disease Control and Prevention; 1997. p. 1–15.

111. Winkel CA. Combined medical and surgical treatment of women with endometriosis. Clin Obstet Gynecol 1999;42:645–663.

112. Berek J, Adashi E, Hillard P. Novak's gynecology. 12th ed. Baltimore: Williams and Wilkins; 1996.

113. Barbieri R. Ambulatory management of uterine leiomyomata. Clin Obstet Gynecol 1999;42:196–205.

114. Marshall LM, Spiegelman D, Barbieri RL, Goldman MB, Hanson JE, Colditz GA, et al. Variation in the incidence of uterine leiomyoma among premenopausal women by age and race. Obstet Gynecol 1997;90:967–973.

115. Marshall LM, Spiegelman D, Goldman MB, Manson JE, Colditz GA, Barbieri RL, et al. A prospective study of reproductive factors and oral contraceptive use in relation to the risk of uterine leiomyomata. Fertil Steril 1998;70:432–439.

116. National Institute of Child Health and Human Development. Uterine fibroids. Washington: National Institutes of Health; 1999.

117. Chiaffarino F, Parazzini F, La Vecchia C, Chatenoud L, DiCintio E, Marsico S. Diet and uterine myomas. Obstet Gynecol 1999;94:395–398.

118. Ravina JH, Herbreteau D, Ciraru-Vigneron N, Bouret JM, Houdart E, Aymard A, et al. Arterial embolization to treat uterine myomata. Lancet 1995;346:671–672.

119. Graves E, Kozak L. National Hospital Discharge Survey: annual summary, 1996. Hyattsville (MD): National Center for Health Statistics; 1998.

120. Brett KM, Marsh JV, Madans JH. Epidemiology of hysterectomy in the United States: demographic and reproductive factors in a nationally representative sample. J Womens Health 1997; 6:309–316.

121. Meilahn EN, Matthews KA, Egeland G, Kelsey SP. Characteristics of women with hysterectomy. Maturitas 1989;11:319–329.

122. Palmer JR, Rao RS, Adams-Campbell LL, Rosenberg L. Correlates of hysterectomy among African-American women. Am J Epidemiol 1999;150:1309–1315.

Chapter 3

Infections

Contents

Introduction

Both women and men are at risk for many infections, but this chapter focuses on the infections that affect women disproportionately, either in terms of numbers or severity. For the most part, that means reproductive tract infections, including sexually transmitted diseases (STDs). Compared to men, women are more easily infected with STDs, more likely to be asymptomatic, are less easily diagnosed, and more likely to experience adverse consequences,[1] including serious, long-lasting repercussions for their health and reproductive capability. Reproductive tract infections that are not necessarily sexually transmitted (e.g., bacterial vaginosis and yeast infections) are also major sources of morbidity that primarily affect women. Also discussed here are data on influenza and pneumonia, two infections that pose a special burden for elderly women.

Reproductive tract infections (RTIs) are a major source of reproductive health morbidity. Most RTIs in women are acquired through sexual activity, but some (e.g., candidiasis) are not necessarily transmitted this way. Most sexually transmitted infections can cause localized symptoms (e.g., chlamydia, genital herpes), and others (e.g., syphilis) begin as localized infections and may, if left untreated, progress to systemic disease. Other sexually transmitted infections, such as HIV and hepatitis B, can cause devastating systemic infections. Some sexually transmitted infections that start in the vagina can have serious, noninfectious consequences (e.g., the association of human papillomavirus with cervical cancer). The ultimate effects of infection often are not realized until years after the infection. For instance, infections are a major cause of infertility in women due both to acute effects and to the subsequent development of pelvic inflammatory disease (PID).[2,3,4,5]

An estimated 15 million new cases of STDs occur each year in the United States.[6] The rates of all sexually transmitted infections are much higher in the United States than in any other developed country, and the rates of many sexually transmitted infections have been increasing.[1] For example, the total number of women diagnosed with acquired immunodeficiency syndrome (AIDS) between 1991 and 1995 increased by 63%, more than in any other group regardless of race or mode of exposure to HIV.[7] Although sexually active women of all ages are susceptible to such STDs, younger women are at the highest risk, with two-thirds of all cases occurring in persons under 25 years of age. Young women are the fastest growing segment of the population infected with HIV.[1] The increased burden of infection for young women is related to both higher-risk behaviors and biologic factors. Differences exist in the bodies of younger women, particularly in the reproductive tract tissues, which may make them biologically more susceptible to these infections.[1] Rates of HIV and other sexually transmitted infections are also higher among poor women and minority women.[1]

Reproductive Tract Infections

Chlamydia trachomatis

Chlamydia is the most prevalent STD in the United States with 657,097 cases reported in 1999, of which 80% were in women.[8] These numbers likely underestimate the true rates because 75% of women with chlamydia infections remain asymptomatic.[9] Experts estimate that there are 2.5 to 3.3 million new cases (men and women) each year.[10] Table 3-1 provides 1999 reported chlamydia rates by age and race/ethnicity.[8] For most women, rates increase with age, peak between age 15 and 24 years, and then decrease sharply. Across all age groups, non-Hispanic black women have the highest rates followed by American Indian/Alaskan Native women and then Hispanic women. Among women under 25 years

Table 3-1

Chlamydia rates per 100,000 U.S. women by age and race/ethnicity, 1999				
Age (years)	White, non-Hispanic	Black, non-Hispanic	Hispanic	Asian/Pacific Islander	American Indian/ Alaskan Native
10–14	57.7	559.2	156.8	47.7	278.5
15–19	1,228.5	8,167.3	2,756.9	1,038.8	4,150.9
20–24	1,044.7	7,080.4	2,754.4	1,107.6	3,983.2
25–29	293.8	2,374.8	1,290.2	436.4	1,753.6
30–34	88.5	794.9	527.4	195.6	756.2
35–39	37.3	315.9	243.4	95.7	391.3
40–44	15.6	128.2	109.3	49.8	202.4
45–54	5.1	48.1	49.4	21.2	102.0
55–64	1.1	17.9	12.5	10.6	25.0
≥65	1.2	14.4	11.0	3.5	55.0

Source: Division of STD Prevention. Sexually transmitted disease surveillance, 1999. Atlanta: Centers for Disease Control and Prevention; 2000. Available from: URL: www.cdc.gov/nchstp/dstd/Stats_Trends/1999SurvRpt.htm.

Figure 3-1

Chlamydia infection rates by gender, United States, 1995–1999*

Rate per 100,000 population

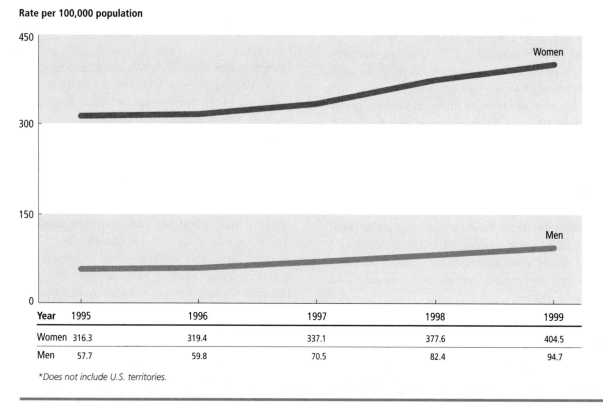

Year	1995	1996	1997	1998	1999
Women	316.3	319.4	337.1	377.6	404.5
Men	57.7	59.8	70.5	82.4	94.7

Does not include U.S. territories.

Source: Division of STD Prevention. Sexually transmitted disease surveillance, 1999. Atlanta: Centers for Disease Control and Prevention; 2000. Available from: URL: www.cdc.gov/nchstp/dstd/Stats_Trends/1999SurvRpt.htm.

of age, the rates for non-Hispanic white and Asian/Pacific Islander women are very similar. After age 25, however, the rates diverge with much higher rates seen among Asian/Pacific Islander women.[8] Within the last few years, the rates of reported chlamydia infections in women and men have increased (Figure 3-1).[8] Expanded screening programs funded by the federal government, use of more sensitive diagnostic tests, and changes to reporting systems primarily explain the increased rates.[8] The rate of reported chlamydia in women is approximately fourfold higher than in men.[8]

Based on data from studies of cohorts of uninfected women, approximately one in ten adolescent girls and one in 20 women of reproductive age in the United States are infected with chlamydia. In a 1997 study conducted of 13,000 female recruits to the U.S. military, the overall prevalence of chlamydia was 9.2%. Chlamydia prevalence sharply declined with increasing age; 17-year-olds had the highest prevalence rate (12.2%) among age groups. Black women had a prevalence of 14.9%, compared to 5.5% in whites and 8.1% in other races.[11]

Nucleic acid amplification assays, such as polymerase chain reaction (PCR) and ligase chain reaction (LCR), are now widely used to screen for and diagnose infection with *Chlamydia trachomatis*. These highly sensitive DNA amplification tests are noninvasive and use urine or vaginal swab samples.[11] Moreover, they allow clinicians to screen larger populations of asymptomatic men and women in virtually any setting.

Table 3-2

Age (years)	White, non-Hispanic	Black, non-Hispanic	Hispanic	Asian/ Pacific Islander	American Indian/ Alaskan Native
Gonorrhea rates per 100,000 U.S. women by age and race/ethnicity, 1999					
10–14	12.7	282.4	24.6	9.1	36.0
15–19	198.3	3,691.0	331.8	117.0	602.6
20–24	178.4	3,273.1	279.6	106.8	590.3
25–29	72.1	1,304.6	137.6	31.1	248.1
30–34	36.4	585.5	66.6	23.3	152.6
35–39	21.8	332.2	38.4	13.1	100.3
40–44	9.1	169.6	23.4	8.0	38.7
45–54	3.3	54.1	8.8	3.2	28.4
55–64	0.8	10.3	3.0	1.1	4.4
≥65	0.2	6.9	1.5	1.2	8.4

Source: Division of STD Prevention. Sexually transmitted disease surveillance, 1999. Table 12B. Atlanta: Centers for Disease Control and Prevention; 2000. Available from: URL: www.cdc.gov/nchstp/dstd/Stats_Trends/1999SurvRpt.htm.

The recent development of a single-dose antibiotic, azithromycin, eliminates the problems caused by a lack of compliance with other prescribed, multidose regimens for treating infections with *Chlamydia trachomatis*. Treatment of sexual partners is also easier to administer. If chlamydia infections are not treated properly and promptly, serious adverse complications can result. Untreated chlamydia increases the risk of developing PID.[2] In a recent study conducted in a managed care setting, routine screening and treatment for chlamydia reduced new cases of PID by 60%.[12] Furthermore, PID[1,13,14] and prior infection with chlamydia[3,13,15,16,17] are strongly associated with an increased risk of ectopic, or tubal, pregnancy.

Gonorrhea

In 1999, 360,076 cases of gonorrhea were reported in the United States. Of these, 179,534 were diagnosed in women.[8] As is true for chlamydia, the high proportion of asymptomatic cases makes estimates of gonorrhea incidence problematic. As many as 80% of gonorrhea infections in women are asymptomatic. Reported rates may underestimate the true rates by 50%.[1] Table 3-2 provides 1999 reported gonorrhea rates by age and race/ethnicity.[8] Rates increase with age, peaking at age 15–19, somewhat earlier than for chlamydia. Rates remain relatively high among women in their twenties and then decline sharply. Across all age groups, non-Hispanic black women have the highest rates followed by American Indian/Alaskan Native women and then Hispanic women. Rates for non-Hispanic white and Asian/Pacific Islander women are very similar and are much lower than for other groups of women at all ages below 45 years.[8] Reported cases of gonorrhea have declined in the last two decades for both men and women.[8] The decline is attributed to national gonorrhea control efforts. Nevertheless, this 20-year trend of decreasing cases appears to have leveled off since 1996 (Figure 3-2).[8]

Figure 3-2

Gonorrhea rates by gender, United States, 1995–1999*

Rate per 100,000 population

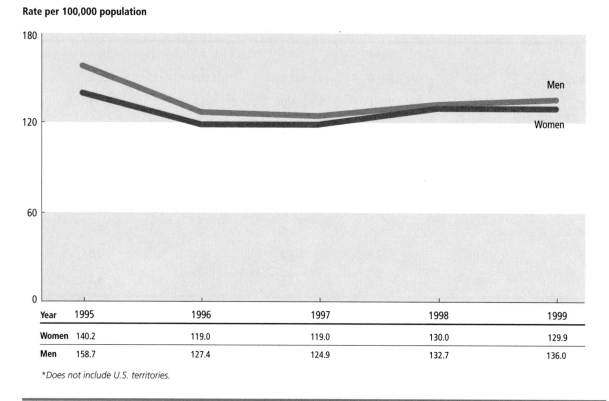

Year	1995	1996	1997	1998	1999
Women	140.2	119.0	119.0	130.0	129.9
Men	158.7	127.4	124.9	132.7	136.0

*Does not include U.S. territories.

Source: Division of STD Prevention. Sexually transmitted disease surveillance, 1999. Atlanta: Centers for Disease Control. Available from: URL: www.cdc.gov/nchstp/dstd/Stats_Trends/1999SurvRpt.htm.

Regardless of declines, gonorrhea is still common within high-density urban areas, among persons less than 24 years old, those who have multiple sexual partners, and those who engage in unprotected sexual intercourse.[18] Presently, as is the case with chlamydia, the highest rate of gonorrhea is found in females between the ages of 15 and 19.[8] African American women have higher gonorrhea rates compared with other women.[8]

Gender differences in gonorrhea rates have narrowed over time. As recently as 1987, gonorrhea was more common among men than among women.[18] At present, little difference exists in the rate of gonorrhea for men compared to women.[8] This is primarily the result of rates in women increasing, rather than rates in men decreasing.

The improvements in screening and testing may have detected cases in women differentially as the proportion of asymptomatic gonorrhea cases is higher in women (30% to 80%) than in men (less than 5%).[9]

As with chlamydia, diagnosis and treatment of gonorrhea have improved with the introduction of highly sensitive, noninvasive DNA amplification assays. Treatment guidelines issued by the Centers for Disease Control and Prevention (CDC) recommend a single dose of ceftriaxone, cefixime, ciprofloxacin, or ofloxacin to be administered as means of improving compliance and managing resistant strains of the bacterial infection. Moreover, this regimen usually is accompanied by a dose of azithromycin, as many

Figure 3-3

Pelvic inflammatory disease hospitalization rates, women aged 15–44 years, United States, 1988–1998

Hospitalizations per 100,000 women aged 15-44 years (x1,000)

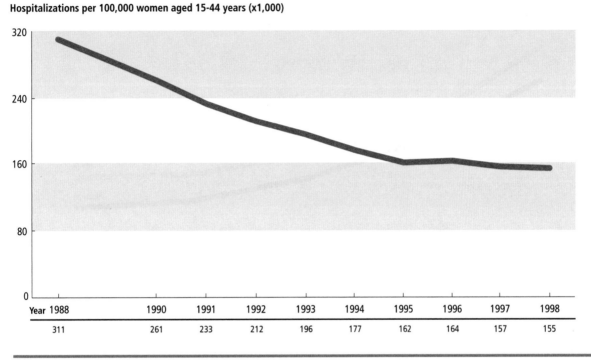

Year	1988	1990	1991	1992	1993	1994	1995	1996	1997	1998
	311	261	233	212	196	177	162	164	157	155

Source: National Center for Health Statistics. National Hospital Discharge Survey. In: Division of STD Prevention. Sexually transmitted disease surveillance, 1999. Atlanta: Centers for Disease Control and Prevention; 2000. Available from: URL: www.cdc.gov/nchstp/dstd/Stats_Trends/1999SurvRpt.htm.

gonorrhea patients also need to be treated for chlamydial infection. In the past, gonorrhea treatment has been complicated by increased prevalence of antibiotic-resistant strains of *Neisseria gonorrhoeae,* the bacterial strain that causes gonorrhea. In 1998, approximately 30% of gonorrhea microorganisms cultured in the Gonococcal Isolates Surveillance Program (GISP) were resistant to penicillin, tetracycline, or both. This surveillance program continues to monitor trends in antimicrobial susceptibility among isolates of *N. gonorrhoeae.*[19]

Pelvic Inflammatory Disease (PID)

More than 750,000 women each year are affected by PID and related complications.[20] In the 1995 National Survey of Family Growth (NSFG), 7.6%

of all women reported ever being treated for PID; rates are similar for Hispanics (7.9%) and non-Hispanic whites (7.2%) but higher for non-Hispanic blacks (10.6%).[21] Most cases of PID are the result of a prior STD having ascended from the vagina or cervix into the upper genital tract (pelvic region). Other infections can also lead to PID. An estimated 10% to 40% of women with untreated chlamydia or gonorrhea will develop PID.[22,23] The major symptoms of PID include lower abdominal pain and abnormal vaginal discharge.[5] A clinician can diagnose PID with a pelvic examination or culture of vaginal and cervical secretions, and the condition can be treated effectively with antibiotics.[5] The rate of hospitalization for PID is declining for women of childbearing age (Figure 3-3). Data on the number of first-time visits to a physician for PID

Figure 3-4

Primary and secondary syphilis rates by gender, United States, 1995–1999*

Rate per 100,000 population

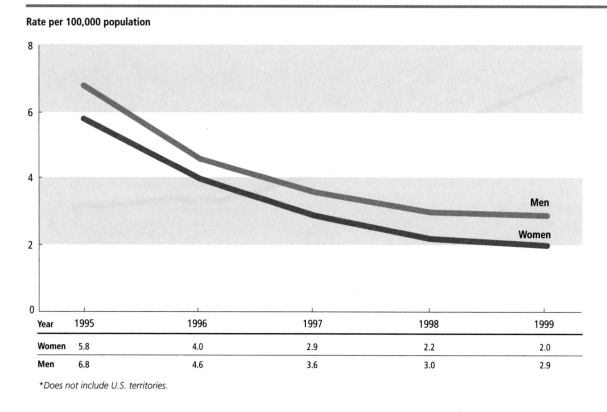

Year	1995	1996	1997	1998	1999
Women	5.8	4.0	2.9	2.2	2.0
Men	6.8	4.6	3.6	3.0	2.9

Does not include U.S. territories.

Source: Division of STD Prevention. Sexually transmitted disease surveillance, 1999. Atlanta: Centers for Disease Control; 2000. Available from: URL: www.cdc.gov/nchstp/dstd/Stats_Trends/1999SurvRpt.htm.

show a similar trend; the number of visits declined from 430,800 in 1989 to 261,000 in 1997.

Approximately 20% of women with PID experience infertility.[5,24] Furthermore, an estimated 30% of female infertility in the United States can be attributed to previous untreated STD infections. Also, PID is strongly associated with an increased risk of ectopic pregnancy[5,13,14] and is a major cause of pelvic pain in women of childbearing age.[20]

Syphilis

In 1999, approximately 6,657 cases of syphilis (primary and secondary) occurred in the United States with 2,796 cases among women.[8] Most women with syphilis do not experience noticeable symptoms. Shortly after exposure, individuals develop a primary lesion, a syphilis ulcer, but it is classically painless. After 6 or more weeks, a rash and other symptoms may develop.[25] In 1999, the reported syphilis infection rate was 2.5 per 100,000 individuals, more than 20% below 1997 and the lowest ever in the United States.[8] Unlike most other STDs, reported cases are believed to represent most of recently acquired cases.[26] Men are slightly more likely to have syphilis than women with a male-to-female ratio of 1.3 in 1998. However, this ratio varies according to race/ethnicity with higher ratios occurring among African American individuals.[27]

Table 3-3

Age (years)	White, non-Hispanic	Black, non-Hispanic	Hispanic	Asian/ Pacific Islander	American Indian/ Alaskan Native
10–14	0.0	1.4	0.1	0.0	0.0
15–19	0.5	20.1	1.5	0.0	6.3
20–24	1.3	26.6	2.7	0.6	6.4
25–29	1.1	29.2	2.1	0.0	11.6
30–34	1.0	28.6	1.9	1.3	6.7
35–39	0.9	26.4	1.1	0.0	6.4
40–44	0.5	15.6	0.9	0.9	2.7
45–54	0.3	6.7	0.4	0.0	2.7
55–64	0.1	1.8	0.6	0.3	0.0
≥65	0.0	0.4	0.0	0.0	0.0

Primary and secondary syphilis rates per 100,000 women by age and race/ethnicity, 1999

Source: Division of STD Prevention. Sexually transmitted disease surveillance, 1999. Table 23B. Atlanta: Centers for Disease Control and Prevention; 2000. Available from: URL: www.cdc.gov/nchstp/dstd/Stats_Trends/1999SurvRpt.htm.

Syphilis appears to follow a pattern of declines followed by epidemics every 7 to 10 years. Since 1990, U.S. syphilis rates overall have declined by 83% in women and by 85% in men. Figure 3-4 shows the declines from 1995 to 1999. Responding to these promising trends, CDC has declared a goal of eliminating syphilis in the United States.[26] Table 3-3 describes syphilis rates for 1999 among women by age and race/ethnicity.[8] In all groups, women aged 20–39 years have the highest incidence of syphilis compared to both older and younger women.[8] Across all age groups, non-Hispanic black women have the highest rates followed by American Indian/Alaskan Native women and then Hispanic women. Rates for non-Hispanic white and Asian/Pacific Islander women are very similar and are much lower than for other groups across most age groups.[8]

Congenital syphilis occurs when a fetus is infected during pregnancy or vaginal delivery. The rate of congenital syphilis generally peaks a year after the peak of adult syphilis within a community. The congenital syphilis rate in the United States peaked in 1991 at 107.3 cases per 100,000 live births and declined by 75% to 26.9 by 1997.[23]

Higher syphilis rates occur in the South. In 1998, 28 of 3,115 counties accounted for half of the syphilis cases, with 19 of those counties in the southern states. Most counties in the U.S. (80%) reported no syphilis cases in 1998.[28] Syphilis rates are also much higher in several U.S. cities (listed in order from highest to lowest): Baltimore, Maryland; Cook County, Illinois (Chicago); Shelby County, Tennessee (Memphis); and Davidson County, Tennessee (Nashville).[28]

Syphilis is usually diagnosed by a serum antibody test. Benzathine penicillin G, an antibiotic, is recommended as the primary treatment for all stages of syphilis.[25]

Hepatitis B Virus (HBV)

The National Health and Nutrition Examination Survey III (NHANES III) reported that approximately 5% of the population has been infected with HBV with an estimated 200,000 infections occurring each year.[29] Approximately half these infections are acquired through sexual transmission; the remainder are acquired through contact with bodily fluids (e.g., blood, saliva).[30] Hepatitis B is diagnosed through a serum (blood) test. Hepatitis B is a highly underreported disease.[26] Of the estimated 200,000 infections (based on NHANES seroprevalence data), only 10,258 were reported in 1998 (3.80 per 100,000).[31] Rates have not been reported separately by gender, but the incidence of acute HBV is reportedly higher in men than in women.[26]

Hepatitis B infection can result in systemic complications such as cirrhosis and liver cancer. No curative treatment is available for hepatitis B, but an effective vaccine is now available. The American Academy of Pediatrics recommends that all infants be immunized as part of routine vaccination schedules.[32] It also recommends that all adolescents not yet immunized be given the series of vaccinations. In addition, further immunization initiatives targeted toward populations at risk may be needed. In 1996, 70% of a population at high risk of HBV infection reported that they had missed an opportunity for immunization in the past. Of these, 42% reported having been treated for an STD at some point.[33]

Human Papillomavirus (HPV)

An estimated 5.5 million new cases of HPV occur each year in the United States.[23] There is no routine surveillance program for this infection, so research studies must be relied upon for estimates of prevalence and incidence. This virus is very common; it is estimated that 75% of the reproductive-age population has been infected with HPV.[34] In a study of female college students in the United States, 43% of the young women in the study became infected with HPV over the

3-year period of observation, yielding an incidence rate of approximately 14%.[35] Data are not as readily available for men, but levels of current infection in men appear similar.[36]

Infection may be asymptomatic or may be manifested as genital warts. It is estimated that 1% of all sexually active adults in the United States have symptomatic genital warts.[37] Among females visiting university health care clinics, the prevalence was approximately 1.5%, compared to rates of 15% in STD clinics.[34] Infection with HPV cannot be cured, but warts can be removed with laser treatment or cryotherapy. Although no curative treatment is available, another study of college students found that HPV infection became undetectable within 2 years.[35] Reinfection or reactivation remains a concern. Most HPV infections spontaneously resolve, but particular strains of HPV can cause cervical cancer. The four types of HPV, which together account for approximately 80% of all cervical cancer cases, are HPV-16, 18, 31, and 45.[34] There are additional types that contribute to cervical cancer cases. Fortunately, adherence to Pap screening guidelines and treatment can cure the cervical cancer caused by HPV[34] (see chapter 4).

Genital Herpes (HSV-2)

Genital herpes is primarily a sexually transmitted infection caused by two serotypes of *Herpes simplex* virus (HSV-1 and HSV-2). Genital herpes is characterized by recurrent, painful, infectious ulcers. Herpes can be fatal in newborns and may be severely debilitating in HIV-positive individuals.[26] No cure exists for herpes infections, but antiviral therapy (e.g., acyclovir) can reduce symptomatic flares. One million new cases of genital herpes occur each year.[23] An estimated 45 million people (22%) have been infected with HSV-2 in the U.S. population.[38] During the late 1980s and early 1990s, sharp increases in HSV-2 infection prevalence were seen among adolescents and young adults.[38] Preliminary data from NHANES now suggest that the prevalence of

Table 3-4

HSV-2 seroprevalence by gender and race/ethnicity, United States, 1976–1994

	Percent seropositive	
	NHANES II 1976–1980* (Age-adjusted)	NHANES III 1988–1994* (Age-adjusted)
All race/ethnic groups**	16.0	20.8
Women	18.4	24.2
Men	13.4	17.1
Whites	12.7	16.5
Women	14.5	18.7
Men	10.7	14.1
Blacks	43.6	47.6
Women	51.4	55.7
Men	34.1	37.5

*Seroprevalence has been adjusted to the 1980 census. The age range is ≥12 years.

**Totals differ from numbers for blacks and whites because other races and ethnic groups are included in the category of all races and ethnic groups.

Source: Division of STD Prevention. Tracking the hidden epidemics. Trends in STDs in the United States, 2000. Atlanta: Centers for Disease Control and Prevention; 2000.

HSV-2 has remained relatively stable over the 1990s.[39] Genital herpes is more common in women that in men. The data from NHANES III indicate that one in four women is infected, but fewer than one in five men is infected (Table 3-4).[26] Rates are higher among blacks than whites for both men and women, but the disparity by gender within racial/ethnic groups is more pronounced among blacks. Most herpes infections are asymptomatic; however, herpes can be transmitted even in the absence of symptoms. The NHANES III found that less than 10% of people with herpes knew that they were infected with the virus.[38]

HIV/AIDS

An estimated 800,000 to 900,000 people in the United States are presently living with HIV.[40] In 1998, the CDC estimated that 28% of those who are HIV-infected are women.[40] Those who are infected with HIV may infect others even before they develop any symptoms. Individuals who are HIV-positive may remain asymptomatic for years and may not develop full-blown AIDS—the most advanced form of the disease—for a decade or longer with aggressive treatment.[5]

As of the end of 1997, a cumulative 641,086 Americans had been diagnosed with AIDS. Women constituted approximately 16% of this cumulative figure and 23% (10,780 of 45,137) of new cases diagnosed in 1999 (Figure 3-5).

Figure 3-5

Percent of new AIDS cases reported in women, United States, 1986–1999*

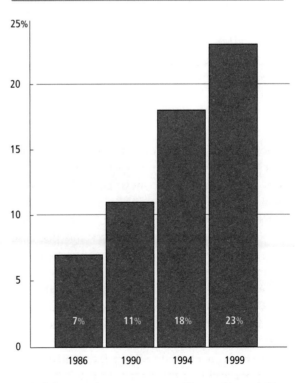

*Includes reported cases among women 13 years of age and older.

Source: Division of HIV/AIDS Prevention. HIV/AIDS surveillance report: 1999 year-end report. Atlanta: Centers for Disease Control and Prevention; 1986, 1990, 1994, 1999.

Figure 3-6

New AIDS cases by gender, United States, 1993–1999*

Number of cases

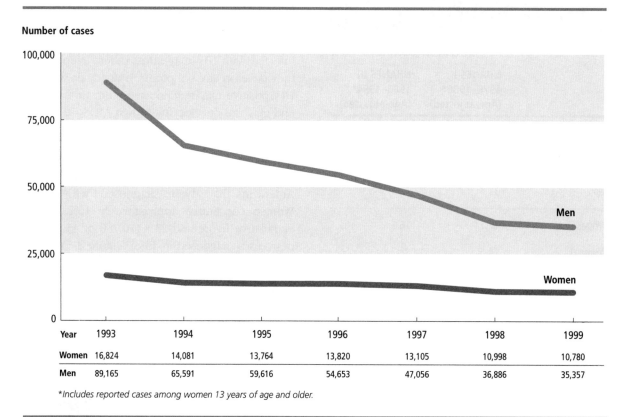

Year	1993	1994	1995	1996	1997	1998	1999
Women	16,824	14,081	13,764	13,820	13,105	10,998	10,780
Men	89,165	65,591	59,616	54,653	47,056	36,886	35,357

*Includes reported cases among women 13 years of age and older.

Source: Division of HIV/AIDS Prevention. HIV/AIDS surveillance report: 1999 year-end report. Atlanta: Centers for Disease Control and Prevention; 1993–1999.

The overall incidence of AIDS has been declining throughout the 1990s. This decrease has been attributed to new combination anti-retroviral therapies to reduce viral loads in HIV-infected individuals and combat the progression of the disease to AIDS.[40] However, this decrease was not as pronounced in women as compared to men.[41] Between 1993 and 1999, the incidence of AIDS was reduced by 60% in men but only 36% in women (Figure 3-6).[40] Some believe that epidemic trends among HIV-infected men and women have diverged because the vast majority of women living with HIV in the United States are poor and lack the resources to obtain necessary treatment.[41,42]

In 1999, heterosexual contact with a person infected with HIV was the most common means for a woman to acquire HIV (approximately 61% of cases).[40] Injection drug use is the next most frequent route of transmission for women. These two transmission routes are not always mutually exclusive and substantial overlap exists.[40]

Most AIDS cases among women are reported among women 30–49 years of age (68% in 1999).[40] As with so many other STDs, racial and ethnic disparities are apparent with HIV/AIDS. Eighty-one percent of women recently diagnosed with AIDS are African American (6,775 women) or Hispanic (2,055 women).[40] The AIDS case rate (new cases per 100,000 population) is

Figure 3-7

AIDS case rates among women by race/ethnicity, United States, 1999*

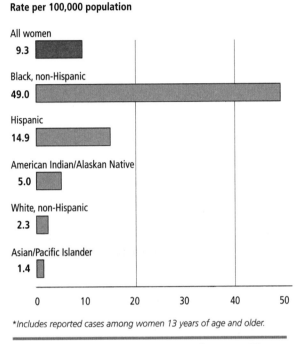

Rate per 100,000 population

All women
9.3

Black, non-Hispanic
49.0

Hispanic
14.9

American Indian/Alaskan Native
5.0

White, non-Hispanic
2.3

Asian/Pacific Islander
1.4

0   10   20   30   40   50

*Includes reported cases among women 13 years of age and older.

Source: Division of HIV/AIDS Prevention. HIV/AIDS surveillance report: 1999 year-end report. Atlanta: Centers for Disease Control and Prevention; 1999; 11(2).

also markedly different by race and ethnicity with higher rates among minority women (Figure 3-7).

For women in the 25–44 age group, AIDS is the third leading cause of death for African Americans, fourth for Hispanics, and tenth for whites (also see Table 4-2 in chapter 4).[40] Due to improved HIV therapies, AIDS deaths have declined dramatically between 1993 and 1998 (Figure 3-8). These declines, however, have been much larger for men than for women.

Prevention strategies frequently focus on behavioral changes. The most prominent is counseling for individuals to use condoms if they are sexually active. Condom use rates have increased in the last few years, presumably as a result of HIV prevention campaigns. The effectiveness of these behavior modifications is limited by women's power, education, and societal level.[41] Health care providers can be a resource for communicating risks of infection, teaching prevention strategies, and providing testing for HIV. However, the majority of women have not talked with their health care provider about HIV/AIDS, although African American women were more likely than Hispanic and white women to report doing so (Figure 3-9).[43] The synergistic relationship between HIV infection and other STDs reinforces the importance of STD prevention. Sexually transmitted diseases can enhance transmission of HIV by a factor of two to five, whereas HIV infection can exacerbate transmission of other STDs.[1] Genital ulcers, cervical ectopy, traumatic sexual intercourse, lack of condom use, anal intercourse, and intercourse during menses are all factors that affect susceptibility.[1] Therefore, other options designed to prevent the sexual transmission of HIV are to treat any underlying STD and to minimize unsafe sexual behavior by promoting abstinence or condom use, or by decreasing the number of sexual partners.[1] Antiretroviral therapy may affect infectivity and is associated with a significant reduction in the sexual transmission of HIV.[1] A combination of these strategies may provide the most effective means of reducing HIV transmission in women in the future.

Trichomoniasis

As one of the most common STDs in the United States, trichomoniasis affects 2–3 million American women annually. No national data exist on the prevalence of trichomoniasis. It is a disease found mostly in women aged 16 to 35 years, is transmitted through sexual activity, and occurs more commonly among women with multiple sexual partners.[1]

Trichomoniasis is asymptomatic for many women, but others experience such symptoms as a foul-smelling or greenish discharge from the

Figure 3-8

AIDS deaths by gender, United States, 1993–1998

Deaths per year

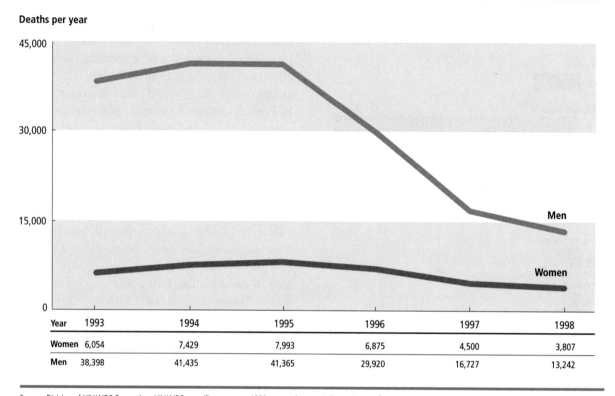

Year	1993	1994	1995	1996	1997	1998
Women	6,054	7,429	7,993	6,875	4,500	3,807
Men	38,398	41,435	41,365	29,920	16,727	13,242

Source: Division of HIV/AIDS Prevention. HIV/AIDS surveillance report: 1999 year-end report. Atlanta: Centers for Disease Control and Prevention; 1999; 11(2).

vagina, vaginal itching, or redness. Other symptoms may include painful sexual intercourse, lower abdominal discomfort, and the urge to urinate. These symptoms commonly develop 6 months from the time of infection. Trichomoniasis is diagnosed through a pelvic exam, during which vaginal samples are taken and examined to diagnose the infection. A single dose of metronidazole is commonly administered to treat this infection.[1] Research is ongoing to examine the potential association between trichomoniasis infection and an increased risk of HIV transmission. In addition, during pregnancy, trichomoniasis infection may be associated with preterm delivery and/or a low-birth-weight baby.[44]

Bacterial Vaginosis (BV)

Bacterial vaginosis is a broadly defined condition in which the benign hydrogen-peroxide-producing lactobacilli, which usually inhabit the vagina, are replaced by other species of bacteria, including *Gardnerella vaginalis, Mycoplasma hominis,* and *Ureaplasma urealyticum.*[45] In essence, the "good" bacteria are wiped out and the "bad" bacteria move in. Episodes of BV during pregnancy are related to increased risk of premature delivery.[46,47,48,49,50,51,52,53] Moreover, women with BV appear to be at much greater risk of acquiring HIV.[54]

No national data exist on the prevalence of BV. Among populations visiting family planning clinics, prevalence rates of BV have been estimated to be 17%.[23] In a multicenter study of over

Figure 3-9

Women's communication with health care providers about HIV/AIDS, United States, 1997

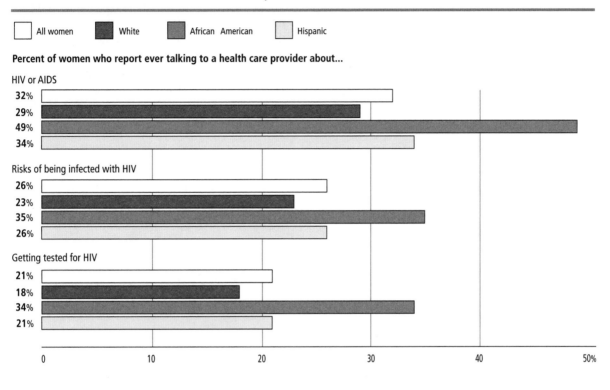

☐ All women   ■ White   ■ African American   ☐ Hispanic

Percent of women who report ever talking to a health care provider about...

HIV or AIDS
- 32%
- 29%
- 49%
- 34%

Risks of being infected with HIV
- 26%
- 23%
- 35%
- 26%

Getting tested for HIV
- 21%
- 18%
- 34%
- 21%

0   10   20   30   40   50%

Source: Henry J. Kaiser Family Foundation. National Survey of Americans on AIDS/HIV, conducted September 19–October 26, 1997.

10,000 pregnant women, the prevalence of BV averaged 16% (ranging from 9% to 28%).[46] This study defined BV based upon a test of a vaginal smear sample. Clinical criteria for diagnosis are much broader and may lead to both false positive and false negative diagnoses.

Women who are black[46,48,55], poor[46], less educated[46], young[46,48], or unmarried[46] have sometimes, but not always, been found to be at increased risk for BV infection. The only behavioral factors that have been identified as possible risk factors are early age at first intercourse[46], smoking[48] and vaginal douching.[56,57]

Bacterial vaginosis can be treated with an antibiotic (metronidazole).[58] Although the treatment is effective, women may acquire the condition repeatedly.

Influenza and Pneumonia

Taken together, influenza (flu) and pneumonia are among the five leading causes of death for people over 65 years of age and are responsible for 7% of deaths for those over the age of 85.[31] Deaths from influenza and pneumonia rise with age, from 42.9 per 100,000 for women ages 65 to 74 years to 933.7 per 100,000 for women over the age of 85 years.[31] Approximately 10% of all hospitalizations for elderly men and women are attributable to pneumonia and bronchitis.[31]

Annual influenza vaccinations can reduce the risk of influenza among older women. The CDC recommends that individuals 65 years and older or those with chronic health conditions receive influenza vaccinations each year to protect themselves against the flu.[31] Influenza vaccines have also proven to be cost effective for healthy, working adults aged 18 to 64 years.[59,60] Additionally, CDC recommends that everyone aged 65 and older should receive a one-time dose of the pneumonia vaccine.[61] In 1997, however, only 64.4% of women aged 65 and older received an influenza vaccine and 45.6% a pneumococcal vaccine in the previous year.[62] Vaccination use increases with age and varies by race and ethnicity, but not by gender.[31,62] For those over the age of 65, non-Hispanic white persons report both higher vaccination rates for influenza and pneumonia as compared to non-Hispanic black or Hispanic persons.[31]

References

1. Eng T, Butler W. The hidden epidemic: confronting sexually transmitted diseases. Washington: Institute of Medicine; 1996.

2. Brunham RC, Binns B, Guijon F, Danforth D, Kosselm ML, Rand F, et al. Etiology and outcome of acute pelvic inflammatory disease. J Infect Dis 1988;158:510–517.

3. Cates W, Wasserheit JN. Genital chlamydial infections: epidemiology and reproductive sequelae. Am J Obstet Gynecol 1991; 164:1771–1781.

4. Grodstein F, Rothman KJ. Epidemiology of pelvic inflammatory disease. Epidemiology 1994;5:234–242.

5. Westrom L, Joesoef R, Reynolds G, Hadgu A, Thompson SE. Pelvic inflammatory disease and fertility: a cohort study of 1,844 women with laparoscopically verified disease and 657 control women with normal laparoscopic results. Sex Trans Dis 1992;19(4):185–192.

6. Cates W Jr. Estimates of the incidence and prevalence of sexually transmitted diseases in the United States. American Social Health Association Panel. Sex Trans Dis 1999;26 (4 Suppl):S2–S7.

7. Wortley PM, Fleming PL. AIDS in women in the United States. Recent trends. JAMA 1997;278:911–916.

8. Division of STD Prevention. Sexually transmitted disease surveillance, 1999. Atlanta: Centers for Disease Control and Prevention; 2000:79,82,83,89,91,92,101,104,105. Available from: URL: www.cdc.gov/nchstp/dstd/Stats_Trends/1999SurvRpt.htm.

9. Judson FN. Gonorrhea. Med Clin North Am 1990;74:1353–1366.

10. Groseclose SL, Zaidi AA, DeLisle S, Levine W, St Louis ME. Estimated incidence and prevalence of genital Chlamydia trachomatis infections in the United States, 1996. Sex Trans Dis 1999;26:339–344.

11. Gaydos CA, Howell MR, Pare B, Clark KL, Ellis DA, Hendrix RM, et al. Chlamydia trachomatis infections in female military recruits. N Engl J Med 1998;339:739–744.

12. Scholes D, Stergachis A, Heidrich FE, Andrilla H, Holmes KK, Stamm WE. Prevention of pelvic inflammatory disease by screening for cervical chlamydial infection. N Engl J Med 1996;334:1362–1366.

13. Brunham RC, Binns B, McDowell J, Paraskevas M. Chlamydia trachomatis infection in women with ectopic pregnancy. Obstet Gynecol 1986;67:722–726.

14. Coste J, Job-Spira N, Fernandez H. Risk factors for ectopic pregnancy: a case-control study in France, with special focus on infectious factors. Am J Epidemiol 1991;133:839–849.

15. Chow JM, Yonekura ML, Richwald GA, Greenland S, Sweet RL, Schachter J. The association between Chlamydia trachomatis and ectopic pregnancy. A matched-pair, case-control study. JAMA 1990;263:3164–3167.

16. Chrysostomou M, Karafyllidi P, Papdimitriou V, Bassiotou V, Mayakos G. Serum antibodies to Chlamydia trachomatis in women with ectopic pregnancy, normal pregnancy, or salpingitis. Eur J Obstet Gynecol Reprod Biol 1992;44:101–105.

17. Phillips RS, Ruomala RE, Feldblum PJ, Schachter J, Rosenberg MJ, Aronson MD. The effect of cigarette smoking, Chlamydia trachomatis infection, and vaginal douching on ectopic pregnancy. Obstet Gynecol 1992;79:85–90.

18. Fox KK, Whittington WL, Levine WC, Moran JS, Zaidi AA, Nakashima AK. Gonorrhea in the United States, 1981–1996. Demographic and geographic trends. Sex Trans Infect 1998; 25:386–393.

19. Division of STD Prevention. Sexually transmitted disease surveillance 1998 supplement: Gonococcal Isolate Surveillance Project (GISP) annual report. Atlanta: Centers for Disease Control and Prevention; 1999.

20. McNeeley SG. Pelvic inflammatory disease. Curr Opin Obstet Gynecol 1992;4:682–686.

21. Abma JC, Chandra A, Mosher WD, Peterson L, Piccinino LJ. Fertility, family planning, and women's health: new data from the 1995 National Survey of Family Growth. Vital Health Stat 1997; 23:1–114.

22. Platt R, Rice P, McCormack W. Risk of acquiring gonorrhea and prevalence of abnormal adnexal findings among women recently exposed to gonorrhea. JAMA 1983;250:3205–3209.

23. Division of STD Prevention. Sexually transmitted disease surveillance. Atlanta: Centers for Disease Control and Prevention; 1998.

24. Pavletic AJ, Wolner-Hanssen P, Paavonen J, Hawes S, Eschenbach, DA. Infertility following pelvic inflammatory disease. Infect Dis Obstet Gynecol 1999;7:145–152.

25. Eschenbach D. Pelvic infections and sexually transmitted diseases. In: Scott J, DiSaia P, Hammond C, Spellacy W, editors. Danforth's obstetrics and gynecology. 6th ed. Philadelphia: JB Lippincott; 1990:933–958.

26. Division of STD Prevention. Tracking the hidden epidemics. Trends in STDs in the United States, 2000. Atlanta: Centers for Disease Control and Prevention; 2000. p 22–23.

27. Centers for Disease Control and Prevention. Primary and secondary syphilis, United States, 1997. MMWR Morb Mortal Wkly Rpt 1998;47:493–497.

28. Centers for Disease Control and Prevention. Primary and secondary syphilis, United States, 1998. MMWR Morb Mortal Wkly Rpt 1999;48:873–878.

29. Coleman PJ, McQuillan GM, Moyer LA, Lambert SB, Margolis HS. Incidence of hepatitis B virus infection in the United States, 1976–1994: estimates from the National Health and Nutrition Examination Surveys. J Infect Dis 1998;178:954–959.

30. Evans A. Viral infections in humans. New York: Plenum Medical Book Company; 1997.

31. Kramarow E, Lentzner H, Rooks R, Weeks J, Saydah S. Health and aging chartbook. Health, United States. (PHS)99–1292. Hyattsville (MD): National Center for Health Statistics; 1999. p 40.

32. Centers for Disease Control and Prevention. Hepatitis B virus: a comprehensive strategy for eliminating transmission in the United States through universal childhood vaccination: recommendations of the Immunization Practices Advisory Committee (ACIP). MMWR Morb Mortal Wkly Rpt 1991;40(no. RR–13).

33. Mast EE, Williams IT, Alter MJ, Margolis HS. Hepatitis B vaccination of adolescent and adult high-risk groups in the United States. Vaccine 1998;16 Suppl:S27–S29.

34. Koutsky L. Epidemiology of genital human papillomavirus infection. Am J Med 1997;102:3–8.

35. Ho GY, Bierman R, Beardsley L, Chang C, Burk RD. Natural history of cervicovaginal papillomavirus infection in young women. N Engl J Med 1998;338:423–428.

36. Division of STD Prevention. Prevention of genital HPV infection and sequelae: report of an external consultants meeting. Atlanta: Centers for Disease Control and Prevention; 1999.

37. Koutsky LA, Galloway DA, Holmes KK. Epidemiology of human papillomavirus infection. Epidemiol Rev 1988;10:122–163.

38. Fleming DT, McQuillan GM, Johnson RE, Nahmias AJ, Aral SO, Lee FK, et al. Herpes simplex virus type 2 in the United States, 1976 to 1994. N Engl J Med 1997;337:1105–1111.

39. McQuillan G. Implications of a national survey for STDs: results from the NHANES Survey. 2000 Infectious Disease Society of America Conference. New Orleans; 2000.

40. Division of HIV/AIDS Prevention. HIV/AIDS surveillance report: 1999 year-end report. Atlanta: Centers for Disease Control and Prevention; 1999;11(2).

41. Gollub EL. Human rights is a U.S. problem, too: the case of women and HIV. Am J Public Health 1999;89:1479–1482.

42. Solomon L, Stein M, Flynn C, Schuman P, Schoenbaum E, Moore J, et al. Health services use by urban women with or at risk for HIV-1 infection: the HIV Epidemiology Research Study (HERS). J Acquir Immune Defic Syndr Hum Retrovirol 1998;17:253–261.

43. Henry J. Kaiser Family Foundation. 1997 national survey of Americans on AIDS/HIV. Washington: The Foundation, 1997.

44. Sobel JD. Vaginitis. N Engl J Med 1997;337:1896–1903.

45. Nugent RP, Krohn MA, Hillier SL. Reliability of diagnosing bacterial vaginosis is improved by a standardized method of gram stain interpretation. J Clin Microbiol 1991;29:297–301.

46. Hillier SL, Nugent RP, Eschenbach DA, Krohn MA, Gibbs RS, Martin DH, et al. Association between bacterial vaginosis and preterm delivery of a low-birth-weight infant. The Vaginal Infections and Prematurity Study Group. N Engl J Med 1995;333:1737–1742.

47. Holst E, Goffeng AR, Andersch B. Bacterial vaginosis and vaginal microorganisms in idiopathic premature labor and association with pregnancy outcome. J Clin Microbiol 1994;32:176–186.

48. Hay PE, Lamont RF, Taylor-Robinson D, Morgan DJ, Ison C, Pearson J. Abnormal bacterial colonisation of the genital tract and subsequent preterm delivery and late miscarriage. Br Med J 1994;308:295–298.

49. Gravett MG, Nelson HP, DeRouen T, Critchlow CW, Eschenbach DA, Holmes KK. Independent associations of bacterial vaginosis and Chlamydia trachomatis infection with adverse pregnancy outcome. JAMA 1986;256:1899–1903.

50. Gravett MG, Hummel D, Eschenbach DA, Holmes KK. Preterm labor associated with subclinical amniotic fluid infection and with bacterial vaginosis. Obstet Gynecol 1986;67:229–237.

51. Kurki T, Sivonen A, Renkonen OV, Savia E, Ylikorkala O. Bacterial vaginosis in early pregnancy and pregnancy outcome. Obstet Gynecol 1992;80:173–177.

52. Martius J, Krohn MA, Hillier SL, Stamm WE, Holmes KK, Eschenbach DA. Relationship of vaginal Lactobacillus species, cervical Chlamydia trachomatis, and bacterial vaginosis to preterm birth. Obstet Gynecol 1988;71:89–95.

53. Riduan JM, Hillier SL, Utomo B, Wiknjosastro G, Linan M, Kandun N. Bacterial vaginosis and prematurity in Indonesia: association in early and late pregnancy. Am J Obstet Gynecol 1993;169:175–178.

54. Taha TE, Hoover DR, Dallabetta GA, Kumwenda NI, Mtimavalye LA, Yang LP, et al. Bacterial vaginosis and disturbances of vaginal flora: association with increased acquisition of HIV/AIDS 1998; 12:1699–1706.

55. Goldenberg RL, Thom E, Moawad AH, Johnson F, Roberts J, Caritis SN. The preterm prediction study: fetal fibronectin, bacterial vaginosis, and peripartum infection. NICHD Maternal Fetal Medicine Unit Network. Obstet Gynecol 1996;87:656–660.

56. Hawes SE, Hillier SL, Benedetti J, Stevens CE, Koutsky LA, Wolner-Hanssen P, et al. Hydrogen peroxide-producing lactobacilli and acquisition of vaginal infections. J Infect Dis 1996;174:1058–1063.

57. Onderdonk AB, Delaney ML, Hinkson PL, DuBois AM. Quantitative and qualitative effects of douche preparations on vaginal microflora. Obstet Gynecol 1992;80:333–338.

58. Centers for Disease Control and Prevention. 1998 guidelines for treatment of sexually transmitted diseases. MMWR Morb Mortal Wkly Rpt 1998;47(RR-1):1–118.

59. Nichol KS, Lind A, Margolis K, Murdoch M, McFadden R, Hauge M, et al. The effectiveness of vaccination against influenza in healthy, working adults. N Engl J Med 1995;333:889–893.

60. Patriarca PA, Strikas RA. Influenza vaccine for healthy adults? N Engl J Med 1995;333:933–934.

61. Centers for Disease Control and Prevention. Prevention of pneumococcal disease: recommendations of the Advisory Committee on Immunization Practices (ACIP). MMWR Morb Mortal Wkly Rep 1997;46:1–24.

62. Centers for Disease Control and Prevention. Influenza and pneumococcal vaccination levels among adults aged greater than or equal to 65 years, United States. MMWR Morb Mortal Wkly Rep 1998;47:797–802.

Chapter 4

Chronic Conditions

Contents

Introduction

Chronic conditions are the leading cause of death and disability for women in the United States. Though no one standard exists to define what constitutes a chronic disorder, *chronic* is defined here as any condition that requires regular medical attention and/or medication. Chronic diseases cannot be cured readily by treatment and, therefore, differ from most acute conditions. Rather, the goal of treatment for chronic conditions is to prevent exacerbation of the condition and minimize adverse consequences. The risk of chronic disease generally increases as a woman ages. Some diseases, such as asthma and type I (juvenile) diabetes, are acquired primarily before adulthood, however.

Some readers may wonder why cancers appear in this chapter. Advances in treatment of cancers have led to increased survival although often without a cure, resulting in many women living with cancer, just as they live with diabetes and other chronic conditions. It will also be evident to some readers that many of the infections discussed in the preceding chapter could also be described as chronic conditions. Until recently, infectious diseases were generally acute conditions with a short duration; the patient either recovered quickly with or without treatment or died proximate to the infection. Recently, however, treatments are extending survival without curing the condition; infections such as HIV/AIDS can now be considered chronic diseases. We have chosen, however, to group infections together within one chapter. Although some infections share features of chronic diseases, the surveillance systems, risk factors, and preventive approaches are generally different.

In this chapter, we provide data on women's experience of several major chronic conditions. These particular disorders were selected for one or more of the following reasons: the disease is a leading cause of mortality among women (e.g., cardiovascular disease, lung cancer); the disease is a leading cause of disability among women (e.g., osteoporosis, arthritis); or the disease is more frequent among women as compared to men (e.g., thyroid disease).

Before examining these specific conditions, it is helpful to examine the data on global indicators of health. These indicators include life expectancy, mortality rates, restricted activity days, activity limitation, and perceived health status.

Life expectancy has dramatically increased for all women over the past century, particularly in the first half of the 20th century (Table 4-1). As with so many indices of health, life expectancy for black women lags behind that of white women. Nevertheless, unlike many other health measures, the gap in life expectancy has narrowed substantially. Life expectancy for women has exceeded that for men over the past century among both blacks and whites.[1]

National mortality statistics indicate that chronic conditions are among the leading causes of death in the United States. To compile such statistics, the National Center for Health Statistics (NCHS) uses the underlying cause of death recorded on the death certificate. In 1998, the age-adjusted death rate for white females was 372.5 per 100,000 and 589.4 per 100,000 for black females.[2] The leading causes of death vary somewhat with the age of the woman (Table 4-2) but are similar by race/ethnicity within age groups (Table 4-3). In older women, cancer and heart disease are the top two causes of death. For younger women, unintentional injuries, homicides, and HIV infection are the leading causes of death. The age-adjusted death rates for many of the leading causes of death are higher for men than they are for women; they are higher for black women than white women (Table 4-4).[2]

A broader measure of disability is captured by measures of activity limitation. The National Health Interview Survey (NHIS) collects self-reported data on the number of days of restricted activity experienced per year (Table 4-

Table 4-1

Life expectancy at birth by gender and race, United States, 1900, 1950, and 1998

| Year | Age (years) | | | |
	White women	White men	Black women	Black men
1900	48.7	46.6	33.5	32.5
1950	72.2	66.5	62.7	58.9
1998	80.0	74.5	74.8	67.6

Source: National Center for Health Statistics. Health, United States, 1999. With health and aging chartbook. (PHS)99–1232. Hyattsville (MD): U.S. Department of Health and Human Services; 1999. Murphy SL. Deaths: final data for 1998. Natl Vital Stat Rep 2000;48(11):1–105.

5). Level of education and family income are both correlated with this measure of health. Both of these factors are associated with many of the major chronic conditions that lead to activity restriction, such as asthma and hypertension. Education and low income correlate most strongly with morbidity among women between the ages of 45 and 64, but the overall impact of low income is stronger that that of low education attainment, in this and in all age groups. In addition, women report more activity-restricted days than do men at all ages. Although income and education both affect morbidity among women, the effect of income is stronger for women than for men, and the effect of education is similar for men and women.[3]

Data are also available from the NHIS on the proportion of women who experience various levels of activity limitation. In 1996, approximately 14.9% of all women reported some degree of activity limitation, but only 4.5% were unable to carry out a major activity of daily living, such as bathing, dressing, or feeding themselves. Among women over 70 years of age, 38.2% have some degree of activity limitation, with 9.1% unable to carry out a major activity of daily living.[4]

Table 4-2

Death rates for women by age for the 10 leading causes of death, United States, 1998

Cause of death	Death rate per 100,000 women*				
	All ages**	15–24 years	25–44 years	45–64 years	≥65 years
All causes	853.5	43.5	107.4	501.9	4,754.9
Malignant neoplasms, including neoplasms of lymphatic and hematopoietic tissues	187.7	3.7	28.0	209.9	912.7
Diseases of heart	268.3	2.1	11.9	101.5	1,658.4
Cerebrovascular diseases	70.4	N/A	3.9	23.3	438.2
Accidents and adverse effects	25.2	19.1	16.5	18.0	83.2
Chronic obstructive pulmonary diseases and allied conditions	40.2	0.5	N/A	21.2	240.2
Pneumonia and influenza	36.8	0.6	1.9	8.2	233.6
Diabetes mellitus	25.4	0.4	2.4	20.1	139.1
Suicide	N/A	3.3	6.0	6.4	N/A
Chronic liver disease and cirrhosis	N/A	N/A	2.9	10.1	N/A
Septicemia	9.8	N/A	N/A	5.2	56.1
Nephritis, nephrotic syndrome, and nephrosis	9.9	N/A	N/A	N/A	59.9
Homicide and legal intervention	N/A	4.3	4.6	N/A	N/A
HIV infection	N/A	0.6	5.1	N/A	N/A
Congenital anomalies	N/A	1.1	N/A	N/A	N/A
Alzheimer's disease	11.3	N/A	N/A	N/A	76.7

*Data available for 10 leading causes of death in each age-race/ethnicity group; no data are available for Asian/Pacific Islander or Native American women.

**Age adjusted.

N/A: the cause of death is not a leading cause in that group.

Source: Murphy, SL. Deaths: final data for 1998. Natl Vital Stat Rep 2000:48(11):1–105.

Table 4-3

Death rates for women by race/ethnicity* and age for the 10 leading causes of death, United States, 1998

| | Death rate per 100,000 women** | | | | | | | | | | | |
| | 15–24 years | | | 25–44 years | | | 45–64 years | | | ≥65 years | | |
Cause of death	White	Black	Hispanic	White	Black	Hispanic	White	Black	Hispanic	White	Black	Hispanic
All causes	41.2	58.0	34.0	92.9	209.2	72.6	465.8	849.1	346.1	4,795.9	5,061.3	2,716.3
Malignant neoplasms, including neoplasms of lymphatic and hematopoietic tissues	3.7	4.0	3.4	26.4	40.4	19.1	205.7	273.4	125.8	918.5	980.0	501.6
Diseases of heart	1.8	3.9	1.3	9.3	30.6	5.7	88.2	221.4	65.6	1,671.9	1,799.1	959.8
Cerebrovascular diseases	0.3	N/A	—	3.0	9.8	3.0	19.4	54.1	20.2	441.0	462.5	225.7
Accidents and adverse effects	20.4	13.0	13.7	16.4	19.4	12.5	17.4	23.7	15.7	85.5	69.1	41.3
Chronic obstructive pulmonary diseases and allied conditions	0.3	1.3	N/A	N/A	3.8	1.0	21.9	21.8	6.4	256.3	123.5	87.7
Pneumonia and influenza	0.4	1.4	—	1.6	4.1	N/A	7.6	14.0	5.4	240.6	190.1	135.9
Diabetes mellitus	0.3	N/A	—	2.1	5.2	1.7	16.4	49.8	25.4	126.1	281.0	183.5
Suicide	3.5	2.2	2.8	6.6	N/A	2.2	7.1	N/A	N/A	N/A	N/A	N/A
Chronic liver disease and cirrhosis	N/A	N/A	N/A	2.7	3.5	2.1	9.8	13.0	12.2	N/A	N/A	36.5
Septicemia	N/A	N/A	N/A	N/A	N/A	N/A	4.2	13.7	N/A	51.9	107.8	N/A
Homicide and legal intervention	2.8	12.6	4.2	3.2	13.0	4.3	N/A	N/A	N/A	N/A	N/A	N/A
HIV infection	N/A	2.9	N/A	1.8	26.1	5.0	N/A	15.5	4.9	N/A	N/A	N/A
Viral hepatitis	N/A	N/A	N/A	N/A	N/A	N/A	N/A	N/A	4.2	N/A	N/A	N/A
Congenital anomalies	1.0	1.4	—	N/A	N/A	N/A	N/A	N/A	N/A	N/A	N/A	N/A
Complications of pregnancy, childbirth, and puerpium	N/A	1.2	—	N/A	N/A	N/A	N/A	N/A	N/A	N/A	N/A	N/A
Alzheimer's disease	N/A	N/A	N/A	N/A	N/A	N/A	N/A	N/A	N/A	81.2	N/A	31.0
Anemias	N/A	1.2	N/A	N/A	N/A	N/A	N/A	N/A	N/A	N/A	N/A	N/A

*Persons of Hispanic origin may be of any race.

**Data available for 10 leading causes of death in each age-race/ethnicity group; data are not available for Asian/Pacific Islander or Native American women.

N/A: the cause is not a leading cause in that group.

—Figure does not meet standards of reliability or precision.

Source: Murphy, SL. Deaths: final data for 1998. Natl Vital Stat Rep 2000:48(11):1–105.

Table 4-4

Ratio of age-adjusted death rates for leading causes of death, United States, 1998

	Age-adjusted death rate	
Cause of death	Male-to-female ratio	Black-to-white female ratio
Heart disease	1.8	1.5
Malignant neoplasms, including neoplasms of lymphatic and hematopoietic tissues	1.4	1.3
Cerebrovascular diseases	1.1	1.8
Chronic obstructive pulmonary diseases	1.4	0.8
Accidents and adverse effects	2.4	1.2
Pneumonia and influenza	1.5	1.4
Diabetes mellitus	1.2	2.4
Suicide	4.3	0.5
Nephritis, nephrotic syndrome, and nephrosis	1.5	2.5
Chronic liver disease and cirrhosis	2.3	1.2
Septicemia	1.2	2.7
Alzheimer's disease	0.9	0.7
Homicide and legal intervention	3.5	5.7
Atherosclerosis	1.3	1.0
Hypertension with or without renal disease	1.1	3.8

Source: Murphy SL. Deaths: final data for 1998. Natl Vital Stat Rep 2000;48(11):1–105.

Table 4-5

Restricted activity days per year among women by education and income, United States, 1996

	Age (years)			
	All Ages	18–44	45–64	65+ years
Total	14.5	22.4	18.7	30.5
Education				
<12 years	27.1	18.2	39.2	39.9
12–15 years	16.1	14.3	19.6	31.1
16 years or more	11.9	10.3	13.5	26.3
Family annual income				
<$10,000	27.9	43.5	51.8	48.0
$10–19,999	21.1	34.4	33.5	34.4
$20,000–34,999	13.0	20.6	18.3	23.6
$35,000+	9.9	17.3	11.9	18.1

Source: Adams P, Hendershot G, Marano M. Current estimates from the National Health Interview Survey, 1996. National Center for Health Statistics. Vital Health Stat 1999;10(200):83–84.

Table 4-6

Women reporting "fair" or "poor" health by race and age, United States, 1996

	Percent		
	18–44 years	45–64 years	65+ years
Total	12	16	27
Black women	19	29	40
White women	11	15	26

Source: Adams P, Hendershot G, Marano M. Current estimates from the National Health Interview Survey, 1996. National Center for Health Statistics. Vital Health Stat 1999;10(200):83–84.

Perceived health status is another important indicator of overall morbidity collected in the 1996 NHIS. Overall, the proportion of women and men who reported their health as "fair" or "poor" is similar.[5] Among women, race has a greater impact on this indicator, with a much higher proportion of black women reporting their health as "fair" or "poor" as compared to white women in all age groups (Table 4-6).

Cardiovascular Disease

As the leading cause of both death and disability for American women, cardiovascular disease (CVD) was implicated in approximately half a million deaths in 1998.[2] The most common manifestations of CVD are heart disease and stroke. The National Institute on Aging estimates that one in 10 women 45 to 64 years of age and one in five women aged 65 years and older have some form of heart disease. Based on 1996 NHIS data, the prevalence of heart disease was 100.3 per 100,000 among women 45–64 years of age and 238.0 per 100,000 among women aged 65 years and older.[4] The age-adjusted death rate for heart disease among women was 93.3 per 100,000 in 1998, a total of 370,962 deaths.[2]

Approximately 1.6 million women in the United State have had a stroke. Furthermore, 97,303 women died from strokes in 1998.[2] Based on 1996 NHIS data, the prevalence of cerebrovascular disease was 9.6 per 100,000 women 45–64 years of age and 44.4 per 100,000 among women 65 years and over.[4] The age-adjusted death rate for cerebrovascular disease among women was 23.6 per 100,000.[2] Certain ethnic minority groups have higher rates of coronary heart disease (CHD) and stroke. This appears to be the result of higher proportions of minority women with standard risk factors for CVD, such as obesity and hypertension, rather than any risk factors unique to minority women.[6]

Risk factors associated with the development of CHD include older age, hypertension, high cholesterol, diabetes, inadequate physical activity, cigarette smoking, and obesity. Coronary events in women who are premenopausal are rare. After menopause, however, the rate rapidly increases.[7] The average age at onset of CHD in women is about 10 years later than in men.

Hypertension is an important risk factor for heart disease[8,9,10,11] as well as the most important risk factor for cerebrovascular disease (e.g., stroke).[8,12] Several factors may influence a woman's risk of hypertension and its severity including alcohol use,[13] physical inactivity,[14,15] diet (particularly salt intake), and obesity.[16,17] Black women are at greater risk for hypertension than white, Asian, and Hispanic women.[18] Rates of hypertension have been declining for all women and for most age groups of women, particularly since 1980 (Figure 4-1). Based on National Health and Nutrition Examination Survey III (NHANES III) age-adjusted data, approximately 19.3% of non-Hispanic white women, 34.2% of non-Hispanic black women, and 22% of Mexican American women have hypertension.[19] A unique concern for women is the elevation of blood pressure that can occur with oral contraceptive use. The risk of oral-contraceptive-induced hypertension increases with age and duration; the older a woman is and the longer she has taken oral contraceptives, the stronger the effect on blood pressure level.[20]

A high blood cholesterol level greatly increases a woman's risk of developing CHD. The National Institute on Aging reports that cholesterol levels in women generally rise after the age of 20 and then increase rapidly at age 40. Cholesterol levels often continue to rise until a woman reaches 60 years of age. The proportion of women with high cholesterol levels (above 240 mg/dL) has been declining over the past four decades overall and in most age groups (Figure 4-2), particularly since 1980. Based on NHANES data, there are no substantial differences among women with high cholesterol by race/ethnicity. Among women 20–74 years of age, approximately 20.4% of whites, 19.4% of blacks, and 17.5% of Mexican Americans have high cholesterol levels.[19] However, these are age-adjusted rates; more than twice as many women over age 55 (40.9%) need

Figure 4-1

Hypertension among women by age, 1960–1994

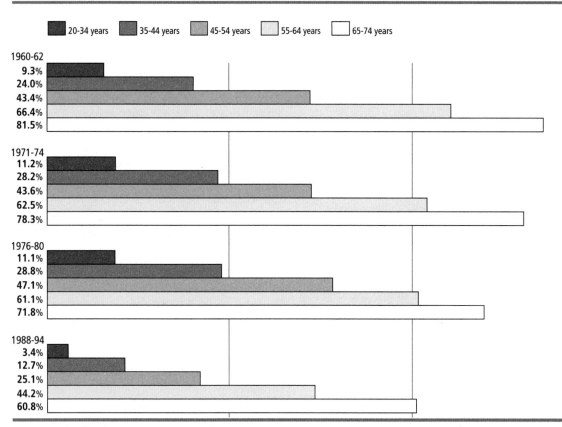

Source: National Health and Nutrition Examination Survey. Table 68. In: Kramarow E, Lentzner H, Rooks R, Weeks J, Saydah S. Health, United States, 1999. With health and aging chartbook. (PHS)99–1232. Hyattsville (MD): National Center for Health Statistics; 1999.

to lower their cholesterol.[19] The higher a person's high-density lipoprotein (HDL) level, often referred to as "good cholesterol," the lower the risk of coronary heart disease. Levels of HDL predict risk more strongly for women than for men.[21] Lowering total cholesterol levels and increasing HDL levels may be accomplished by altering diet, increasing activity, losing excess weight, and using medication.

Obesity may be an independent risk factor, or it may influence CHD risk solely through its effects on related factors such as blood pressure, glucose tolerance, and cholesterol.[6] The prevalence of obesity (defined as a body mass index greater than or equal to 30) was greater among

black women than among white women: 37.6% versus 23.5% in 1994.[19] In contrast to improvements seen for hypertension and high cholesterol levels, the proportion of women who are obese has been steadily increasing over the past four decades among all races and ages (Figure 4-3).[19]

Epidemiologic observational studies have shown that women who use postmenopausal hormone replacement therapy (HRT), such as estrogen or estrogen-progesterone, have an approximate 50% reduction in the risk of developing coronary artery disease.[22] However, black women and other nonwhite groups have been underrepresented in studies of this type.[23] Data on the proportion of women who use HRT are

Figure 4-2

High cholesterol among women by age, 1960–1994

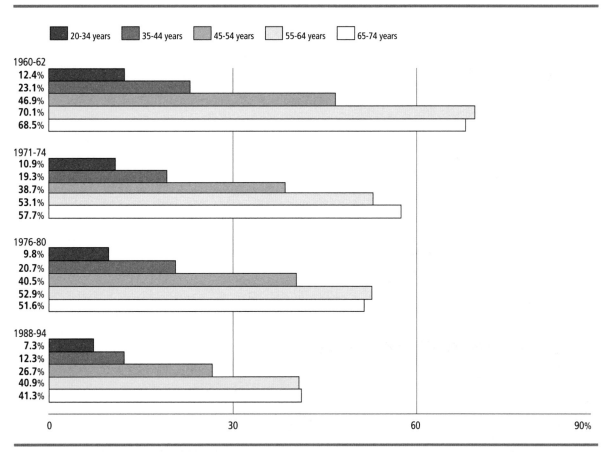

Source: National Health and Nutrition Examination Survey. Table 69. In: Kramarow E, Lentzner H, Rooks R, Weeks J, Saydah S. Health, United States, 1999. With health and aging chartbook. (PHS)99–1232. Hyattsville (MD): National Center for Health Statistics; 1999.

discussed in chapter 6. Hormone replacement therapy is most effective in reducing risk among women who are at highest risk of developing coronary artery disease.[24,25] However, these studies are observational and may be biased (i.e., women who use postmenopausal HRT are also generally healthier and have healthier lifestyles).

Women who have diabetes are approximately three times more likely to develop heart disease than those who do not.[26,27] It is hypothesized that diabetes reduces the protective effects of female hormones against CHD.[28] In addition, women with diabetes who have myocardial infarctions are more likely to die than women who do not

have diabetes or men.[28] Rates of diabetes among women are provided in the next section.

Physical activity reduces the risk of CHD, which is most likely due to the effects of exercise on cholesterol, obesity, and hypertension.[14,15,29] The Nurses' Health Study recently reported that less vigorous exercise, such as walking, may be as useful for reducing the number of CHD events as is vigorous exercise.[30] Data on physical activity behaviors in women are discussed in chapter 6.

Smoking is a strong and modifiable risk factor for CHD.[9,10,11] The Nurses' Health Study found that the women who reported smoking the most

Figure 4-3

Obesity among women by age, 1960–1994

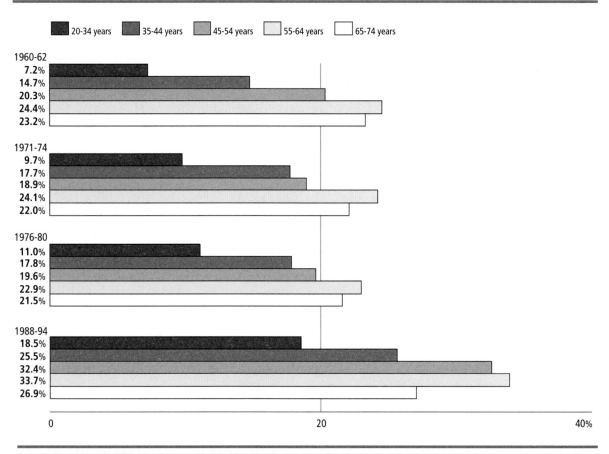

Source: National Health and Nutrition Examination Survey. Table 68. In: Kramarow E, Lentzner H, Rooks R, Weeks J, Saydah S. Health, United States, 1999. With health and aging chartbook. (PHS)99–1232. Hyattsville (MD): National Center for Health Statistics; 1999.

were more than six times as likely to be at risk for developing CHD than nonsmoking women. However, women who stop smoking for at least 3–5 years are able to reduce their risk of CHD to nearly that of nonsmokers.[31] This risk factor is particularly important for women because more adolescent and young women are smoking in the United States than ever before.[32] Also, estrogen levels are reduced among women who smoke; therefore, the known beneficial effects of estrogen on preventing CHD are reduced.[11] Smoking rates are discussed in chapter 6.

A woman's socioeconomic status (SES) may also be related to her cardiovascular health. Women at

lower socioeconomic levels have consistently higher blood pressure than do those in the highest socioeconomic levels.[33] These associations with socioeconomic status are magnified and observed more consistently among women than among men, perhaps a reflection of the higher rates of obesity among women of lower socio-economic levels. Furthermore, lower SES women have higher rates of poor cardiovascular health. [33]

Psychological factors may also be related to cardiovascular health. However, studies investigating psychological risk factors have focused primarily on men, and psychosocial risk factors that are relevant to men may not be relevant to women. For example, women with type A personality who were enrolled in the Framingham study were not at increased risk for a coronary event.[34] The same study, however, concluded that stress does play a major role in a woman's coronary health. Other psychosocial risk factors that may affect women differently than men include anger, hostility, hopelessness, depression, social support/networks, education, occupation, stressful life events, job control, and chronic fatigue.[35]

Diabetes Mellitus

Generally, diabetes mellitus, a chronic metabolic condition which results in abnormal regulation and production of insulin, is diagnosed by a blood test to measure the level of glucose or sugar in the blood and is classified into three types: insulin-dependent diabetes (type I), non-insulin dependent diabetes (type II), and gestational diabetes. Type I diabetes is an autoimmune disease characterized by onset and diagnosis in childhood or adolescence and the requirement of insulin injections for survival. Conversely, type II diabetes develops in adults and is often controlled through nutrition and exercise but may require insulin or oral medications. Gestational diabetes is characterized by onset during pregnancy and is similar to type II diabetes; it can usually be controlled through proper nutrition.[36]

In 1998, diabetes was ranked the sixth leading cause of death among women overall and the fourth leading cause of death among black and Hispanic women.[2] For all women, the age-adjusted death rate due to diabetes in 1998 was 25.4 per 100,000 women.[2]

Based on the results of the NHANES III survey of 1988–94, the overall prevalence of diabetes among women 20 years of age or older in the United States was 5.4% (5.6 million when applied to 1997 projections of U.S. population).[37] Table 4-7 describes the prevalence of diabetes for

Table 4-7

Diabetes prevalence in U.S. women, 1988–1994				
	Prevalence* of diabetes (percent)			
Age (years)	**All women**	**White, non-Hispanic**	**Black, non-Hispanic**	**Mexican American**
≥20	7.8	7.1	11.8	10.2
20–39	1.7	1.3	3.3	2.7
40–49	6.0	4.8	10.4	14.1
50–59	12.4	9.7	23.0	24.0
60–74	17.8	16.0	32.4	32.5
≥75	17.5	16.6	26.6	31.2

*Prevalence includes both previously diagnosed diabetes (table 1 in source) and undiagnosed diabetes (table 2 in source, defined as fasting plasma glucose ≥126 mg/dL, age-adjusted).

Source: Adapted from NHANES III (1988–1994). Harris M, Flegal K, Cowie C. Prevalence of diabetes, impaired fasting glucose, and impaired glucose tolerance in the U.S. adults: the Third National Health and Nutrition Examination Survey. Diabetes Care 1998;21:518–524.

women by age and race/ethnicity based upon NHANES III data. The prevalence among all groups increased with age with a slight decline in women 75 years of age or older overall and among blacks and Mexican Americans (rates for other Hispanic groups were not estimated). The rates are higher for minority women in all age groups but the differences are more pronounced among older women, as prevalence increases with age.[37] Prevalence rates were higher for non-Hispanic black women than for non-Hispanic black men, whereas rates were higher for the non-Hispanic white and Mexican American men.[37] Overall, the prevalence of diabetes for all individuals has been rising in the United States in the past decade. The prevalence increased from 28 in 1986-88 to 31 per 1,000 persons in 1996. Data on gestational diabetes are provided in chapter 2.

People with diabetes experience an increased risk of developing heart, kidney, peripheral vascular, and eye disease, as well as complications during pregnancy. Diabetes is the leading cause of end-stage renal disease (ESRD) accounting for an estimated 40% of new cases each year. Diabetes is also the leading cause of blindness in adults aged 20 to 74 years old.[38,39] The risk of death due to stroke and heart disease is approximately two to four times higher in diabetics than in those without diabetes and an estimated 60% to 65% of diabetics have hypertension.[40,41] In 1997, the estimated years of potential life lost before the age of 75 for women with diabetes were 318.3 per 100,000 among blacks, 306.4 per 100,000 among American Indian/Alaskan Natives, 167.9 per 100,000 among Hispanics, and 111.1 per 100,000 non-Hispanic whites.[42] Overall, for men and women, the age-adjusted death rate from diabetes has increased from 38 in 1986 to 41 per 100,000 persons in 1996.[19]

Being obese; having a family history of diabetes; being black, Hispanic, or American Indian; and/or having complications known to be related to diabetes are risk factors for type II diabetes. Approximately 78% of nondiabetic adults in the United States have at least one of these risk factors and 23% have three or more.[43] Family history of a sibling or parent with type I diabetes is the major known risk factor for this type of diabetes. Children born to women with type I diabetes have a 1 in 40 chance of developing the disease and a 1 in 20 chance if their father has the disease.[44] Women who are obese, have a first-degree relative with diabetes, a history of glucose intolerance, or are black, Hispanic, Native American, or Asian/Pacific Islander are at increased risk of developing gestational diabetes.[45]

Referred to by many as the silent killer, diabetes is often detected after the onset of a life-threatening condition. Nearly half of adults diagnosed with type II diabetes report experiencing symptoms that led to testing while the other half report the detection of diabetes through routine physical exams.[43] Rates of screening for diabetes are higher among high-risk groups. However, it is estimated that one-third of people with diabetes go undiagnosed.[37]

Primary prevention of type II and gestational diabetes may be achieved through maintenance of ideal body weight over the course of a woman's lifetime. Control of blood glucose levels and maintenance of normal body weight through diet and exercise are key to preventing complications due to diabetes.[36] Screening is now recommended for all adults.

Family planning and attention to reproductive health is important for all women, but this is especially true for women with diabetes. Women who are overweight and have diabetes have a two-fold increased risk of developing endometrial cancer when compared to non-overweight diabetic women and therefore should undergo yearly routine pelvic examinations.[46] Tight glycemic control by a diabetic woman prior to conception and in early pregnancy can practically eliminate the excess risk of birth defects associated with maternal diabetes. Pregnancy may also necessitate adjustment in medication and diet to maintain control of blood glucose levels.[47,48,49] Additionally, women with cardiovascular or renal disease secondary to diabetes may experience various difficulties from the increased metabolic and vascular demands due to the pregnancy.[50,51] Finally, pregnancy may unmask susceptibility to this disease. Pregnant women who develop gestational diabetes experience a 33% increase in risk of developing type II diabetes within 5 years following pregnancy.[52]

Cancers

There are no national sources of data that provide the actual number or rate of new cases of cancer diagnosed each year. Estimates of the incidence of cancer are made from the Surveillance, Epidemiology, and End Results (SEER) program of the National Cancer Institute. National vital statistics data provide numbers and rates of cancer

Figure 4-4

Age-adjusted cancer death rates*, females by site, United States, 1930–1997

Rate per 100,000 female population

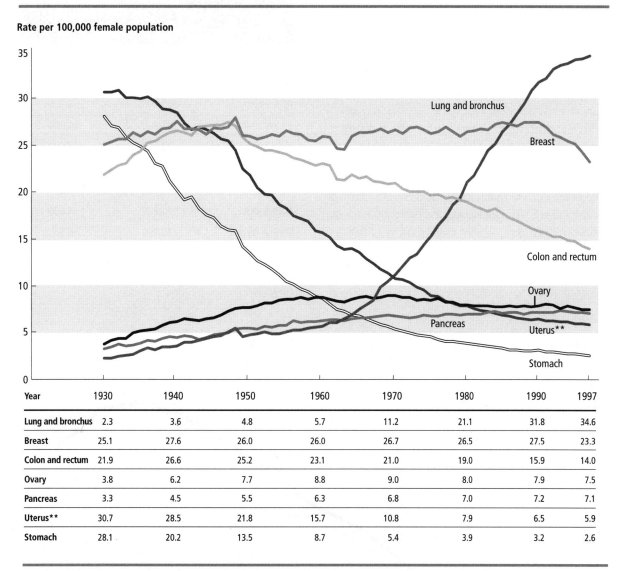

Year	1930	1940	1950	1960	1970	1980	1990	1997
Lung and bronchus	2.3	3.6	4.8	5.7	11.2	21.1	31.8	34.6
Breast	25.1	27.6	26.0	26.0	26.7	26.5	27.5	23.3
Colon and rectum	21.9	26.6	25.2	23.1	21.0	19.0	15.9	14.0
Ovary	3.8	6.2	7.7	8.8	9.0	8.0	7.9	7.5
Pancreas	3.3	4.5	5.5	6.3	6.8	7.0	7.2	7.1
Uterus**	30.7	28.5	21.8	15.7	10.8	7.9	6.5	5.9
Stomach	28.1	20.2	13.5	8.7	5.4	3.9	3.2	2.6

*Per 100,000, age-adjusted to the 1970 U.S. standard population. Due to changes in ICD coding, numerator information has changed over time. Rates for cancer of the uterus, ovary, lung and bronchus, and colon and rectum are affected by these coding changes.

**Uterus cancer death rates are for uterine cervix and uterine corpus combined.

Source: National Center for Health Statistics. U.S. mortality public use data tapes, 1960–1997, U.S. mortality volumes, 1930–1959. Hyattsville (MD): U.S. Department of Health and Human Services; 2000. In: American Cancer Society. Cancer facts and figures 2001. Atlanta: The Society. Reprinted by the permission of the American Cancer Society, Inc.

related deaths in the United States. The age-adjusted cancer death rates for women by site of the cancer are shown in Figure 4-4. This section discusses cancers that affect primarily women (breast), exclusively women (cervical, ovarian, and endometrial), and other cancers (lung and colorectal) that are leading causes of death among women. Death rates for lung cancer have been rising among women, but death rates from other cancers have dropped or are unchanged.

Breast Cancer

An estimated 182,800 new cases of invasive breast cancer were expected to be diagnosed in women in 2000, with an estimated 40,800 deaths occurring in that year (Table 4-8).[53] The incidence of breast cancer in the United States has remained constant since 1990, yet it represented 29% of the newly diagnosed cancer cases for 1999.[54] Like most cancers, the incidence of breast cancer increases with age; the risk increases from 0.43% in women less than 40 years to 4.00% in women 40–59 and 6.88% in women 60–79.[55] Figure 4-5 depicts rates of invasive breast cancer by age. (Rates of invasive breast cancer are much lower than overall rates of breast cancer.) The incidence and mortality rates of breast cancer also vary by race/ethnicity (Table 4-9). At most ages, the incidence rate is higher for white women, but the mortality rate is higher for

Table 4-8

Estimated new cancer cases and deaths from selected sites of cancer for women, United States, 2000

Site	Number of new cases	Number of deaths
All sites	600,400	268,100
Breast	182,800	40,800
Lung and bronchus	74,600	67,600
Colon and rectum	66,600	28,500
Pancreas	14,600	14,500
Uterine cervix	12,800	4,600
Uterine corpus	36,100	6,500
Ovarian	23,100	14,000

Source: American Cancer Society. Cancer facts and figures, 2000. Atlanta: The Society; 2000.

Figure 4-5

Breast cancer (invasive) incidence by age and race, 1992–1996

Incidence rate per 100,000 women

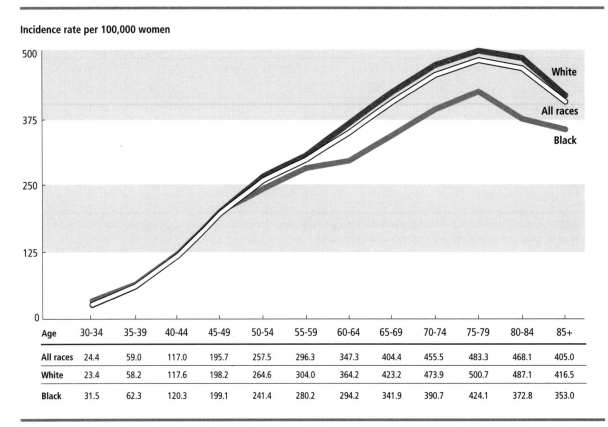

Age	30-34	35-39	40-44	45-49	50-54	55-59	60-64	65-69	70-74	75-79	80-84	85+
All races	24.4	59.0	117.0	195.7	257.5	296.3	347.3	404.4	455.5	483.3	468.1	405.0
White	23.4	58.2	117.6	198.2	264.6	304.0	364.2	423.2	473.9	500.7	487.1	416.5
Black	31.5	62.3	120.3	199.1	241.4	280.2	294.2	341.9	390.7	424.1	372.8	353.0

Source: Ries L, Kosary C, Hankey B, Miller B, Clegg L, Edwards B, editors. SEER cancer statistics review, 1973–1996. Table IV-2. Bethesda (MD): National Cancer Institute; 1999.

Table 4-9

Age-adjusted cancer incidence and mortality rates for women by race/ethnicity, United States, 1990–1997*

| Site | Incidence per 100,000 women** | | | | |
	All	White	Black	Asian/Pacific Islander	Hispanic
Breast	109.7	114.0	100.2	74.6	68.9
Lung and bronchus	41.6	43.3	45.8	22.5	19.4
Colon and rectum	37.1	36.6	45.2	30.9	23.6
Cervical	8.9	8.4	11.7	10.2	15.3
Endometrial, uterine, and not otherwise specified	21.2	22.5	15.0	13.9	13.4
Ovarian	14.7	15.2	10.3	10.7	11.5

| Site | Mortality per 100,000 women** | | | | |
	All	White	Black	Asian/Pacific Islander	Hispanic
Breast	25.6	25.3	31.4	11.2	15.1
Lung and bronchus	33.4	34.0	33.0	14.9	11.0
Colon and rectum	14.7	14.3	19.9	8.9	8.3
Cervical	2.8	2.4	5.9	2.7	3.4
Endometrial, uterine, and not otherwise specified	3.3	3.1	5.8	1.8	2.4
Ovarian	7.6	7.9	6.4	4.0	4.8

*Rates are from the SEER program and are based on data from population-based registries in Connecticut, New Mexico, Utah, Iowa, Hawaii, Atlanta, Detroit, Seattle-Puget Sound, and San Francisco-Oakland.

**Incidence and mortality rates are per 100,000 and are age-adjusted to the 1970 U.S. standard population.

Source: Ries L, Eisner M, Kosary C, Hankey B, Miller B, Clegg L, Edwards B, editors. SEER cancer statistics review, 1973–1997. Bethesda (MD): National Cancer Institute; 2000.

black women (Figure 4-6).[56] Between 1990 and 1995, overall breast cancer mortality rates declined.[57] This decline may be attributable to a variety of factors, including lifestyle changes, early diagnosis, and/or the quality of treatment available.[53] Mammography screening, for instance, has been shown to reduce the mortality rate by at least 30% in women who are age 50 or older.[58]

Many potential risk factors for breast cancer have been explored, ranging from personal health behaviors to the use of hormones. Several risk factors relate to a woman's hormone levels, suggesting that estrogen level may play a role in the initiation or progression of this cancer. The risk of developing breast cancer increases with age and is higher in women who experience early menarche, late menopause, higher education and socioeconomic status, or a personal family history of the disease.[53,55] Women who have never borne children are at an increased risk for

Figure 4-6

Breast cancer (invasive) mortality by age and race, 1992–1996

Rate per 100,000 women

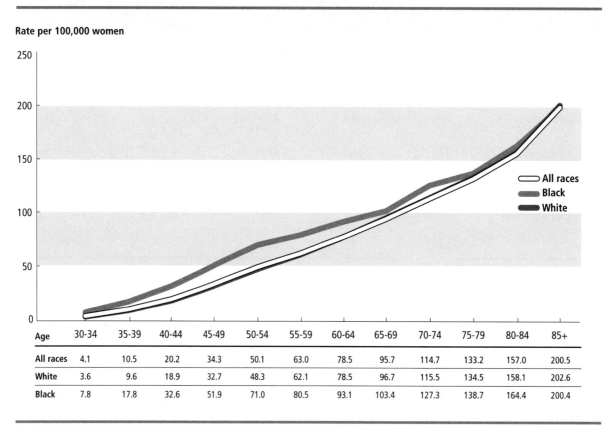

Age	30-34	35-39	40-44	45-49	50-54	55-59	60-64	65-69	70-74	75-79	80-84	85+
All races	4.1	10.5	20.2	34.3	50.1	63.0	78.5	95.7	114.7	133.2	157.0	200.5
White	3.6	9.6	18.9	32.7	48.3	62.1	78.5	96.7	115.5	134.5	158.1	202.6
Black	7.8	17.8	32.6	51.9	71.0	80.5	93.1	103.4	127.3	138.7	164.4	200.4

Source: Ries L, Kosary C, Hankey B, Miller B, Clegg L, Edwards B, editors. SEER cancer statistics review, 1973–1996. Table IV-3. Bethesda (MD): National Cancer Institute; 1999.

breast cancer, as are women who delay having their first birth until after age 30.[59,60,61] Long-term use of oral contraceptives may slightly increase the risk of premenopausal breast cancer but has no effect on or only slightly increases the risk of postmenopausal breast cancer.[59,60,61,62,63,64]

Other factors may be associated with increased risk of developing breast cancer, but the published literature is inconsistent or weak. The duration of breast-feeding, for example, is associated with a decreased risk of breast cancer in some studies (the longer one breast-feeds the lower the risk),[65,66,67] and with no difference in risk in others.[68,69] Recent studies, however, suggest that extended lactation may protect against post-menopausal breast cancer.[70,71]

The relationship between HRT and breast cancer continues to be debated. It appears that the combination of progesterone with estrogen may increase risk of breast cancer.[72] A few studies suggest that long-term use of postmenopausal hormones may be associated with increased incidence of breast cancer.[73] It appears that the cancers associated with HRT are less invasive and have a more favorable prognosis than those that are not associated with HRT.[74,75] Data on HRT are included in chapter 6.

Obesity increases the risk of postmenopausal, but not premenopausal, breast cancer.[76,77] Weight gain also appears to influence risk in a dose-response fashion, but the effect seems to be confined to women who have never used hormones.[77] The association between dietary fat intake and the development of breast cancer is quite controversial, with some investigators asserting an increased risk associated with increased intake[78] and others arguing that there is no effect.[76] Recent reports from the Nurses' Health Study have examined the effect of dietary factors other than fat. Premenopausal women who consume five or more servings of fruits and vegetables per day have a moderately lower risk of breast cancer than those who consume fewer than two servings per day.[79] Some studies suggest that women who engage in regular physical activity have a reduced risk of breast cancer. As shown in a recent meta-analysis, recreational exercise appears to reduce the risk of breast cancer by 12% to 60%.[80,81,82] The intensity and frequency of physical activity required to reduce risk are not yet clear, as few conclusive studies have been done. Alcohol consumption may increase one's risk of developing breast cancer,[61,76] although current research

suggests that any increase in risk could be counteracted by folate supplementation.[83]

New research about BRCA1 and BRCA2 genes for breast cancer is exploring the familial risks of breast cancer. General screening of the population is not recommended at this time. Currently, researchers are in the process of gathering information in an effort to assess the characteristics of these genes and review their role in the incidence of breast cancer.[53]

Prevention of breast cancer is compromised by the absence of clearly identified, modifiable risk factors. The evidence is mixed about whether measures such as reducing alcohol and fatty food intake and increasing physical activity can reduce rates of breast cancer, but clearly these changes offer other benefits (e.g., reducing CHD).[84] Although early childbearing and breast-feeding are linked to a decrease in risk of breast cancer, these are not behaviors that can be recommended

Table 4-10

Five-year relative survival rates for women for selected sites by stage of cancer, United States, 1989–1996*

Site	Percent of women surviving > 5 years				
	All stages	Local**	Regional***	Distant†	Unstaged
Breast	85.0	96.5	77.0	21.4	54.0
Lung and bronchus	16.3	52.5	22.7	2.7	9.9
Colon and rectum	61.2	90.1	65.4	8.5	31.1
Cervix	69.9	91.5	48.6	12.6	60.3
Corpus and uterus, not otherwise specified	83.7	95.7	63.5	26.4	52.1
Ovarian	50.4	94.6	79.0	28.2	28.0

*Rates are from the SEER program and are based on data from population-based registries in Connecticut, New Mexico, Utah, Iowa, Hawaii, Atlanta, Detroit, Seattle-Puget Sound, and San Francisco-Oakland.

**Cancer has not spread beyond tumor site.

***Cancer has spread beyond initial tumor but all cells are connected to original site.

†Cancer has spread to sites not connected to initial tumor, usually lung, bone, or brain.

Source: Ries L, Eisner M, Kosary C, Hankey B, Miller B, Clegg L, Edwards B, editors. SEER cancer statistics review, 1973–1997. Bethesda (MD): National Cancer Institute; 2000.

for all women to adopt. If a woman chooses to have children, however, breast-feeding should be encouraged to reduce her risk of cancer, benefit the infant's health, prevent osteoporosis, and return to her pre-pregnancy weight.

Another approach to prevention involves the use of drugs that target estrogen receptors in the body. Recent research suggests that the risk of developing breast cancer may be reduced with the drugs tamoxifen and raloxifene. The Breast Cancer Prevention Trial, for example, reported that tamoxifen reduced the risk of invasive and noninvasive breast cancer by 50% among high-risk women after 5 years of use, compared to those who took a placebo.[85] However, tamoxifen was found to increase the risk of endometrial cancer.[85,86] Raloxifene, a related drug, may reduce the risk of breast cancer without increasing the risk of endometrial cancer. In a study of post-menopausal women with osteoporosis, raloxifene reduced the risk of invasive breast cancer by 76%.[87] The Study of Tamoxifen and Raloxifene (STAR), one of the largest breast cancer prevention studies ever funded by the National Cancer Institute, is comparing these two drugs among postmenopausal women who have been identified as being at increased risk of breast cancer.[53,88]

The rise of breast cancer incidence rates from 1975 to 1990 is due at least in part to improved screening. If performed correctly, monthly breast self-examinations and annual clinical breast exams improve the likelihood of detecting breast cancer in its early stages.[89] However, this screening tool should be in addition to, not a substitute for, mammography. For women over age 50, mortality from breast cancer is significantly reduced by early detection with mammography. Whether the benefits of mammography outweigh its risks among younger women (40 to 49 years old) is currently a subject of intense debate.[90] The potential benefits of mammography for women in their forties include earlier diagnosis and the option to choose breast-conserving therapy. These benefits must be weighed against the risks of false-positive results (e.g., unnecessary biopsies, surgery), the lower sensitivity of mammography for women in their

Table 4-11

Age-adjusted 5-year relative cancer survival rates for U.S. women by race, 1989–1996

Site	Percent of women attaining 5-year survival	
	White	Black
All sites	63.0	49.3
Breast	86.4	71.4
Lung and bronchus	16.6	13.5
Colon and rectum	62.0	51.9
Reproductive	71.0	55.5
Cervix	71.6	58.6
Corpus	86.4	58.6
Uterine, not otherwise specified	24.5	24.9
Ovarian	50.1	47.5

Source: Ries L, Eisner M, Kosary C, Hankey B, Miller B, Clegg L, Edwards B, editors. SEER cancer statistics review, 1973–1997. Bethesda (MD): National Cancer Institute; 2000.

forties, and the costs incurred in providing this screening method to more women. Early detection of breast cancer in younger women is an elusive goal at present. Given the lower efficacy of mammography in younger women[91], improvements in early detection depend on the development of an effective screening method for women less than 50 years old.

Treatment options vary depending on the stage of the disease but include lumpectomy or mastectomy with lymph node dissection, radiation therapy, chemotherapy, or hormone therapy. Typically, two or more methods are used in combination. Overall, 5-year survival rates were approximately 85% for the period 1989–1996 (Table 4-10). Survival rates decline when the disease has metastasized to distant organ systems. Racial differences in survival persist; 5-year survival rates for black women are significantly lower than for white women (Table 4-11). These differences have yet to be

Figure 4-7

Cervical cancer (invasive) incidence by age and race, 1992–1996

Rate per 100,000 women

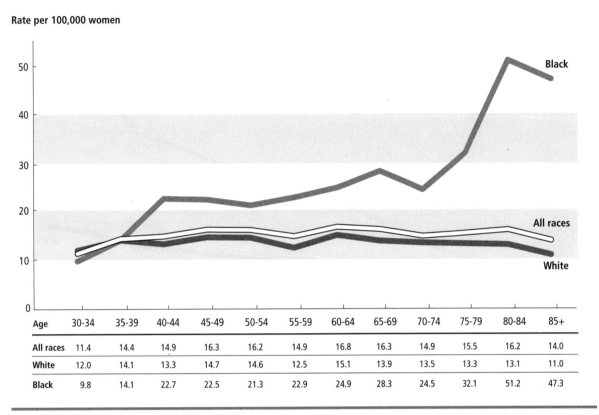

Age	30-34	35-39	40-44	45-49	50-54	55-59	60-64	65-69	70-74	75-79	80-84	85+
All races	11.4	14.4	14.9	16.3	16.2	14.9	16.8	16.3	14.9	15.5	16.2	14.0
White	12.0	14.1	13.3	14.7	14.6	12.5	15.1	13.9	13.5	13.3	13.1	11.0
Black	9.8	14.1	22.7	22.5	21.3	22.9	24.9	28.3	24.5	32.1	51.2	47.3

Source: Ries L, Kosary C, Hankey B, Miller B, Clegg L, Edwards B, editors. SEER cancer statistics review, 1973–1996. Table V-2. Bethesda (MD): National Cancer Institute; 1999.

explained by research on treatment, insurance coverage, or socioeconomic status.[92,93,94,95,96]

Cervical Cancer

Approximately 12,800 new cases of invasive cervical cancer were diagnosed in U.S. women in 2000, leading to approximately 4,600 deaths.[53]

Unlike many other cancers, the risk of invasive cervical cancer does not dramatically increase with age, except for black women (Figure 4-7). Although the incidence of invasive cervical cancer has been declining overall, the rate among Asian/Pacific Islander women has increased approximately 1.5% from 1990 to 1995.

Rates for white, black, Hispanic, and Native American women have decreased.[97] Despite overall declines in incidence and mortality, the incidence rate for black women (11.7 per 100,000) remains much higher than that for white women (8.4 per 100,000).[98] Although the death rate for black women (5.9 per 100,000) has declined more rapidly than for white women, it remains more than twice the rate for white women (2.4 per 100,000). It appears that a higher death rate among older black women accounts for this gap (Figure 4-8).[99]

Sexual activity and related behaviors strongly influence a woman's risk for cervical cancer. The most important risk factor is sexually transmitted

Figure 4-8

Cervical cancer (invasive) mortality by age and race, 1992–1996

Rate per 100,000 women

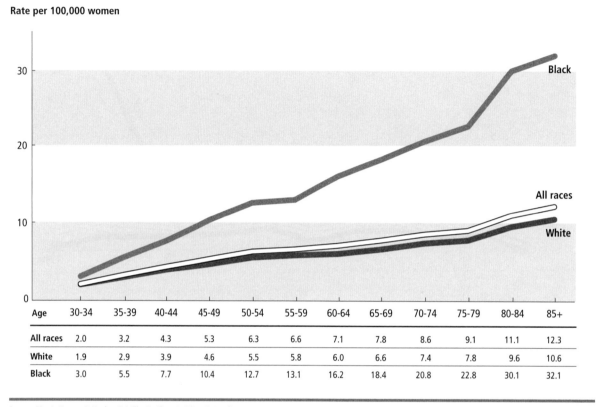

Age	30-34	35-39	40-44	45-49	50-54	55-59	60-64	65-69	70-74	75-79	80-84	85+
All races	2.0	3.2	4.3	5.3	6.3	6.6	7.1	7.8	8.6	9.1	11.1	12.3
White	1.9	2.9	3.9	4.6	5.5	5.8	6.0	6.6	7.4	7.8	9.6	10.6
Black	3.0	5.5	7.7	10.4	12.7	13.1	16.2	18.4	20.8	22.8	30.1	32.1

Source: Ries L, Kosary C, Hankey B, Miller B, Clegg L, Edwards B, editors. SEER cancer statistics review, 1973–1996. Table V-2. Bethesda (MD): National Cancer Institute; 1999.

infection with specific subtypes of human papillomavirus (HPV), chiefly HPV-16, 18, 31, 33, 35, and 45.[59,100,101,102,103,104] In a recent cohort study, investigators estimated that up to 46% of all college-age women are infected with HPV,[105] although not necessarily the subtypes leading to cervical cancer. Having first intercourse at an early age, multiple sexual partners, or a partner who has had multiple sexual partners all increase a woman's risk of HPV and cervical cancer.[53,59] See chapter 3 for data on HPV.

Smoking may increase the risk of cervical cancer, as it exposes the body to many cancer-causing chemicals.[105,106,107] Tobacco by-products (which may damage the DNA of cells in the cervix) have been found in the cervical mucus of women smokers.[98,108] Cigarette smoking is also associated with an increased risk of high-grade cervical intraepithelial neoplasia among women with mildly abnormal cervical smears.[109] The use of oral contraceptives may also increase the risk of cervical cancer, albeit through an indirect route. Women who use oral contraceptives without barrier contraception may be at an increased risk of developing HPV, which is a risk factor for cervical cancer.[110]

Primary prevention of cervical cancer fundamentally depends upon stopping transmission of HPV. Promoting healthy sexual behaviors (e.g., abstinence, use of condoms, fewer sexual partners) and increasing public awareness about the link between HPV and cervical cancer could reduce cervical cancer risk substantially. Prophylactic vaccination against HPV-16, the strain thought to be responsible for half of all cases of cervical cancer, will enter phase III of human testing in 2001. A therapeutic vaccine that will trigger an immune response against cells that are already infected, but where invasive neoplasia has not developed, is also in phase I trials.[111]

Much of the mortality due to cervical cancer is preventable through Pap test screening.[112] The primary goal of cervical cancer screening is to increase detection and treatment of precancerous cervical lesions and thus prevent the occurrence of cervical cancer. Cervical cancer in situ (a precancerous condition) now occurs more frequently than invasive cervical cancer; this shift is likely due to the increased rates of Pap screening.[113] Pap testing has increased in recent years, but promoting the participation of women in screening programs is a persistent challenge in cervical cancer control.

Survival rates are comparatively good for cervical cancer across all stages, but significant differences exist across racial and ethnic groups. When detected in the early stages, the survival rate is greater than 90%. Nearly 100% of women diagnosed with cervical cancer in situ (detected primarily by the Pap test) survive. Survival rates decline when the disease is detected in its later stages. Treatment options vary depending on the stage of the disease but include surgery, radiation, chemotherapy, or all three for invasive cervical cancers.[114,115] For in situ cancers, changes in the cervix can be treated with cryotherapy, which uses extreme cold to destroy cancer cells; laser ablation; electrocoagulation, which uses intense heat by electric current to destroy cancerous tissue; or local surgery.[113]

Ovarian Cancer

In 2000, an estimated 23,100 women were diagnosed with ovarian cancer, and approximately 14,000 women died from the disease.[53] Ovarian cancer accounts for 4% of all cancers and is the fifth leading cause of cancer death among females.[116]

Between 1990 and 1997, ovarian cancer incidence rates for white women (15.2 per 100,000) were approximately 50% greater than those for black women (10.3 per 100,000) and 34% higher than those for Hispanic women (11.5 per 100,000).[116]

In 1996, the 1-year and 5-year survival rates for women with ovarian cancer were 77.7% and 49.6%, respectively.[116] The age-adjusted mortality rate in women is 7.6 per 100,000. However, there is considerable variation by age. The rate in women 65 years and older was 43.3 per 100,000, nearly 11 times higher than the rate of 3.7 per 100,000 in women under 65 years of age.[116]

The risk of developing ovarian cancer increases with age but also appears to be closely tied to the number of ovulation cycles that a woman experiences over the course of her lifetime.[117,118,119,120,121] Current research suggests that ovarian cancer may be caused, in part, by mutations in the epithelial surface after multiple ovulation cycles and exposure to ovulation stimulating hormones.[122,123]

The lifetime risk of developing ovarian cancer is 1 in 55[124], making this a relatively rare cancer. Risk factors for ovarian cancer include no prior live births, infertility, history of endometriosis, and family history of breast or ovarian cancer.[125,126] Although white women have higher ovarian cancer incidence rates than black women, there are no apparent risk factors unique to white women. The higher rates for white women may actually be related to an increased prevalence of risk factors.[116,127] Higher socioeconomic status among women of all ethnicities is associated with higher risk of ovarian cancer that may be due in part to lower parity (number of live births) or nulliparity (no live births) among women with higher education.[126]

Among women who use oral contraceptives, there is a 50% reduction in the risk of developing ovarian cancer after 5 years of use and a 60% reduction after 10 years of use. Similarly, parity is associated with a decrease in risk, with a reduction of 61% for one pregnancy and 22% for each subsequent pregnancy regardless of the age of the mother. Women who have breast-fed have a slight decrease in risk of 1% for each month of lactation.[118] These reductions of risk associated with the use of oral contraceptives, pregnancy, and lactation may be due, in part, to the reduced number of lifetime ovulation cycles and the amount of exposure to ovulation stimulating hormones.

A positive family history of a mother or sister with ovarian cancer or breast cancer with mutation of the BRCA genes increases the lifetime risk of cancer to 9.4% and 16%, respectively.[119,128] Similarly, women with endometriosis have an increased risk of 4.2%.[129] Women who have used infertility drugs (e.g., clomiphene citrate) appear to have an increased lifetime risk of 4.6% for developing ovarian cancer, although there have been some studies suggesting no effect. It is hypothesized that risk associated with infertility drugs may be due to an increase in number of ovulation cycles and level of hormones.[130] Incomplete pregnancy due to induced or spontaneous abortion, alcohol, smoking, and HRT do not appear to change the risk of developing ovarian cancer.[121,131,132]

Many factors associated with a reduction in risk are not modifiable or they represent significant life choices (e.g., childbearing) and, therefore, cannot be readily converted into prevention efforts. For women who choose contraception, oral contraceptives may offer some advantages depending on the woman's level of risk for this disease. Certainly breast-feeding could be recommended for women who bear children.

Unlike breast and cervical cancer, there is no generally recommended annual screening test for ovarian cancer. In addition, the symptoms of ovarian cancer, which include swelling of the abdomen, intestinal gas, and cramping, are often vague and lead to delayed detection and a high case-fatality rate.[125] The inability to detect this cancer in its early, largely asymptomatic, treatable stage is the primary reason why survival has

not improved substantially over the past few decades. Periodic transvaginal ultrasounds and CA-125 blood tests, in addition to annual pelvic exams, are being investigated.[133] These tests are much more sensitive—likely to give a positive result when disease is truly present—and specific—likely to give a negative result if the disease is truly absent—in postmenopausal women. Specificity may be better because many of the other conditions that can lead to a false positive are less frequent in postmenopausal women.[134,135]

Because no test is available to detect ovarian cancer and because of its nonspecific symptoms, all women should undergo a thorough, annual pelvic examination. Women who are at increased risk due to family history of ovarian or breast cancer may benefit from the use of oral contraceptives or prophylactic removal of the ovaries when they have completed child bearing.[125,136]

Treatment for ovarian cancer depends on the stage and the invasiveness of the tumor and age of the woman and may include removal of one or both ovaries, lymph nodes, fallopian tubes, and a hysterectomy in conjunction with chemotherapy and/or radiation.[125] Survival could also be dramatically improved if a sensitive and specific screening test were developed to detect the cancer in the early, more treatable stages of the disease, although failure to identify a precursor lesion makes this difficult.

Uterine Corpus Cancer (Endometrial)

Uterine cancer is the fourth leading cause of cancer in women after breast, lung, and colon, and is the eighth leading cause of death in women; it will affect one of every 45 women during her lifetime.[116,137] The incidence of endometrial cancer increased rapidly in the early 1970s due to the increased use of unopposed estrogens in postmenopausal women. With the decline in the use of exogenous estrogens in the late 1970s and the change in the composition of

HRT administered to postmenopausal women, the incidence of endometrial cancer declined.[138] Over the past decade, the incidence has changed little. In 2000, an estimated 36,100 cases were diagnosed and approximately 6,500 deaths due to endometrial cancer occurred.[53] Between 1990 and 1997, the incidence rate for white women (22.5 per 100,000) was 51% greater than for black women (15 per 100,000) and 67% greater than for Hispanic women (13.4 per 100,000).[124]

The 5-year relative survival rates for all women diagnosed with endometrial cancer is 83.7%. The 5-year survival rate for black women (58.6%) is substantially lower than that for white women (86.4%). Although the time to medical consultation after the onset of initial symptoms appears similar, black women present with a more aggressive grade and stage of tumor and have a significantly poorer survival rate even when treatments are the same as those given white women.[139,140,141] Parity has a positive effect on 5-year survival, with women who have had a live birth having a 30% higher likelihood of survival.[142]

The lifetime risk of being diagnosed with endometrial cancer is 2.69% for all women and increases with age.[116] The risk for white women (2.83%) is 1.5 times that for black women (1.71%).

Risk factors for endometrial cancer include nulliparity, infertility, obesity, use of estrogen-only HRT, and a family history of breast and ovarian cancer.[137,143] Among women who have given birth, there is a 10% reduction in the risk of endometrial cancer regardless of age at first birth.[144] Women who have diabetes have a twofold greater risk of endometrial cancer; obese women with diabetes have a threefold greater risk than do obese nondiabetic women.[46]

The risk of endometrial cancer increases with socioeconomic status (SES) in white, black, and Hispanic women.[126] It is theorized that this increase may be due to greater use of estrogen replacement therapy among more highly educated women and due to later menopause in women of higher SES.[145,146]

There are no easily modifiable risk factors, making primary prevention efforts elusive. Obesity increases risk, but changes in this factor alone might not achieve appreciable reductions in the rate of this cancer. However, adding a progestin to any exogenous estrogen treatment regimen reduces the incidence.

The symptoms of endometrial cancer are abnormal uterine bleeding, in both pre- and postmenopausal women, and pelvic pain. No general screening test is available to detect the disease.[137] Women who are symptomatic may undergo transvaginal ultrasound and/or endometrial biopsy.[133]

Choice of treatment for endometrial cancer depends on age at diagnosis and stage of disease and may include surgery to remove the uterine corpus, cervix, and lymph nodes, as well as radiation, chemotherapy, or hormonal therapy. Five-year survival rates have changed little over time.

Lung Cancer

The American Cancer Society projected 74,600 new cases of lung cancer and 67,600 deaths from lung and bronchial cancer for women in 2000.[53] Although the incidence rate for men is declining (from 81.7 per 100,000 in 1990 to 70.0 per 100,000 in 1996), it is increasing for women (from 41.5 per 100,000 in 1990 to 42.3 per 100,000 in 1996).[124] As with incidence rates, mortality rates for men have declined from 75.2 per 100,000 in 1990 to 68.2 per 100,000 in 1996. Lung cancer mortality rates continue to rise in women, from 31.6 per 100,000 in 1990 to 34.3 per 100,000 in 1996.[124] The Centers for Disease Control and Prevention's (CDC) Tobacco Information and Prevention Source reports that between 1960 and 1990, lung cancer deaths among women increased by more than 400%.[147] Mortality and incidence rates in whites and blacks are similar and are much higher than for other racial/ethnic groups.

The current trends in lung cancer mortality among women (Figure 4-9) are comparable to

Figure 4-9

Age-adjusted rates of death from lung and breast cancer among U.S. women by race, 1975–1997

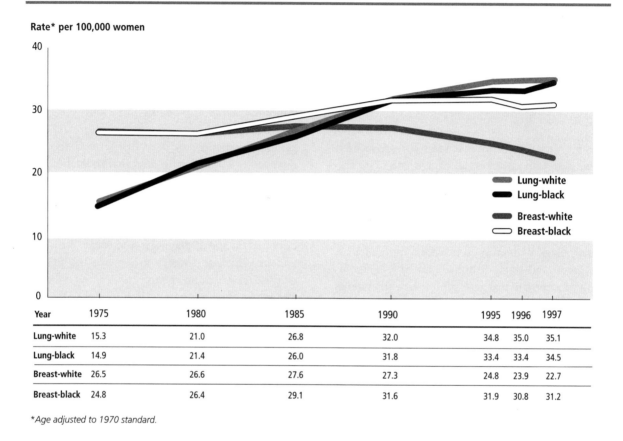

Rate* per 100,000 women

Year	1975	1980	1985	1990	1995	1996	1997
Lung-white	15.3	21.0	26.8	32.0	34.8	35.0	35.1
Lung-black	14.9	21.4	26.0	31.8	33.4	33.4	34.5
Breast-white	26.5	26.6	27.6	27.3	24.8	23.9	22.7
Breast-black	24.8	26.4	29.1	31.6	31.9	30.8	31.2

*Age adjusted to 1970 standard.

Source: Ries L, Eisner M, Kosary C, Hankey B, Miller B, Clegg L, Edwards B, editors. SEER cancer statistics review, 1973–1997. Bethesda (MD): National Cancer Institute; 2000.

those observed in men more than 20 years ago.[148] Despite present attention directed toward breast cancer, lung cancer has been the leading cause of cancer deaths in women in the United States since 1987.[149]

A review of SEER data identified an age-specific relationship between lung cancer mortality and race. White women have experienced higher lung cancer mortality rates in the age group 65 years and older, but black women have higher rates among women less than 65 years of age.[150] This difference in mortality rates widens as black women have lower 5-year survival rates compared to white women at any age of diagnosis.[124]

Exposure to radon, asbestos, and ionizing radiation has been associated with lung cancer in women.[148,150] Cigarette smoking, however, is the most important risk factor for developing lung cancer.[150] Approximately 80% of lung cancer cases in women are thought to be attributable to cigarette smoking.[150,151] The level of increased risk depends upon a number of factors including age at initiation, number of cigarettes smoked, type of product smoked, and inhaling pattern.[148] One study found that women were more likely to develop lung cancer than men, given the same level of exposure to cigarette smoke.[149] An increased susceptibility may relate to genetic risk factors.[152,153,154] Smoking rates and risk factors for smoking are discussed in further detail in chapter 6.

Exposure to environmental tobacco smoke (ETS) has emerged as another important risk factor for women. Studies have mostly focused on nonsmoking women who have developed lung cancer. Between 9% and 13% of female lung cancer cases occur in women who never smoked.[155] The Environmental Protection Agency identified ETS as a human lung carcinogen in adults in 1992 and a recent meta-analysis of research demonstrated a statistically significant excess risk of 24% among nonsmokers who lived with a smoker.[156]

Primary prevention for lung cancer begins with public health education and promotion efforts on the dangers of smoking. Recent legislative efforts have led to the designation of smoke-free environments, changes in cigarette advertising and marketing, and financial settlements. Other preventive measures include reducing exposure to environmental tobacco smoke, radiation, radon, and asbestos.[148,150] Early detection of lung cancer is difficult, as symptoms often do not appear until the disease is advanced. Diagnosis may be aided through chest X-ray and sputum cytology.[148] Treatment depends on the type and stage of cancer; it may involve surgery, radiation therapy, or chemotherapy.

Smoking cessation is beneficial regardless of the time of initiation. The American Cancer Society's Cancer Prevention Study II reported a reduction in risk of developing lung cancer after smoking cessation. For instance, a 75-year-old woman who may have quit smoking in her thirties has only 10% the risk of lung cancer of current smokers, whereas if she quit later in her fifties she would have 23% the risk of current smokers.[157]

Additional efforts are directed toward harm reduction strategies, such as reducing the number of cigarettes an individual smokes per day by introducing nicotine replacement therapeutic methods, such as nicotine gum, patches, or prescription medication. It has been observed, however, that clinical trials with nicotine replacement are less effective in women than in men trying to quit smoking; further research is needed to identify the reasons and implications of this distinction.[158]

Colorectal Cancer

Colorectal cancer is the fourth most commonly diagnosed cancer and ranks second in cancer deaths in the United States.[159] The American Cancer Society projected 51,700 new cases of colon cancer and 15,300 cases of rectal cancer in women in 1999.[98] The American Cancer Society also estimated 24,900 deaths from colon cancer and 3,900 deaths from rectal cancer in women in 1999.[97] However, the incidence and mortality rates for colorectal cancer among women are declining. Incidence rates have fallen from 30.3 per 100,000 in 1990 to 26.6 per 100,000 in 1996. Mortality rates have also fallen from 15.6 per 100,000 to 14.0 per 100,000 during the same years.[124] Incidence rates may have been affected by lifestyle changes (e.g., diet), and mortality rates may have been reduced by early detection.[160] Although mortality rates are declining, the preponderance of cases are detected at later stages, which results in deaths among approximately 50% of all colorectal cancer cases within 5 years of diagnosis.[161]

Among women, the incidence and mortality rates are highest among blacks, followed by whites, and Asian/Pacific Islanders.[116] However, across each racial/ethnic group, both incidence and mortality rates for colorectal cancer are higher in men compared to women.[159] Early detection of colorectal cancer in a localized stage is associated with a 90.1% 5-year survival rate. After colorectal cancer has spread regionally, 5-year survival rates drop to 65.4%. For women with distant metastases, 5-year survival is only 8.5%.[116]

The risk of developing colorectal cancer increases with age and can be divided into two categories: average risk and increased risk.[116] Among average-risk women, age is the primary risk factor, with women 50 years of age and older at increased risk. The incidence of colorectal cancer is six times higher among people aged 65 and older versus those aged 40 to 64. Furthermore, 73% of the newly diagnosed cases occur in people aged 65 and older.[53] Women at an increased risk for developing colorectal cancer include those with a family history of familial adenomatous polyposis (FAP) and/or hereditary non-polyposis colon cancer (HNPCC), and those with a personal history of colorectal cancer, adenomatous polyps, or inflammatory bowel disease.[161]

Epidemiologic studies show that several dietary factors can influence all stages of carcinogenesis. A diet low in fat and red meat has been shown to have a protective effect.[162,163] The role of dietary fiber, once thought to have a protective effect against colorectal cancer, has recently been disputed in the literature. Using data from the Nurses' Health Study, one study showed no protective effect from dietary fiber among the participants,[164] and other investigators found that folate from dietary sources led to a reduction in colon cancer risk and that long-term use of multivitamins may reduce this risk more extensively.[165] The use of nonsteroidal anti-inflammatory drugs appears to have a protective effect against colorectal cancer.[166] The use of calcium has reduced recurrence of colorectal adenomas, the precursor lesion to colorectal cancer;[166] current postmenopausal hormone use may decrease the risk of colorectal cancer.[167,168] An inactive lifestyle[169] appears to increase one's risk as well.

Primary prevention methods presumably include changes in diet and levels of physical activity. Currently most attention is directed toward secondary prevention by early detection, which is difficult as many women are asymptomatic. Because the majority of colorectal cancers develop from premalignant adenomatous polyps,[161] early detection of polyps may change the natural history of the disease.[170] In 1997, the Agency for Health Care Policy and Research recommended the use of a fecal occult blood test (FOBT) and periodic sigmoidoscopy as effective screening tests for women and men aged 50 and older. Alternatives included double contrast barium enema every 5–10 years or colonoscopy every 10 years.[171] Unfortunately, the 1997 Behavioral Risk Factor Surveillance System (BRFSS) indicated that only 21% of female respondents 50 years of age and older have had a FOBT in the past year, and only 27% reported having a sigmoidoscopy/proctoscopy in the past 5 years.[172] Computed tomography colonography (CTC) and virtual colonoscopy are emerging tests that have the potential to increase screening in women, because they are minimally invasive.[173] Treatment options for colorectal cancer include chemotherapy, radiation therapy, and surgery.

Disorders of Connective Tissue and Skeleton

Arthritis

Arthritis and other rheumatic conditions are the leading causes of disability in the United States. An estimated 43 million people are currently affected, but this number is expected to rise to 60 million by 2020 as the U.S. population ages.[174,175] The prevalence of arthritis and other rheumatic conditions is greater in women than in men.[174,176] Almost two-thirds of women over 70 years of age reported experiencing arthritis in a national survey, as compared to approximately half of men of the same age.[19] Based on 1997 National Hospital Discharge Survey (NHDS) data, there were approximately 451,000 hospital discharges among women who had been admitted because of arthritis with an average length of stay of 5.6 days.[174]

Surveillance systems in the United States currently gather only self-reported data that lump together all arthritic conditions. Therefore, estimates of the prevalence of specific types of arthritis, such as osteoarthritis, are not available. Furthermore, self-reported data may underestimate the prevalence of these conditions, as they are often undiagnosed.[177] The Arthritis Foundation and CDC recommend that surveillance efforts be improved at both state and national levels to accurately measure prevalence for each specific type of arthritis (e.g., rheumatoid), and both organizations also recommend the inclusion of such objectives for Healthy People 2010.[174] This would provide a means to estimate and monitor the prevalence and associated morbidity of these conditions.

Osteoarthritis. A degenerative joint disease, osteoarthritis predominantly affects the hips, knees, and hands. Osteoarthritis specifically is believed to affect 20 million of the 43 million people with arthritis in the United States.[174]

Much of the existing research on osteoarthritis developed out of the Framingham Heart Study cohort and constitutes the Framingham Osteoarthritis Study. This body of research focuses on the etiology of knee osteoarthritis.[178] It is important to note that the majority of all research on osteoarthritis focuses on the knee, with a limited number of longitudinal studies focusing on other sites in the body.

The risk of developing osteoarthritis increases with age, although the mechanism involved is unclear.[179] Women are more likely to suffer from osteoarthritis than men, especially after women reach menopause.[179] This finding has led researchers to examine how hormonal changes in women affect cartilage metabolism and the onset of osteoarthritis. Preliminary results suggest that estrogen replacement therapy may have a protective effect on knee and, to a lesser extent, hip osteoarthritis,[180,181] but further study is needed. Other risk factors include joint trauma, obesity, and repetitive joint use, all of which may relate to osteoarthritis through excessive stress to the knee and hip joints.[175,179]

Primary prevention strategies include weight control, exercise,[179] and the avoidance of occupational and sports-related injuries.[174,175,179] There is no screening test for early detection. Diagnosis is made by examining radiographic changes in the affected joint.[179] For most individuals with osteoarthritis, treatment options are designed to control symptoms and reduce pain. Physical therapy, exercise, and weight reduction are used as both preventive and treatment strategies.[179,182] Medication may also alleviate symptoms, particularly pain.[174,179] No data are available on the proportion of women with arthritis who apply these nonsurgical treatment strategies. Joint replacement is a surgical treatment option that can improve the quality of life of individuals debilitated by osteoarthritis.[179,183,174,184] The 1996 National Ambulatory Surgery Survey reported that 112,000 women underwent replacement operations or other knee repair in the United States during 1996.[185]

Rheumatoid Arthritis. Rheumatoid arthritis is a systemic autoimmune disease characterized by an inflammation of joints resulting in stiffness, swelling, and pain. It also affects internal organs such as the heart, lungs, kidneys, and eyes.[186,187] In autoimmune diseases such as rheumatoid arthritis and lupus, the woman's own immune system attacks healthy cells, tissues, and organs as a result of a breakdown of the immune system's ability to distinguish between foreign agents and native cells.[188]

Applying 1971–1975 NHANES I prevalence rates to the 1990 U.S. population, the National Arthritis Data Workgroup estimated that 1.5 million women in the United States currently have rheumatoid arthritis. The NHANES I data are based on clinical diagnosis; tests for rheumatoid factor and hand and foot radiographs were not obtained. The prevalence of rheumatoid arthritis increases with age in both men and women, ranging from 1 per 1,000 in those aged 25 to 35 years to 15 per 1,000 in those aged 65 to 74 years.[177] More prevalent in women than men, the female-to-male ratio is estimated to be 5:1 during the childbearing years (15 to 45 years) and 2:1 in children.[189] The median age for the development of rheumatoid arthritis is 45 years in women.[188]

In addition to age, low levels of the hormone dehydroepiandrosterone sulfate (DHEAS) in young, premenopausal women may be a risk factor for development of the disease.[190] Fertility is not impaired by rheumatoid arthritis. Women experience an improvement in symptoms during pregnancy and may have a reduced risk of pre-eclampsia.[191] However, the disease is exacerbated in almost all women a month or two after delivery.[192]

The cause of rheumatoid arthritis is unknown. Possible causes of rheumatoid arthritis may include a genetic susceptibility combined with environmental factors such as bacteria or viruses.[188]

Osteoporosis

Osteoporosis is a metabolic bone disease that makes bones fragile and susceptible to fracture because of low bone mass density. Between the ages of 20 and 30 years, a woman reaches her peak bone mass, which usually remains stable until ages 35–40; bone mass decreases after age 40.[193]

It is estimated that 8 million individuals in the United States have osteoporosis and an additional 20 million have osteopenia, or low bone mass.[194] Table 4-12 shows rates for women 65 years and older, the group at highest risk. Osteopenia is defined as a bone mineral density (BMD) of at least one but no more than 2.5 standard deviations (SD) below the mean peak bone mass. Osteoporosis is defined as a BMD more than 2.5 SD below the mean peak bone mass. Severe osteoporosis is defined as a BMD more than 2.5 SD below the mean peak bone mass coupled with the occurrence of one or more fractures. The NHANES, one of the best sources of data on diseases that require diagnostic tests, has not previously included total BMD measurements, and few women and men have had their BMD measured. Rather, diagnoses of osteoporosis and osteopenia were based on hip bone density alone.

A more readily available measure of the burden of osteoporosis in the United States is the rate of osteoporosis-related fractures. The National Institutes of Health and the National

Table 4-12

Prevalence of osteoporosis and osteopenia* among U.S. women aged 65 years and older, 1988–1994

| Age (years) | Percent** | |
	Osteoporosis	Osteopenia
65+	26.1	45.9
65–74	19.0	46.9
75–84	32.5	45.8
85+	50.5	39.6

*Based on hipbone density alone.

**Standard error estimates reported in source.

Source: Kramarow E, Lentzner H, Rooks R, Weeks J, Saydah S. Health, United States, 1999. With health and aging chartbook. (PHS)99-1232. Hyattsville (MD): National Center for Health Statistics; 1999.

Osteoporosis Foundation report that one out of every two women and one in eight men aged 50 and above will have an osteoporosis-related fracture.[195] Osteoporosis leads to more than 1.5 million fractures annually, including 300,000 hip, 700,000 vertebral, and 250,000 wrist fractures.[196] Of the approximately 300,000 hip fractures in 1996 among individuals 65 years and older, 80% occurred in women.[197]

Gender, race, age, and family history are non-modifiable risk factors for osteoporosis.[193,194,195,198] Women have a greater risk of developing osteoporosis than men, possibly because they have less bone tissue and lose bone more rapidly due to menopause and also because men do not have the dramatic drop in testosterone that women have with estrogen.[194] White and Asian American women develop osteoporosis more often than black women.[195,199] The risk of osteoporosis also increases with age as bone mass decreases from peak bone mass. However, it is important to note that risk factors can be identified but account for only 30% of the prevalence of the disease.

Estrogen levels, dietary intake, absorption of calcium and vitamin D, and tobacco use are all modifiable risk factors for osteoporosis.[193,194,195,198,200,201] The rate of bone mass loss accelerates after menopause without hormone replacement.[193] Bone mass appears to drop 3% to 5% a year at the time of menopause, regardless of diet or lifestyle activity, suggesting a link to lower estrogen.[202] Premature menopause, as a consequence of ovary removal or dysfunction, may therefore increase lifetime risk of developing osteoporosis.

Estrogen depletion accelerates loss of bone density, regardless of intake and absorption of calcium and vitamin D, but dietary factors do play an important role in the prevention of osteoporosis. A diet rich in calcium and vitamin D, especially in a woman's twenties, will increase her likelihood of reaching her peak bone mass but will not prevent bone loss, particularly in early menopause. Maintenance of this diet can slow the rate of bone loss and the risk of osteoporotic fractures.[203] Tobacco use appears to reduce bone density and places women at greater risk of osteoporotic fractures.[204]

Primary prevention for osteoporosis must begin at an early age. Young women in their teens and twenties should be educated about the importance of a diet rich in calcium and vitamin D, the benefits of weight-bearing exercise, and the roles that low body weight and cigarette smoking play in reducing bone mass.[193,200,201] Effective health education earlier in life might allow more women to include calcium and vitamin D in their diet and weight-bearing exercise into their weekly physical activity, increasing their potential of reaching peak bone mass in their twenties and of maintaining a healthier lifestyle as they grow older.

Screening typically begins with a complete physical exam and may involve bone mineral density testing, such as single photon absorptiometry, dual photon absorptiometry, ultrasound, quantitative computed tomography, and dual-energy X-ray absorptiometry (DEXA), currently the "gold standard" of testing.[194,198,205] In 1996, the U.S.

Preventive Services Task Force reported, "there is insufficient evidence to recommend for or against screening for osteoporosis or decreased bone density in asymptomatic, postmenopausal women."[206] The American College of Obstetricians and Gynecologists does not recommend routine screening for osteoporosis.[207] However, more recent guidelines from the National Osteoporosis Foundation advise a risk-factor-based screening strategy for women willing to begin a therapy for prevention or treatment, if indicated. The Centers for Medicare and Medicaid Services (CMS), formerly called the Health Care Financing Administration, has approved payment for testing for all women enrolled in Medicare.

Lupus Erythematosus

Systemic lupus erythematosus (lupus) is an incurable inflammatory autoimmune disease that strikes women at a median age of 25 years and may cause weight loss, fever, fatigue, aching, and/or weakness and may involve different organ systems such as the central nervous system, the heart, lungs, kidneys, muscles, and joints.[188]

The National Arthritis Data Work Group has estimated that 239,000 men and women in the United States have suspected or definite lupus.[177] Results of longitudinal studies and data from the NHANES I survey estimate the overall prevalence of lupus to be between 14.6 and 50.8 cases per 100,000 people.[177,191,208,209] For both whites and blacks, the prevalence of lupus is higher for females than males with an estimated female-to-male ratio of 12:1 during the childbearing years (age 15 to 45 years) and 9:1 overall.[177,191,208,209] Lupus affects black women at a rate four times higher than for white women, with an estimated age-specific prevalence of 408 per 100,000 black females age 15–64 years and 100 per 100,000 white females age 15–64 years.[177,210] Survival among women with lupus has improved, but 15% of women die within 10 years of diagnosis.[211] A recent study examined the effect of autoimmune diseases overall (including lupus) on mortality among women and found that when counts of autoimmune disease deaths (e.g., multiple sclerosis, rheumatoid arthritis, systemic lupus erythematosus) were compared to frequencies of the 10 leading causes of death among women, autoimmune disease deaths exceeded the frequency of the tenth leading cause in every age category of women.[212]

Due to the strong preponderance of the disease among women, the etiology of lupus is suspected to be related to both genetics and the female hormones estrogen and progesterone.[188] Inadequate production of the female hormone progesterone and a gene on chromosome 6 have been linked with susceptibility to lupus. The use of certain medications, most notably procainamide and hydralazine, may cause a reversible "drug-induced lupus."[213]

Pregnancy and oral contraceptive use may exacerbate the condition.[214,215] Women with lupus have normal fertility, although they have a doubled risk of miscarriage or fetal loss during pregnancy.[216,217] Women with lupus have an increased risk of developing CVD due to steroid medications, which they must take to prevent progression of their disease.[191] Additionally, women with lupus have an increased risk of developing low bone mass and a fivefold increase in the number of bone fractures as compared to women without lupus.[218]

As there are no known modifiable causes or risk factors for lupus, it is infeasible at this time to address prevention of the disease itself. Attention should be given, however, to the prevention of the adverse consequences of the disease (tertiary prevention). There is a high risk of developing organ-related disease if inflammation is left untreated. Generally, treatment includes the use of anti-inflammatory medications (e.g., nonsteroidal anti-inflammatory drugs, corticosteroids) and drugs that suppress the immune system. Additional types of medications may be prescribed depending on which organ systems are involved.[188]

Thyroid Disorders

Hashimoto's thyroiditis is an organ-specific autoimmune disease that leads to damage of the thyroid gland and results in hypothyroidism (underactivity of the thyroid gland). It is characterized by relatively nonspecific symptoms such as fatigue, weight gain, intolerance of cold temperatures, and muscle cramps.[187,219] Conversely, Graves' disease is an autoimmune disease of the thyroid gland resulting in hyperthryoidism (overactivity of the thyroid gland). It is characterized by symptoms such as weight loss, heat intolerance, heart palpitations, insomnia, sweating, bulging eyes, and bowel disorders.[187] Postpartum thyroiditis is an inflammation of the thyroid gland that develops in the first year after pregnancy causing hypothyroidism. This condition usually resolves spontaneously.[220]

Thyroid dysfunction affects approximately 10% of the general population in the United States.[221] Hashimoto's thyroiditis affects women 8.5 times more frequently than men and Graves' disease four to eight times more frequently.[188] In white and black women older than 55 years, the prevalence of hyperthyroidism is estimated to be 3.6% and 0.7%, respectively. In that same population, the prevalence of hypothyroidism is estimated to be 9.5% in white women and 6.6% in black women.[222] Based upon a review of the literature that identified methodologically sound studies, the best estimate of the prevalence of postpartum thyroiditis is 4.9%, with a range of 3.7 to 5.5%.[220]

Thyroiditis is thought to be inherited; up to 50% of first-degree relatives of those affected also have thyroid antibodies.[223] Additionally, increased iodine intake is an environmental risk factor for the development of postpartum thyroiditis.[224] Smoking has been shown to increase the risk of developing overt hypothyroidism among women with subclinical disease.[225]

Women with hypothyroidism may have reduced fertility and experience a twofold increase in the risk of spontaneous abortion during pregnancy.[226]

Untreated hypothyroidism may lead to CVD due to associated high levels of cholesterol and triglycerides.[187] Women with Graves' disease are at increased risk of developing osteoporosis.[187] Among women with Graves' disease, diabetes mellitus and cigarette smoking increase a woman's risk for developing complications of the eye.[227] In older patients, hyperthyroidism may exacerbate underlying heart problems, including irregular heartbeat, atrial fibrillation, and heart attack.

Asymptomatic or minimally symptomatic patients with early hypothyroidism can be identified with an inexpensive screening test for thyroid stimulating hormone (TSH).[228] There are no known modifiable factors related to hypothyroidism and hyperthyroidism, and, consequently, no preventive measures can be recommended. Treatment of thyroid disorders appears to limit the damage caused by these conditions.[187]

Alzheimer's Disease

Alzheimer's disease is the most common cause of dementia among the elderly. Alzheimer's disease affects the parts of the brain that control thought, memory, and language. An estimated 4 million people in the United States have Alzheimer's disease.[229] As the current nonelderly population in the United States steadily ages and life expectancy increases, the prevalence of Alzheimer's disease is also expected to increase substantially.[230] Alzheimer's disease disproportionately affects women because they live longer than men.[230]

Diagnosis requires a wide array of techniques. Neuropsychological tests are used by physicians to measure a patient's problems with memory, problem solving, attention, counting, and language skills. Brain scans are frequently used to view the patient's brain. Computed tomography (CT), positron emission tomography (PET), and MRI scans are used to help establish a diagnosis of Alzheimer's disease.

Alzheimer's disease can only be diagnosed definitively upon finding disease-related plaques

and fiber tangles in the brain at autopsy. Diagnosis remains challenging. First, the clinical natural history of the disease varies greatly. Second, due to the cognitive impairment associated with Alzheimer's disease, much of the patient's history must be collected from proxy sources such as spouses, family, friends and caretakers. In most people with Alzheimer's disease, the first symptoms do not appear until after age 60. The prevalence of disease doubles every 5 years after age 65.[229]

The two most prominent risk factors are age and family history of Alzheimer's disease. Other risk factors under study are history of serious head injury, lower level of education, a type of a protein called apolipoprotein E (APOE), and environmental exposure to certain metals (such as aluminum and zinc).[231,232,233]

There may also be some biologic differences in Alzheimer's disease in women as compared to men. It has been found that women who are postmenopausal are at higher risk for Alzheimer's disease as compared to premenopausal women. This may be due to older age but there is evidence to suggest that the drop in estrogen also plays a role.[234] In addition, women who have developed Alzheimer's disease seem to have a different natural history as compared to men. Women experience greater cognitive impairment and a more rapid decline in their status. Curiously, despite seemingly more severe disease, women with Alzheimer's are less likely to die from the disease compared to men.[235]

Due to tremendous variability in the progression of Alzheimer's disease, researchers find it difficult to describe the natural history of the disease. There is no cure for Alzheimer's disease. Some medications can alleviate symptoms such as impaired cognition, sleeplessness, agitation, anxiety and depression. On average, people live for 8 to 10 years after they are diagnosed.[229] Women tend to live longer than men after diagnosis which may not be due to the disease itself but, rather, due to coexisting diseases that affect men more.[229]

References

1. National Center for Health Statistics. Health, United States, 1999. With health and aging chartbook. (PHS)99–1232. Hyattsville (MD): U.S. Department of Health and Human Services; 1999.

2. Murphy SL. Deaths: final data for 1998. Natl Vital Stat Rep 2000;48:1–105.

3. Feinleib M, Ingster L. Socioeconomic gradients in health among men and women. In: Ness R, Kuller L, editors. Health and disease among women: biological and environmental influences. New York: Oxford University Press; 1999:3–32.

4. Adams P, Hendershot G, Marano M. Current estimates from the National Health Interview Survey, 1996. National Center for Health Statistics. Vital Health Stat 1999; 10(200):83–84.

5. Summer L, O'Neill G, Shirey L. Challenges for the 21st century: chronic and disabling conditions. Washington: National Academy on an Aging Society; 1999. Available from: URL: http://www.aging-society.org/profiles.htm.

6. Rosenberg L, Palmer JR, Rao RS, Adams-Campbell LL. Risk factors for coronary heart disease in African American women. Am J Epidemiol 1999;150:904–909.

7. Samsioe G. Cardiovascular disease in postmenopausal women. Maturitas 1998;30:11–18.

8. O'Donnell CJ, Kannel WB. Cardiovascular risks of hypertension: lessons from observational studies. J Hypertens Suppl 1998; 16:S3–S7.

9. Sharp PC, Koenen JC. Women's cardiovascular health. Prim Care 1997;24:1–14.

10. Hennekens CH. Risk factors for coronary heart disease in women. Cardiol Clin 1998;16:1–8.

11. Holdright DR. Risk factors for cardiovascular disease in women. J Hum Hypertens 1998;12:667–673.

12. Hall WD, Ferrario CM, Moore MA, Hall JE, Flack JM, Cooper W, et al. Hypertension-related morbidity and mortality in the southeastern United States. Am J Med Sci 1997;313:195–209.

13. van Leer EM, Seidell JC, Kromhout D. Differences in the association between alcohol consumption and blood pressure by age, gender, and smoking. Epidemiol 1994;5:576–582.

14. Berlin JA, Colditz GA. A meta-analysis of physical activity in the prevention of coronary heart disease. Am J Epidemiol 1990;132:612–628.

15. Limacher MC. Exercise and rehabilitation in women. Indications and outcomes. Cardiol Clin 1998;16:27–36.

16. Solomon CC, Manson JE. Obesity and mortality: a review of the epidemiologic data. Am J Clin Nutr 1997;66 Suppl:1044S–1050S.

17. Colombel A, Charbonnel B. Weight gain and cardiovascular risk factors in the post-menopausal woman. Hum Reprod Suppl 1997;12:134–145.

18. Benson V, Marano M. Current estimates from the National Health Interview Survey, 1995. Vital Health Stat 1998;10(199):1–428.

19. Kramarow E, Lentzner H, Rooks R, Weeks J, Saydah S. Health, United States, 1999. With health and aging chartbook. (PHS)99–1232. Hyattsville (MD): National Center for Health Statistics; 1999.

20. Brady WA, Kritz-Silverstein D, Barrett-Connor E, Morales AJ. Prior oral contraceptive use is associated with higher blood pressure in older women. J Womens Health 1998;7:221–228.

21. LaRosa JC. Lipids and cardiovascular disease: do the findings and therapy apply equally to men and women? Womens Health Issues 1992;2:102–111.

22. van der Mooren MJ, Mijatovic V, van Baal WM, Stehouwer CO. Hormone replacement therapy in postmenopausal women with specific risk factors for coronary artery disease. Maturitas 1998; 30:27–36.

23. Nicholson WR, Brown AF, Gathe J, Grumbach K, Washington AJ, Perez-Stable EJ. Hormone replacement therapy for African American women: missed opportunities for effective intervention. Menopause 1999;6:147–155.

24. Wenger NK. Postmenopausal hormone therapy. Is it useful for coronary prevention? Cardiol Clin 1998;16:17–25.

25. American College of Physicians. Guidelines for counseling postmenopausal women about preventive hormone therapy. Ann Intern Med 1992;117:1038–1041.

26. Barrett-Connor EL, Wingard DL. Sex differential in ischemic heart disease mortality in diabetics: a prospective population-based study. Am J Epidemiol 1983;118:489–496.

27. Barrett-Connor EL, Cohn BA, Wingard DL, Edelstein SL. Why is diabetes mellitus a stronger risk factor for fatal ischemic heart disease in women than in men? The Rancho Bernardo study. JAMA 1991;265:627–631.

28. Hanes DS, Weir MR, Sowers JR. Gender considerations in hypertension pathophysiology and treatment. Am J Med 1996; 101:10S–21S.

29. Centers for Disease Control and Prevention. Public health focus: physical activity and the prevention of coronary heart disease. MMWR Morb Mortal Wkly Rep 1993;42:669–672.

30. Manson JE, Hu FB, Rich-Edwards JW, Colditz GA, Stampfer MJ, Willett WC, et al. A prospective study of walking as compared with vigorous exercise in the prevention of coronary heart disease in women. N Engl J Med 1999;341:650–658.

31. Kawachi I, Colditz GA, Stampfer MJ, Willett WC, Manson JE, Rosner B, et al. Smoking cessation and time course of decreased risks of coronary heart disease in middle-aged women. Arch Intern Med 1994;154:169–175.

32. Peto R, Lopez AD, Boreham J, Thun M, Heath Jr C. Mortality from tobacco in developed countries: indirect estimation from national vital statistics. Lancet 1992;339:1268–1278.

33. Colhoun HM, Hemingway H, Poulter NR. Socio-economic status and blood pressure: an overview analysis. J Human Hypertens 1998;12:91–110.

34. Eaker ED. Psychological factors in the epidemiology of coronary heart disease in women. Psychiatr Clin North Am 1989; 12:167–173.

35. Eaker ED. Psychosocial risk factors for coronary heart disease in women. Cardiology Clin 1998;16:103–111.

36. National Diabetes Data Group. Diabetes in America, 2nd ed. Bethesda, MD: National Institutes of Health, 1995.

37. Harris M, Flegal K, Cowie C. Prevalence of diabetes, impaired fasting glucose, and impaired glucose tolerance in the U.S., adults. The Third National Health and Nutrition Examination Survey. Diabetes Care 1998;21:518–524.

38. U.S. Renal Data System. USRDS 1997 annual data report. Bethesda (MD): National Institutes of Health, National Institutes of Diabetes and Digestive and Kidney Disease; 1997.

39. Klein R, Klein B. Vision disorder in diabetes. Diabetes in America. 2nd ed. Bethesda (MD): National Institutes of Health; 1995: 293–338.

40. Wingard D, Barrett-Connor E. Heart disease and diabetes. Diabetes in America. 2nd ed. Bethesda (MD): National Institutes of Health; 1995:429–448.

41. Kuller L. Stroke and diabetes. Diabetes in America. 2nd ed. Bethesda (MD): National Institutes of Health; 1995:449–456.

42. Benson V, Marano M. Current estimates from the National Health Interview Survey, 1995. Series 10, number 199. Hyattsville (MD): National Center for Health Statistics; 1998.

43. Harris M. Classification, diagnostic criteria, and screening for diabetes. Diabetes in America. 2nd ed. Bethesda (MD): National Institutes of Health; 1995:15–36.

44. Tuomilehto J, Podar T, Tuomilehto-Wolf E, Virtala E. Evidence for importance of gender and birth cohort for risk of IDDM in offspring of IDDM parents. Diabetologia 1995;38:975–982.

45. Metzger BE, Coustan DR. Summary and recommendations of the Fourth International Workshop-Conference on Gestational Diabetes Mellitus. The Organizing Committee. Diabetes Care 1998;21 Suppl 2:B161–B167.

46. Shoff SM, Newcomb PA. Diabetes, body size and risk of endometrial cancer. Am J Epidemiol 1998;148:234–240.

47. Garner P. Type I diabetes mellitus and pregnancy. Lancet 1995; 346:157–161.

48. Barr Jr M. Teratogen update: angiotensin-converting enzyme inhibitors. Teratology 1994;50:399–409.

49. Elwood JM, Little J, Elwood JH. Epidemiology and control of neural tube defects. Monogr Epidemiol Biostat 1992;20:424–433.

50. Landon MB, Gabbe SG. Fetal surveillance in the pregnancy complicated by diabetes mellitus. Clin Obstet Gynecol 1991;34:535–543.

51. York R, Brown L, Swank A, Samuels P, Robbins D, Armstrong C. Diabetes mellitus in pregnancy: clinical review. J Perinatol 1990; 10:285–293.

52. Dornhorst A, Rossi M. Risk and prevention of type 2 diabetes in women with gestational diabetes. Diabetes Care 1998;21 Suppl 2:B43–B49.

53. American Cancer Society. Cancer facts and figures, 2000. Atlanta: The Society; 2000.

54. Landis SH, Murray T, Bolden S, Wingo PA. Cancer statistics, 1999. CA Cancer J Clin 1999;49:8–31.

55. National Cancer Institute. SEER program: breast cancer. Bethesda (MD): U.S. Department of Health and Human Services; 1998.

56. McDonald CJ. Cancer statistics, 1999: challenges in minority populations. CA Cancer J Clin 1999;49(1):6–7.

57. Wingo PA, Ries LA, Rosenberg HM, Miller DS, Edwards BK. Cancer incidence and mortality, 1973–1995: a report card for the United States. Cancer 1998;82:1197–1207.

58. Fletcher SW, Black W, Harris R, Rimer BK, Shapiro S. Report of the International Workshop on Screening for Breast Cancer. J Natl Cancer Inst 1993;85:1644–1656.

59. Hulka BS. Epidemiologic analysis of breast and gynecologic cancers. Progress Clin Biol Res 1997;396:17–29.

60. Velentgas P, Daling JR. Risk factors for breast cancer in younger women. J Natl Cancer Inst Monogr 1994;16:15–24.

61. Kelsey JR. Breast cancer epidemiology: summary and future directions. Epidemiol Rev 1993;15:256–263.

62. Rosenberg L, Palmer JR, Rao RS, Strom BL, Zauber AG, Warshauer ME, et al. Case-control study of oral contraceptive use and risk of breast cancer. Am J Epidemiol 1996;143:25–37.

63. Van Os WA, Edelman DA, Rhemrev PE, Grant S. Oral contraceptives and breast cancer risk. Adv Contracept 1997;13:63–69.

64. Collaborative Group on Hormonal Factors in Breast Cancer. Breast cancer and hormonal contraceptives: further results. Contraception 1996;54:1S–106S.

65. Katsouyanni K, Lipworth L, Trichopoulou A, Samole E, Stuver S, Trichopoulos, D. A case-control study of lactation and cancer of the breast. Br J Cancer 1996;73:814–818.

66. Brinton LA, Potischman NA, Swanson CA, Schoenburg JB, Coates RJ, Gammon MD, et al. Breastfeeding and breast cancer risk. Cancer Causes Control 1995;6:199–208.

67. Layde PM, Webster LA, Baughman AL, Wingo PA, Rubin GL, Ory HW. The independent associations of parity, age at full term pregnancy, and duration of breastfeeding with the risk of breast cancer: Cancer and Steroid Hormone Study group. J Clin Epidemiol 1989; 42:963–973.

68. Thomas DB, Noonan EA. Breast cancer and prolonged lactation: The WHO Collaborative Study of Neoplasia and Steroid Contraceptives. Int J Epidemiol 1993;22:619–626.

69. Michels KB, Willett WC, Rosner BA, Manson JE, Hunter DJ, Colditz GA, et al. Prospective assessment of breastfeeding and breast cancer incidence among 89,887 women. Lancet 1996; 347:431–436.

70. Newcomb PA, Egan KM, Titus-Ernstoff L, Trentham-Dietz A, Greenberg ER, Baron JA, et al. Lactation in relation to postmenopausal breast cancer. Am J Epidemiol 1999;150:174–182.

71. Gilliland F, Hunt W, Baumgartner K, Crumley D, Nicholson C, Fetherolf J, et al. Reproductive risk factors for breast cancer in Hispanic and non-Hispanic white women. Am J Epidemiol 1998;148:683–692.

72. Ross R, Paganini-Hill A, Wan P, Pike M. Effect of hormone replacement therapy on breast cancer risk: estrogen versus estrogen plus progestin. J Natl Cancer Inst 2000;92:328–332.

73. Colditz GA. Hormones and breast cancer: evidence and implications for consideration of risks and benefits of hormone replacement therapy. J Womens Health 1999;8:347–357.

74. Gapstur SM, Morrow M, Sellers TA. Hormone replacement therapy and risk of breast cancer with a favorable histology. Results of the Iowa Women's Study. JAMA 1999;281:2091–2097.

75. Bush TL, Whiteman MK. Hormone replacement therapy and risk of breast cancer. JAMA 1999;281:2140–2141.

76. Willett WC. Diet and human cancer. In: Brugge J, editor. Origins of human cancer: a comprehensive review. New York: Cold Spring Harbor Laboratory Press; 1991.

77. Huang Z, Hankinson SE, Colditz GA, Stampfer MJ, Hunter DJ, Manson JE, et al. Dual effects of weight and weight gain on breast cancer risk. JAMA 1997;278:1407–1411.

78. Greenwald P, Clifford C. Dietary prevention. In: Kramer BS, Weed KL, editors. Cancer prevention and control. New York: Marcel Dekker; 1995.

79. Zhang S, Hunter DJ, Forman MR, Rosner BA, Speizer FE, Colditz GA, et al. Dietary carotenoids and vitamins A, C, and E and risk of breast cancer. Natl Cancer Inst Monogr 1999;91:547–556.

80. Bernstein L, Henderson BE, Hanisch R, Sullivan-Halley J, Ross RK. Physical exercise and reduced risk of breast cancer in young women. J Natl Cancer Inst 1994;86:1403–1408.

81. Gammon M, John E, Britton J. Recreational and occupational physical activities and risk of breast cancer. J Natl Cancer Inst 1998;90:100–117.

82. Thune I, Brenn T, Lund E, Gaard M. Physical activity and the risk of breast cancer. N Engl J Med 1997;336:1269–1275.

83. Zhang S, Hunter DJ, Hankinson S, Giovannucci EL, Rosner BA, Colditz GA, et al. A prospective study of folate intake and the risk of breast cancer. JAMA 1999;281:1632–1637.

84. Swanson GM. Cancer prevention and control: a science-based public health agenda. J Public Health Manag Pract 1996;2:1–8.

85. Fisher B, Costantino JP, Wickerham DL, Redmond CK, Kavanah M, Cronin WM, et al. Tamoxifen for prevention of breast cancer: report of the National Surgical Adjuvant Breast and Bowel Project P-1 study. J Natl Cancer Inst 1998;90:1371–1388.

86. Fisher B, Constantino JP, Redmond CK, Fisher ER, Wickerham DL, Cronin WM. Endometrial cancer in tamoxifen-treated breast cancer patients: findings from the National Surgical Adjuvant Breast and Bowel Project (NSABBP) B-14. J Natl Cancer Inst 1994;86:527–537.

87. Cummings SR, Eckert SK, Krueger KA, Grady D, Powles TJ, Cauley JA, et al. The effect of raloxifene on risk of breast cancer in postmenopausal women: results from the MORE randomized trial. JAMA 1999;281:2189–2197.

88. Fisher B. Highlights from recent National Surgical Adjuvant Breast and Bowel Project studies in the treatment and prevention of breast cancer. CA Cancer J Clin 1999;49:159–177.

89. Hacker N. Breast disease: a gynecologic perspective. In: Hacker N, Moore J, editors. Essentials of obstetrics and gynecology. 3rd ed. Philadelphia: WB Saunders Company; 1998:737.

90. Ernster VL. Mammography screening for women aged 40 through 49. A guidelines saga and a clarion call for informed decision making. Am J Public Health 1997;87:1103–1106.

91. Dickersin K. Breast screening in women aged 40–49 years: what next? Lancet 1999;353:1896–1897.

92. Roetzheim RG, Pal N, Tennant C, Voti L, Ayanian JZ, Schwabe A, et al. Effects of health insurance and race on early detection of cancer. J Natl Cancer Inst 1999;91:1409–1415.

93. Velanovich V, Yood MK, Bawle U, Nathanson SD, Strand VF, Talpos GB, et al. Racial differences in the presentation and surgical management of breast cancer. Surgery 1999;125:375–379.

94. Flaws JA, Newschaffer CJ, Bush TL. Breast cancer mortality in black and in white women: a historical perspective by menopausal status. J Womens Health 1998;7:1007–1015.

95. Klonoff-Cohen HS, Schaffroth LB, Edelstein SL, Molgaard C, Saltzstein SL. Breast cancer histology in Caucasians, African Americans, Hispanics, Asians, and Pacific Islanders. Ethn Health 1998;3:189–198.

96. Lannin DR, Mathews HF, Mitchell J, Swanson MS, Swanson FH, Edwards MS. Influence of socioeconomic and cultural factors on racial differences in late-stage presentation of breast cancer. JAMA 1998;279:1801–1807.

97. American Cancer Society. Cervical cancer: prevention and risk factors. Atlanta: The Society; 1998.

98. American Cancer Society. Facts and figures. Atlanta: The Society; 1999.

99. National Cancer Institute. NCI cancer trials: cervical cancer background: Bethesda (MD): U.S. Department of Health and Human Services; 1999.

100. Beutner KR, Tyring S. Human papillomavirus and human disease. Am J Med 1997;102:9–15.

101. Verdon ME. Issues in the management of the human papillomavirus genital disease. Am Fam Physician 1997; 55:1813–1816,1819,1822.

102. Munoz N, Bosch FX. The causal link between HPV and cervical cancer and its implications for prevention of cervical cancer. Bull Pan Am Health Organ 1996;30:362–377.

103. Turek LP, Smith EM. The genetic program of genital human papillomaviruses in infection and cancer. Obstet Gynecol Clin North Am 1996;23:735–758.

104. Stoler MH. A brief synopsis of the role of human papillomaviruses in cervical carcinogenesis. Am J Obstet Gynecol 1996; 175:1091–1098.

105. Eng T, Butler W. The hidden epidemic: confronting sexually transmitted diseases. Washington: Institute of Medicine; 1996.

106. Phillips AN, Smith GD. Cigarette smoking as a potential cause of cervical cancer: has confounding been controlled? Int J Epidemiol 1994;23:42–49.

107. Simons AM, Mugica van Herckenrode C, Rodriguez JA, Maitland N, Anderson M, Phillips DH, et al. Demonstration of smoking-related damage in cervical epithelium and correlation with human papillomavirus type 16, using exfoliated cervical cells. Br J Cancer 1996;71:246–249.

108. Prokopczyk B, Cox JE, Hoffmann D, Waggoner SE. Identification of tobacco-specific carcinogen in the cervical mucus of smokers and nonsmokers. J Natl Cancer Inst 1997;89:868–873.

109. Daly SF, Doyle M, English J, Turner M, Clinch J, Prendiville W. Can the number of cigarettes smoked predict high-grade cervical intraepithelial neoplasia among women with mildly abnormal cervical smears? Am J Obstet Gynecol 1998;179:399–402.

110. Ylitalo N, Sorensen P, Josefsson A, Frisch M, Sparen P, Ponten J, et al. Smoking and oral contraceptives as risk factors for cervical carcinoma in situ. Int J Cancer 1999;81:357–365.

111. Murakami M, Gurski KJ, Steller MA. Human papillomavirus vaccines for cervical cancer. J Immunother 1999;22:212–218.

112. U.S. Preventive Services Task Force. Guide to clinical preventive services: an assessment of the effectiveness of 160 interventions. Baltimore: Williams and Wilkins; 1989.

113. American Cancer Society. Cervical cancer: treatment. Atlanta: The Society; 1999.

114. Rose PG, Bundy BN, Watkins EB, Thigpen JT, Deppe G, Maiman MA, et al. Concurrent cisplatin-based radiotherapy and chemotherapy for locally advanced cervical cancer. N Engl J Med 1999; 340:1144–1153.

115. Morris M, Eifel PJ, Lu J, Grigsby, PW, Levenback C, Stevens, RE. Pelvic radiation with concurrent chemotherapy compared with pelvic and para-aortic radiation for high-risk cervical cancer. N Engl J Med 1999;340:1137–1143.

116. Ries L, Eisner M, Kosary C, Hankey B, Miller B, Clegg L, Edwards B, editors. SEER cancer statistics review, 1973–1997. Bethesda (MD): National Cancer Institute; 2000.

117. Gross TP, Schlesselman JJ. The estimated effect of oral contraceptive use on the cumulative risk of epithelial ovarian cancer. Obstet Gynecol 1994;83:419–424.

118. Risch H, Marrett L, Howe G. Parity, contraception, infertility, and the risk of epithelial ovarian cancer. Am J Epidemiol 1994; 140:585–597.

119. Hartge P, Whittemore AS, Itnyre J, McGowan L, Cramer D and the Collaborative Ovarian Cancer Group. Rates and risks of ovarian cancer in subgroups of white women in the United States. Obstet Gynecol 1994;84:760–764.

120. Hankinson SE, Colditz GA, Hunter DJ, Willett WC, Stampfer MJ, Rosner B, et al. A prospective study of reproductive factors and risk of epithelial ovarian cancer. Cancer 1995;76:284–290.

121. Chen MT, Cook LS, Daling JR, Weiss NS. Incomplete pregnancies and risk of ovarian cancer. Cancer Causes Control 1996; 7:415–420.

122. Fathalla MF. Incessant ovulation—a factor in ovarian neoplasia? Lancet 1971;7716:163.

123. Whittemore A, Harris R, Itnyre J. Collaborative Ovarian Cancer Group. Characteristics relating to ovarian cancer risk: collaborative analysis of 12 U.S. case-control studies IV. The pathogenesis of epithelial ovarian cancer. Am J Epidemiol 1992;136:1212–1220.

124. Reis L, Kosary C, Hankey B, Miller B, Clegg L, Edwards B, editors. SEER cancer statistics review, 1973–1996. Bethesda (MD): National Cancer Institute; 1999.

125. Kuo D, Jones J, Runowica C. Diseases of the ovary and fallopian tubes. In: Scott RJ, ed. Danforth's obstetrics and gynecology. Philadelphia: Lippincott, Williams and Wilkins; 1999:847–907.

126. Liu L, Deapen D, Bernstein L. Socioeconomic status and cancer of the female breast and reproductive organs: a comparison across racial/ethnic populations in Los Angeles County, California. Cancer Causes Control 1998;9:369–380.

127. John EM, Whittemore AS, Harris R, Itnyre J. Characteristics relating to ovarian cancer risk: collaborative analysis of seven U.S. case-control studies. Epithelial ovarian cancer in black women. Collaborative Ovarian Cancer Group. J Natl Cancer Inst 1993; 85:142–147.

128. Struewing J, Hartge P, Wacholder S, Baker SM, Berlin M, McAdams M, et al. The risk of cancer associated with specific mutations of BRCA1 and BRCA2 among Ashkenazi Jews. N Engl J Med 1997;336:1401–1408.

129. Brinton L, Gridley G, Persson I, Baron J, Bergqvist A. Cancer risk after a hospital discharge diagnosis of endometriosis. Am J Obstet Gynecol 1997;176:572–579.

130. Glud E, Kjaer SK, Troisi R, Brinton L. Fertility drugs and ovarian cancer. Am J Epidemiol 1998;20:237–257.

131. Hempling RE, Wong C, Piver MS, Natarajan N, Meltlin CJ. Hormone replacement therapy as a risk factor for epithelial ovarian cancer: results of a case-control study. Obstet Gynecol 1997; 89:1012–1016.

132. Whittemore AS, Wu ML, Paffenbarger RS, Sarles DL, Kampert JB, Grosser S, et al. Personal and environmental characteristics related to epithelial ovarian cancer. II. Exposure to talcum powder, tobacco, alcohol and coffee. Am J Epidemiol 1988;128:1228–1240.

133. Zweizig S. Office screening for gynecologic cancer. Clin Obstet Gynecol 1999;42:267–275.

134. Cane P, Azen C, Lopez E. Tumor marker trends in asymptomatic women at risk for ovarian cancer: relevance for ovarian cancer screening. Gynecol Oncol 1995;57:240–245.

135. Karlan B, Platt L. The current status of ultrasound and color doppler imaging in screening for ovarian cancer. Gynecol Oncol 1994; 55:28–33.

136. Shureiqi I, Breener D. Chemoprevention of epithelial cancers. Curr Opin Oncol 1999;11:408–411.

137. Brady P. Diseases of the uterus. In: Scott JR, editor. Danforth's obstetrics and gynecology. Philadelphia: Lippincott, Williams and Wilkins; 1999:837–856.

138. Persky V, Davis F, Barrett R, Ruby E, Sailer C, Levy P. Recent time trends in uterine cancer. Am J Public Health 1990;80:935–939.

139. Liu J, Conaway M, Rodriguez G, Soper J, Clarke-Pearson D, Berchuck A. Relationship between race and interval to treatment in endometrial cancer. Obstet Gynecol 1995;86:486–490.

140. Coates RJ, Click LA, Harlan LC, Robboy S, Barrett RJ, Eley JW, et al. Differences between black and white patients with cancer of the uterine corpus in interval from symptom recognition to initial medical consultation. Cancer Causes Control 1996;7:328–336.

141. Hill HA, Coates RJ, Austin H, Correa P, Robboy SJ, Chen V, et al. Racial differences in tumor grade among women with endometrial cancer. Gynecol Oncol 1995;56:154–163.

142. Salvesen HB, Akslen LA, Albrektsen G, Iversen OE. Poorer survival of nulliparous women with endometrial carcinoma. Cancer 1998; 82:1328–1333.

143. Rubin GL, Peterson HB, Lee WL, Maes EF, Wingo PA, Becker S. Estrogen replacement therapy and the risk of endometrial cancer: remaining controversies. Am J Obstet Gynecol 1990;162:148-154.

144. Parazzini F, Negri E, La Vecchia C, Benzi G, Chiaffarino F, Polatti A, et al. Role of reproductive factors on the risk of endometrial cancer. Int J Cancer 1998;76:784–786.

145. Shapiro S, Kaufman DW, Slone D, Rosenberg L, Miettinen OS, Stolley PD, et al. Recent and past use of conjugated estrogens in relation to adenocarcinoma of the endometrium. N Engl J Med 1980;303:485–489.

146. Weiss NS, Szekely DR, English DR, Schweid AI. Endometrial cancer in relation to patterns of menopausal estrogen use. JAMA 1979; 242:261–264.

147. CDC Tobacco Information and Prevention Source. Facts on women and tobacco. Atlanta: Centers for Disease Control and Prevention, Office on Smoking and Health; 1998.

148. Samet J. Lung cancer. In: Greenwald P, Kramer B, Weed D, editors. Cancer Prevention and Control. New York: Marcel Dekker; 1996. p. 561–579.

149. Zang E, Wynder E. Differences in lung cancer risk between men and women: examination of the evidence. J Natl Cancer Inst 1996;88:183–192.

150. Ernster VL. Female lung cancer. Ann Rev Public Health 1996; 17:97–114.

151. Baldini EH, Strauss GM. Women and lung cancer: waiting to exhale. Chest 1997;112(4 Suppl):229S–234S.

152. Bennett WP, Alavanja MC, Blomeke B, Vahakangas KH, Castren K, Welsh JA, et al. Environmental tobacco smoke, genetic suscepti- bility, and risk of lung cancer in never-smoking women. J Natl Cancer Inst 1999;91:2009–2013.

153. Shriver SP, Bourdeau HA, Gubish CT, Tirpak DL, Davis AL, Luketich JD, et al. Sex-specific expression of gastrin-releasing peptide receptor: relationship to smoking history and risk of lung cancer. J Natl Cancer Inst 2000;92:24–33.

154. Gauderman WJ, Morrison JL. Evidence for age-specific genetic rela- tive risks in lung cancer. Am J Epidemiol 2000;151:41–49.

155. Brownson R, Alavanja M, Caporaso N, Simoes E, Chang J. Epidemiology and prevention of lung cancer in nonsmokers. Epidemiol Rev 1998;20:218–235.

156. Hackshaw A, Law M, Wald N. The accumulated evidence on lung cancer and environmental tobacco smoke. Br Med J 1997;315:980–988.

157. Halpern M, Gillespie B, Warner K. Patterns of absolute risk of lung cancer mortality in former smokers. J Natl Cancer Inst 1993; 85:457–464.

158. Perkins KA. Nicotine discrimination in men and women. Pharmacol Biochem Behav 1999;64:295–299.

159. Miller BA, Kolonel LN, Bernstein L, Young, Jr. JL, Swanson GM, West D, et al. Racial/ethnic patterns of cancer in the United States, 1988–1992. NIH Pub. No. 96-4104. Bethesda (MD): National Cancer Institute; 1996.

160. Donovan J, Syngal S. Colorectal cancer in women: an underappreci- ated but preventable risk. J Womens Health 1998;7:45–48.

161. Winawer S, Shike M. Prevention and control of colorectal cancer. In: Greenwald P, Kramer B, Weed D, editors. Cancer prevention and control. New York: Marcel Dekker; 1995:537–555.

162. Willett WC, Stampfer MJ, Colditz GA, Rosner BA, Speizer FE. Relation of meat, fat, and fiber intake to the risk of colorectal cancer in a prospective study among women. N Engl J Med 1990;323:1664–1672.

163. Jain M, Cook GM, Davis FG, Grace MG, Howe GR, Miller AB. A case-control study of diet and colorectal cancer. Int J Cancer 1980;26:757–768.

164. Fuchs CS, Giovannucci EL, Colditz GA, Hunter DJ, Stampfer MJ, Rosner B, et al. Dietary fiber and the risk of colorectal cancer and adenoma in women. N Engl J Med 1999;340:169–176.

165. Giovannucci E, Stampfer MJ, Colditz GA, Hunter DJ, Fuchs C, Rosner BA, et al. Multivitamin use, folate, and colon cancer in women in the Nurses' Health Study. Ann Intern Med 1998; 129:517–524.

166. Potter JD. Colorectal cancer: molecules and populations. J Natl Cancer Inst 1999;91:916–932.

167. Grodstein F, Martinez ME, Platz EA, Giovannucci E, Colditz GA, Kautzky M, et al. Postmenopausal hormone use and risk for colorectal cancer and adenoma. Ann Intern Med 1998; 128:705–712.

168. Grodstein F, Newcomb P, Stampfer MJ. Postmenopausal hormone therapy and the risk of colorectal cancer: a review and meta-analysis. Amer J Med 1999;106:574–582.

169. Lee I, Paffenbarger Jr R, Hsieh C. Physical activity and risk of developing colorectal cancer among college alumni. J Natl Cancer Inst 1991;83:1324–1329.

170. Bond JH. Screening guidelines for colorectal cancer. Amer J Med 1999;106:7S–10S.

171. Winawer SJ, Fletcher RH, Miller L, Godlee F, Stolar MH, Mulrow CD, et al. Colorectal cancer screening: clinical guidelines and rationale. Gastroenterology 1997;112:594–642.

172. Centers for Disease Control and Prevention. Screening for colorectal cancer, United States, 1997. MMWR Morb Mortal Wkly Rpt 1999;48:116–121.

173. Morrin M, Farrell R, Kruskal J, LaMont J. Virtual colonoscopy: a kindler, gentler colorectal cancer screening test? Lancet 1999;354:1048–1049.

174. Centers for Disease Control and Prevention. Targeting arthritis: the nation's leading cause of disability. Atlanta: U.S. Department of Health and Human Services; 1999.

175. Callahan LF, Rao J, Boutaugh M. Arthritis and women's health: prevalence, impact, and prevention. Amer J Prev Med 1996; 12:401–409.

176. National Center for Health Statistics. Healthy people 2000 review, 1998–99. Hyattsville (MD): U.S. Department of Health and Human Services; 1999.

177. Lawrence RC, Helmick CG, Arnett FC, Deyo RA, Felson DT, Giannini EH, et al. Estimates of the prevalence of arthritis and selected musculoskeletal disorders in the United States. Arthritis Rheum 1998;41:778–799.

178. Felson DT, Zhang Y, Hannan MT, Naimark A, Weissman BN, Aliabadi P, et al. The incidence and natural history of knee osteoarthritis in the elderly: The Framingham Osteoarthritis Study. Arthritis Rheum 1995;38:1500–1505.

179. Creamer P, Hochberg MC. Osteoarthritis. Lancet 1997; 350:503–508.

180. Felson D, Nevitt M. The effects of estrogen on osteoarthritis. Curr Opin Rheum 1998;10:269–272.

181. Nevitt M, Felson D. Sex hormones and the risk of osteoarthritis in women: epidemiological evidence. Ann Rheum Dis 1996; 55:673–676.

182. Minor MA. Exercise in the treatment of osteoarthritis. Rheum Dis Clin North America 1999;25:397–415.

183. NIH Consensus Development Program. Total hip replacement. NIH consensus statement online. Bethesda (MD): National Institutes of Health; 1994 Sep 12–14;12(5):1–31. Available from: URL: http://odp.od.nih.gov/consensus/cons/098/098_statement.htm

184. Di Cesare PE. Surgical management of osteoarthritis. Clin Geriatr Med 1998;14:613–631.

185. Hall M, Lawrence L. Ambulatory surgery in the United States, 1996. Advance data from vital and health statistics. Hyattsville (MD): National Center for Health Statistics; 1998:1–16.

186. Manzi S, Ramsey-Goldman R. Autoimmune diseases. In: Ness R, Kuller L, eds. Health and disease among women: biological and environmental influences. New York: Oxford University Press; 1999:343–372.

187. Carlson K, Eisenstat S, Ziporyn T. The Harvard guide to women's health. Cambridge (MA): Harvard University Press; 1996.

188. Lahita RG. Collagen disease: the enemy within. Int J Fertil Womens Med 1998;43:229–234.

189. Masi A. Incidence of rheumatoid arthritis: do the observed age-sex interaction patterns support a role of androgenic-anabolic steroid deficiency in its pathogenesis? Br J Rheumatol 1994;33:697–699.

190. Masi AT, Feigenbaum S, Chatterton R. Hormonal and pregnancy relationships to rheumatoid arthritis: convergent effect with immunologic and microvascular systems. Semin Arthritis Rheum 1995;25:1–27.

191. Manzi S, Selzer F, Sutton-Tyrrell K, Fitzgerald S, Rairie J, Tracy R, et al. Prevalence and risk factors of carotid plaque in women with systemic lupus erythematosus. Arthritis and Rheum 1999; 42:51–60.

192. Unger A, Kay A, Griffin J, Panayi, GS. Disease activity and pregnancy associated alpha-2 glycoprotein in rheumatoid arthritis during pregnancy. Br Med J 1983;286:750–752.

193. Butler R. Osteoporosis: prevention and treatment. Practitioner. 1999;243:176–188.

194. Watts N. Postmenopausal osteoporosis. Obstet Gynecol Surv 1999;54:532–537.

195. National Institutes of Health. Osteoporosis overview. Washington: National Institutes of Health, National Osteoporosis Foundation; 1999:1–9.

196. Ray N, Chan J, Thamer M, Melton L III. Medical expenditures for the treatment of osteoporotic fractures in the United States in 1995: report from the national osteoporosis foundation. J Bone Miner Res 1997;12:24–35.

197. National Center for Health Statistics. National Hospital Discharge Survey. Atlanta: Centers for Disease Control and Prevention; 1996.

198. Bowman MA, Spangler JG. Osteoporosis in women. Primary Care 1997;24:27–36.

199. Bohannon AD. Osteoporosis and African American women. J Womens Health Gen Based Med 1999;8:609–615.

200. Dawson-Hughes B. Calcium and vitamin D nutritional needs of elderly women. J Nutr 1996;126:1165S–1167S.

201. LeBoff MS, Kohlmeier L, Hurwitz S, Franklin J, Wright J, Glowacki J. Occult vitamin D deficiency in postmenopausal U.S. women with acute hip fracture. JAMA 1999;281:1505–1511.

202. NIH Consensus Development Panel on Optimal Calcium Intake. Optimal calcium intake. JAMA 1994;272:1942–1947.

203. Fox B, Cameron A. Food science, nutrition and health. 6th ed. London: Arnold; 1995. p. 388.

204. Hopper JE, Seeman E. The bone density of female twins discordant for tobacco use. N Engl J Med 1994;330:387–392.

205. Kanis JA. Diagnosis of osteoporosis. Osteoporos Int 1997;7 Suppl 7:S108–S116.

206. U.S. Preventive Services Task Force. Guide to clinical preventive services. 2nd ed. Baltimore: Wilkins and Wilkins; 1996.

207. American College of Obstetricians and Gynecologists. Guidelines for women's health care. Washington: American College of Obstetricians and Gynecologists; 1996.

208. Mitchet CJ, McKenna C, Elveback L, Kaslow R, Kurland L. Epidemiology of systemic lupus erythematosus and other connective tissue disease in Rochester, Minnesota, 1950 through 1979. Mayo Clin Proc 1985;60:105–113.

209. Fessel WJ. Systemic lupus erythematosus in the community: incidence, prevalence, outcome, and first symptoms, the high prevalence in black women. Arch Intern Med 1974;134:1027–1035.

210. McCarty DJ, Manzi S, Medsger TA, Ramsey-Goldman R, LaPorte RE, Kwoh CK. Incidence of systemic lupus erythematosus. Race and gender differences. Arthritis Rheum 1995;38:1260–1270.

211. Ward M, Pyun E, Studenski S. Long-term survival in systemic lupus erythematosus: patient characteristics associated with poorer outcomes. Arthritis Rheum 1995;38:274–83.

212. Walsh S, Rau L. Autoimmune diseases: a leading cause of death among young and middle-aged women in the United States. Am J Public Health 2000;90:1463–1466.

213. Yung RL, Richardson BC. Drug-induced lupus. Rheum Dis Clin North Am 1994;20:61–86.

214. Jungers P, Dougados M, Pelissier C, Kuttenn F, Tron F, Lesavre P, et al. Influence of oral contraceptive therapy on the activity of systemic lupus erythematosus. Arthritis Rheum 1982;25:618–623.

215. Mintz G, Niz J, Gutierrez G, Garcia-Alonso A, Karch S. Prospective study of pregnancy in systemic lupus erythematosus. Results of a multidisciplinary approach. J Rheumatol 1986;13:732–739.

216. Hardy CJ, Palmer BP, Morton SJ, Muir KR, Powell RJ. Pregnancy outcome and family size in systemic lupus erythematosus: a case-control study. Rheumatology 1999;38:559–563.

217. Fraga A, Mintz G, Orozco J. Sterility and fertility rates, fetal wastage and maternal morbidity in systemic lupus erythematosus. J Rheumatol 1974;1:293–298.

218. Ramsey-Goldman R, Dunn JE, Huang CF, Dunlop D, Raine JE, Fitzgerald S, et al. Frequency of fractures in women with systemic lupus erythematosus. Comparison with U.S. population data. Arthritis Rheum 1999;42:882–890.

219. Dayan C, Daniels G. Chronic autoimmune thyroiditis. N Engl J Med 1996;335:99–107.

220. Gerstein HC. How common is postpartum thyroiditis? A methodologic overview of the literature. Arch Intern Med 1990;150:1397–1400.

221. Sawin CJ, Castelli WP, Hershman JM, McNamara P, Bacharach P. The aging thyroid: thyroid deficiency in the Framingham study. Arch Intern Med 1985:1386–1388.

222. Bahehi N, Brown T, Parish R. Thyroid dysfunction in adults over age 55 years. Arch Intern Med 1990;150:785–787.

223. Phillips D, McLachlan S, Stephenson A, Roberts D, Moffitt S, McDonald D, et al. Autosomal dominant transmission of autoantibodies to thyroglobulin and thyroid peroxidase. J Clin Endocrinol Metab 1990;70:742–746.

224. Terry AJ, Hague WH. Postpartum thyroiditis. Semin Perinatol 1998;22:497–502.

225. Muller B, Zulewski H, Huber P, Ratcliffe J, Staub J. Impaired action of thyroid hormone associated with smoking in women with hypothyroidism. N Engl J Med 1995;333:964–969.

226. Stagnaro-Green A, Roman S, Cobin R, el-Harazy E, Alvarez-Marfany M, Davies T. Detection of at-risk pregnancy by means of highly sensitive assays for thyroid autoantibodies. JAMA 1990; 264:1422–1425.

227. Kalmann R, Mourits MP. Diabetes mellitus: a risk factor in patients with Graves' orbitopathy. Br J Ophthalmol 1999;83:463–465.

228. Danese MD, Powe NR, Sawin CT, Ladenson PW. Screening for mild thyroid failure at the periodic health examination: a decision and cost-effectiveness analysis. JAMA 1996;276:285–292.

229. National Institute on Aging. Progress report on Alzheimer's disease, 1998. (NIH)99–3616. Bethesda (MD): National Institutes of Health; 1999.

230. McCann J, Hebert L, Bennett D, Skul V, Evans D. Why Alzheimer's disease is a women's health issue. J Am Med Womens Assoc 1997;52:132–137.

231. Bullido MJ, Artiga MJ, Recuero M, Sastre I, Garcia MA, Aldudo J, et al. A polymorphism in the regulatory region of APOE associated with risk for Alzheimer's dementia. Nat Genet 1998;18:69–71.

232. Farrer LA, Cupples LA, Haines JL, Hyman B, Kukull WA, Mayeux R, et al. APOE and Alzheimer Disease Meta Analysis Consortium. Effects of age, sex, and ethnicity on the association between apolipoprotein E genotype and Alzheimer's disease. A meta-analysis. JAMA 1997;278:1349–1356.

233. Duara R, Barker WW, Lopez-Alberola R, Loewenstein DA, Grau LB, Gilchrist D, et al. Alzheimer's disease: interaction of apolipoprotein E genotype, family history of dementia, gender, education, ethnicity, and age of onset. Neurology 1996;46:1575–1579.

234. Solerte S, Fioravanti M, Racchi M, Trabucchi M, Zanetti O, Govoni S. Menopause and estrogen deficiency as a risk factor in dementing illness: hypothesis on the biological basis. Maturitas 1999;31:95–101.

235. Gambassi G, Lapane KL, Landi F, Sgadari A, Mor V, Bernabie R. Systematic Assessment of Geriatric drug use via Epidemiology (SAGE) Study Group. Gender differences in the relation between comorbidity and mortality of patients with Alzheimer's disease. Neurology 1999;53:508–516.

Chapter 5

Mental Health

Contents

Introduction

Health is defined by the World Health Organization as a "complex state of physical, mental, and social well-being;" it is not simply the absence of disease. Most of the chapters in this book address factors relating to women's physical health, but this chapter focuses on women's mental health. Certain mental disorders disproportionately affect women, namely major depression, postpartum depression, anxiety, and eating disorders. Women do not experience more mental illness than men; they simply are more likely to develop different types of mental disorders. Men are more likely to have addictive disorders and antisocial personality disorder.

Recently, the Global Burden of Disease study, a collaboration of the World Health Organization, the World Bank, and the Harvard School of Public Health, reported that mental disorders are responsible for more of the global burden of disease than all cancers combined.[1] This landmark study was the first to show the profound impact that mental illness is having on the health and well-being of people in the United States and the world. In 1992, about 40 million people in the United States had a diagnosable mental illness,[2] and one in five women will experience a mental disorder during her lifetime.[2]

Estimating rates of mental illness is difficult because of the complexity of defining who has mental disorders. Mental disorders are diagnosed based on clusters of symptoms. The symptoms of many mental disorders overlap, making diagnosis somewhat subjective. The subjective nature of psychiatric diagnosis makes it difficult to determine and compare the true rates of mental illness in subgroups of the population. Psychiatric research is further complicated because only a small percentage of individuals with mental illness ever seek treatment. Individuals who seek treatment for psychiatric disorders are very different from those who do not seek treatment; therefore, population-based studies are needed to assess the true prevalence of and risk factors for mental illness. Such studies are difficult and expensive, as they require trained individuals to conduct long, in-depth interviews with a large sample.

To date, there have been only two nationally representative, population-based studies of mental health disorder prevalence in the United States: the Epidemiologic Catchment Area (ECA) study, conducted in the early 1980s, and the National Comorbidity Survey (NCS), conducted in the early 1990s. The ECA was a multisite, prospective study that involved conducting successive interviews to assess prevalence, incidence, and service use for mental health disorders among adults in communities, prisons, and psychiatric hospitals.[3] The NCS was a cross-sectional study designed to update prevalence figures and to clarify the patterns of comorbidity in mental and addictive disorders.[2] This study included adolescents but excluded adults over age 54.[2] Much of what is known about the prevalence and distribution of mental disorders in the United States is derived from these two studies. New data are needed because the most recent data were collected nearly 10 years ago. Furthermore, little has been published on the prevalence of mental health conditions in the elderly. The co-occurrence of chronic illness and frequent use of medications in this age group also make measurement of mental illness more difficult in this population. The aging of the U.S. population lends urgency to monitoring this issue more closely in the future.

Given the profound impact that mental illness can have on one's health and well-being, the increased prevalence of depression, anxiety, and eating disorders among women in the United States are public health issues that we cannot afford to ignore. Despite what has been learned in the past century about the etiology of mental disorders, these conditions continue to be plagued with stigmatization. Studies have shown that nearly two-thirds of all people with a diagnosable mental disorder do not seek treatment and that stigma is a commonly noted barrier to care.[2] (Issues around access are discussed in detail in chapter 8.) Future efforts should focus on increasing awareness, reducing stigma, increasing access, and improving insurance coverage for behavioral health services.

Mood Disorders

Currently, at least 7 million women in the United States have a diagnosable mood disorder.[4] These disorders are characterized by disturbances in one's emotional state.

Major Depression

In any given year, about 13% of women will have a diagnosable depressive disorder.[5] Major depression is roughly characterized as a period of at least 2 weeks during which a person loses pleasure in nearly all activities and/or exhibits a depressed mood.[6] About one in five women will experience an episode of major depression during her lifetime, twice the rate seen in men (Figure 5-1).[5,7] The estimated cost of depression in the United States, including treatment and loss of productivity, is $40 billion annually.[8]

The symptoms of major depression can limit physical and social functioning even more than other chronic medical conditions, such as diabetes and arthritis.[9] Some common symptoms of major depression include feelings of sadness and hopelessness, changes in appetite, sleep disturbances, and physical complaints.[6,10,11] If left untreated, the symptoms can persist for 6 months or more and can become severely disabling. Although most cases of major depression resolve without treatment, about 5% to 10% of individuals will experience symptoms for at least 2 years.[6]

Recent studies suggest that the prevalence of depression is increasing worldwide.[12] A cohort analysis of data from the NCS suggests that the lifetime prevalence of depression among U.S. women aged 20 to 24 years increased from about 6% in the early 1960s to around 28% in the early 1990s.[13] Researchers suggest that this is evidence of the influence of the changing environment on depressive symptoms, as neither the gene pool

Figure 5-1

Lifetime prevalence* of selected mental disorders in U.S. women and men aged 15–54 years

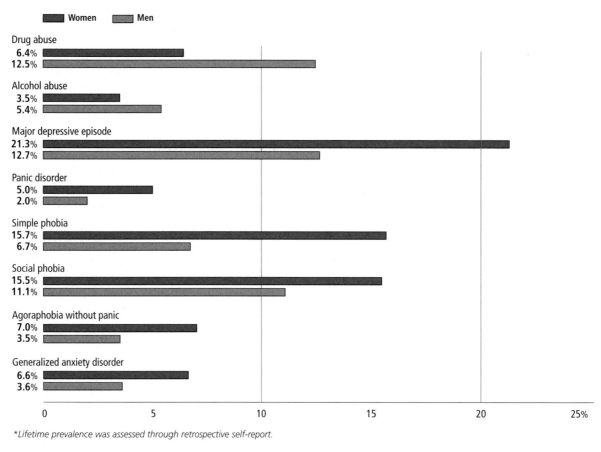

Lifetime prevalence

Women ■ Men ■

Drug abuse
6.4%
12.5%

Alcohol abuse
3.5%
5.4%

Major depressive episode
21.3%
12.7%

Panic disorder
5.0%
2.0%

Simple phobia
15.7%
6.7%

Social phobia
15.5%
11.1%

Agoraphobia without panic
7.0%
3.5%

Generalized anxiety disorder
6.6%
3.6%

0   5   10   15   20   25%

*Lifetime prevalence was assessed through retrospective self-report.

Source: Kessler RC. Sex differences in DSM-III-R psychiatric disorders in the United States: results from the National Comorbidity Survey. J Am Womens Assoc 1998;53:148-157.

nor the distribution of sex hormones could have changed significantly during that period of time.[14] It should be noted, however, that women who were older at the time of the NCS simply may have been less likely than younger women to remember having had depressive symptoms, not less likely to have experienced depressive symptoms, in their early twenties.

The average age of first onset of major depression is in the mid-twenties, with the peak prevalence occurring between 25 and 44 years of age.[6] The prevalence of major depression decreases substantially after age 65, although depression is the most common mental health problem for older women.[6,7]

Depressive symptoms are also prevalent among America's youth. Figure 5-2 presents the prevalence of depressive symptoms among adolescents by race and gender. As with adult women, depression is almost twice as likely to be reported by female adolescents than by male adolescents. This gender difference does not become apparent until puberty, leading some to suggest that hormones may play a role.[15,16,17] In addition, several hypotheses have been advanced to examine the importance of women's social roles. The sex-role theory proposes that women are more likely to be depressed than men because gender stereotypes lead them to experience more stress and less fulfillment in their daily lives than men.[18]

Figure 5-2

U.S. adolescents in grades 9–12 who reported feeling sad or hopeless* by race/ethnicity and gender, 1999

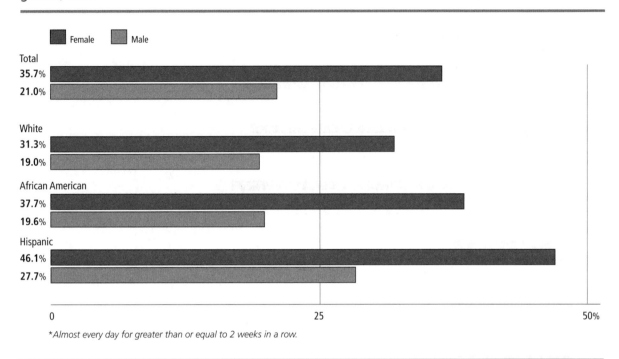

*Almost every day for greater than or equal to 2 weeks in a row.

Source: Centers for Disease Control and Prevention. Youth risk behavior surveillance—United States, 1999. June 09, 2000/49(SS05);1–96. Table 12. Atlanta: U.S. Department of Health and Human Services; 1999.

The numerous research studies examining the association between race/ethnicity and depression are inconclusive. In most studies, African American women typically report depressive symptoms more often than white women do.[19] It should be noted that researchers have questioned whether this finding is due to true racial differences or whether it is a result of low socioeconomic status, because African American women are more likely to be poor and poor women are at greater risk for depression. A recent study reported an apparent interaction between race and socioeconomic status, with race effects found only among nonpoor women.[20] Finally, in contrast to the smaller studies, the two largest epidemiological studies of mental disorders in the United States to date (ECA and NCS) have reported that African Americans are less likely to have major depression (Figure 5-3).[2,7]

Major depression is multicausal and is associated with a number of well-established risk factors. A family history of major depression increases a woman's risk by a factor ranging from 1.5 to 3.[6] Prior history of a major depressive episode is a significant risk factor, with at least half of the women with an initial episode experiencing a recurrence within 5 years.[10] Serious medical conditions, such as cancer and heart disease, are strongly associated with the development of major depression. It is estimated that up to half of all hospitalized patients have diagnosable depression.[10]

There are also a number of psychological and social risk factors. As mentioned, low socioeconomic status is a risk factor for depression, presumably as a result of the psychological impact of having limited access to economic and social resources.[21] Married women are at greater

Figure 5-3

Lifetime prevalence of major depression and generalized anxiety disorder among U.S. women aged 15–54 years by race/ethnicity

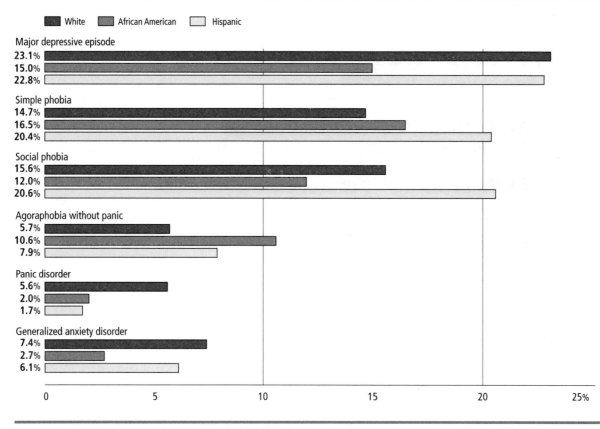

| | White | African American | Hispanic |

Major depressive episode
- 23.1%
- 15.0%
- 22.8%

Simple phobia
- 14.7%
- 16.5%
- 20.4%

Social phobia
- 15.6%
- 12.0%
- 20.6%

Agoraphobia without panic
- 5.7%
- 10.6%
- 7.9%

Panic disorder
- 5.6%
- 2.0%
- 1.7%

Generalized anxiety disorder
- 7.4%
- 2.7%
- 6.1%

Source: Unpublished data from the 1992 National Comorbidity Survey (DSM-III-R Diagnostic Criteria); 1992.

risk for developing depression compared to single women, presumably because of the many roles that married women are expected to play in both the workplace and at home.[11] Personality, apparently, plays little role in the development of depression among women as the differences that are seen with personality type disappear when one takes into account prior history of mental illness.[14,22]

Several treatment options are available to depressed patients. The two most common therapies used in the United States are psychotherapy and drug therapy. Currently, there are over 20 antidepressant medications marketed in the United States.[23] Most of the clin-

ical trials that have been done in the United States have shown that psychotherapy with medication is more effective than psychotherapy alone.[24,25,26] A woman's reproductive status should be considered when developing a plan of treatment, because some antidepressant medications have not yet been tested in pregnant or breast-feeding mothers.[27]

Although the course of the illness is variable, major depressive disorders are associated with high morbidity and mortality. The average major depressive episode lasts about 9 months in the absence of treatment, and about half of individuals who have one episode will experience a recurrence later in life.[6,28,29]

Postpartum Depression

One particularly important type of major depression that affects women is postpartum depression. Between 30% and 75% of all women will experience mild "baby blues" after any given pregnancy, a condition that typically peaks 4 to 5 days after delivery and resolves without treatment within 2 weeks.[23,30] About 10% of childbearing women, however, will experience severe postpartum depression during their lifetime. Postpartum depression is characterized by disabling depressive symptoms that begin anywhere from 24 hours to a month after delivery.[31] Although often thought of as a distinct illness, the symptoms of postpartum depression are the same as the symptoms of major depression; the time of onset is the only factor that distinguishes the two diagnoses.[6,32]

Postpartum depression is particularly difficult to diagnose because some of its symptoms, such as weight loss and fatigue, are what one might expect a normal postpartum mother to experience during the postpartum adjustment period.[33] In addition, women who have just given birth may be less likely to report depressive symptoms because of a fear of being viewed as a "bad mother."[33] This condition, if left untreated, can have lasting effects on both the mother and infant.[32,34,35,36,37,38] About one-third of women who have a postpartum depressive episode experience episodes in subsequent pregnancies.[39,40]

Suicide

In severe cases, people with major depressive disorder may contemplate suicide; up to 15% of severely affected individuals will eventually commit suicide.[6] Suicide is the eighth leading cause of death in the United States, with a death rate of 11.4 per 100,000 population.[41] It is of particular concern to women of reproductive age; suicide is the fourth leading cause of death

Figure 5-4

U.S. adolescent females in grades 9–12 who reported seriously considering attempting suicide or attempting suicide by race/ethnicity, 1999

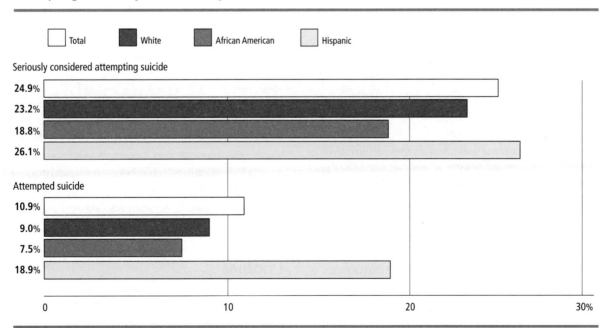

Source: Centers for Disease Control and Prevention. Youth risk behavior surveillance—United States, 1999. June 09, 2000/49(SSO5);1–96. Table 12. Atlanta: U.S. Department of Health and Human Services; 1999.

among women aged 15 to 24 years and the fifth leading cause of death among women aged 25 to 44 years (see Table 4-3 for additional data by race and age).[41] Individuals aged 65 years and older have the highest risk of committing suicide, with a suicide rate more than twice that seen in the general population.[42] Despite this trend, suicide is not a leading cause of death in the elderly because other causes of death, such as heart disease and cancers, are much more common.

More than nine out of 10 suicides can be linked to depression.[43] Alcohol and/or drug use also greatly increase one's risk; alcoholics have a lifetime suicide risk of about 3%, and heroin addicts have a suicide rate twice that of the general population.[42] One newly identified risk factor for suicide is homosexuality. Recent studies have demonstrated that homosexuals are much more likely than heterosexuals to attempt suicide.[44,45]

Women are more likely to attempt suicide than men, but men are four times more likely to be successful in the attempt.[46,47] Males typically attempt suicide with a firearm, whereas women tend to use less lethal methods, such as self-poisoning.[47] At every age, white females are more likely to commit suicide than African American females, with death rates of 4.9 and 1.9 per 100,000 population, respectively.[41]

The pattern of suicide among America's youth is very similar to the pattern seen among adults. The 1999 Youth Risk Behavior Survey (YRBS) reported that adolescent females (24.9%) in grades 9–12 were significantly more likely than adolescent males (13.7%) to have reported considering attempting suicide.[48] Within the subset of adolescents enrolled in school, female students were also significantly more likely than male students to have reported attempting suicide: 10.9% compared to 5.7%, respectively.[48] In 1999, Hispanic females (18.9%) were more than twice as likely as either African American or white females to have reported attempting suicide, 7.5% and 9.0%, respectively (Figure 5-4).[48]

Anxiety Disorders

Like depressive disorders, anxiety disorders are more common among women than they are among men.[5] Although they often receive less attention than depressive disorders, anxiety disorders are the most common psychiatric disorders in the United States.[5,49] Slightly more than one-third of women in the United States (34.3%) will experience an anxiety disorder during her lifetime; in any given year, almost a quarter of American women (24.7%) will be affected by a disorder of this kind.[2] Anxiety disorders can be difficult to diagnose because women with anxiety problems often present to their primary care physician with vague physical complaints and may be reluctant to discuss mental symptoms.[50]

Although it is normal for women to occasionally experience mild feelings of anxiety, when the feelings become persistent and begin to interfere with a woman's daily activities, an anxiety disorder may be present. Three of the major types of anxiety disorders are panic, phobias, and generalized anxiety disorder.[6] Anxiety disorders often co-occur with depression.[51] Among individuals with at least one psychiatric disorder, nearly 80% will experience two or more diagnosable disorders at the same time.[2] Despite years of research, relatively little is known about the causes of these disorders.[51]

Although an estimated 20 million people have an anxiety disorder, only about 6 million receive treatment.[52] Pharmacotherapy and psychotherapy, alone or in combination, have been shown to be effective for the treatment of anxiety disorders.[53] Presently, at least 15 medications have been approved for the treatment of these disorders.[51] Self-help methods, such as relaxation techniques, have also been shown to be effective.[54]

Phobias

Phobias are the most common anxiety disorders experienced by U.S. women.[2] There are three main types of phobias: specific phobia, social phobia, and agoraphobia.[6] American women are more than two times as likely men to experience specific phobia, characterized by fear of a particular object (e.g., spiders) or situation (e.g., heights) that causes social or occupational impairment or significant emotional distress.[6] About 16% of women will experience a specific phobia during their lifetime.[2] More than 80% of people with a specific phobia develop the disorder before age 25.[55] Individuals often alter their lifestyle to avoid exposure to the feared object or situation, but few seek professional treatment.[56]

Social phobias are also more common in women than in men, with more than 15% of U.S. women experiencing the disorder during their lifetime.[2] Social phobia is characterized by the persistent fear of social situations in which the individual feels that he or she will be scrutinized by others.[6] A fear of public speaking is the most common type of social phobia.[6] The most important risk factors for social phobia are family history of social phobia, female gender, being unmarried, low socioeconomic status, and a low level of education.[57,58] Although social phobia can be effectively treated with psychotherapy and/or medication, only about 5% of people seek treatment.[53,57]

Agoraphobia is a less common but disabling phobia. Individuals with agoraphobia fear public places, particularly crowded places.[6] It differs from social phobia in that individuals with agoraphobia fear crowds, regardless of whether they fear being scrutinized. The disorder can be severely disabling and, in some cases, can cause individuals to become housebound.[59] Women are twice as likely as men to experience agoraphobia without panic symptoms; about 7% of women will experience this type of agoraphobia during their lifetime as compared with 3.5% of men.[2] In more than 70% of cases, the illness begins before age 25.[60] Agoraphobia is more common in African Americans than among whites or Hispanics.[54] Low socioeconomic status is also a risk factor.[54]

Panic Disorder

Panic disorder is two to three times more common in women than in men.[2] Although only about one in 20 women will experience panic disorder during their lifetime, the disorder can cause significant disability.[2,56] A panic attack is characterized by the simultaneous occurrence of at least four of the following symptoms: shortness of breath, sweating, trembling, choking, nausea, dizziness, chills or flushes, heart palpitations, feeling of being detached from one's self, numbness or tingling, and tightness in the chest.[6] Individuals with panic disorder sometimes present to the emergency room complaining of a heart attack. The diagnostic criteria for panic disorder include frequent, unexpected panic attacks, followed by at least 1 month of worry about having another attack.[6] Panic disorder often begins early in life and onset after age 45 is rare.[6,51] Approximately one-third to one-half of individuals with panic disorder experience comorbid agoraphobia.[6] There are no significant differences in the prevalence of panic disorder by race/ethnicity.[54]

Generalized Anxiety Disorder

Generalized anxiety disorder (GAD) is slightly more common than panic disorder, with a lifetime prevalence of 6.6% among American women.[2] As with all other anxiety disorders, it is more common in women than in men.[53] The main feature of GAD is excessive worry about a number of events or activities, occurring on more days than not for at least 6 months.[6] Women with GAD may present to their primary care physician with general physical complaints such as urinary frequency, pelvic pain, nausea, or diarrhea.[53] The frequency of physical complaints may explain why women with GAD have been shown to utilize health care services more frequently than women without the disorder.[61] The disorder is most frequently seen in people aged 25 and older.[46] The most important risk factors known to date include unemployment or being divorced or separated.

Eating Disorders

Studies have shown that the prevalence of eating disorders is increasing in America.[62,63] Eating disorders affect an estimated 5 million Americans each year; more than 90% of those affected are female.[6,64] The two main types of eating disorders, anorexia nervosa and bulimia nervosa, are characterized by eating disturbances and excessive concern about body shape or body weight.[6] Studies are currently underway to determine if binge-eating disorder should be added as a specific diagnostic category.[65] Although only about 3% of young women meet the strict diagnostic criteria for these disorders, they are associated with substantial morbidity and mortality.[64]

Although excessive dieting in and of itself is not sufficient evidence of the presence of an eating disorder, studies have shown that excessive dieting is a major risk factor.[66,67] In addition, recent population-based studies have shown between 29% and 38% of normal-weight U.S. women are dieting at any one time.[68] Given the apparent obsession in the United States with obtaining the "perfect" body, it is more important than ever to understand the etiology of these disorders.

Although the specific cause of eating disorders is not known, they are associated with several well-documented risk factors. Nearly all cases of eating disorders are initiated by dieting.[69] Certain individuals are particularly prone to pathological dieting, including ballet dancers, gymnasts, and wrestlers. Other risk factors are perfectionism, poor family communication, and a family history of eating disorders.[65,67] Times of transition, such as puberty and leaving home for college, are known to be particularly vulnerable periods.[46]

As with other mental disorders, the two main types of treatment for eating disorders are psychotherapy and pharmacotherapy. The standard treatment for anorexia nervosa includes nutritional restoration as well as cognitive and behavioral therapy.[66] Although most anorectics (see below) can be treated successfully in an outpatient setting, hospitalization may be needed in severe cases.[65] Hospitalization is often required for the treatment of individuals with bulimia nervosa (see below), particularly when individuals are bingeing and purging several times a day.[70] Antidepressants have been shown to be effective in the treatment of both disorders.[66]

Anorexia Nervosa

Anorexia nervosa affects approximately 1% of young women.[71] The major diagnostic criteria for anorexia nervosa are a failure to maintain at least 85% of normal body weight based on height; an intense fear of gaining weight; preoccupation with one's body weight or shape; and amenorrhea (loss of a period for at least 3 consecutive months).[6]

The two main types of anorexia nervosa are the restricting type and the binge-purge type.[6] Restrictors achieve weight loss through dieting, fasting, or excessive exercise. They control their intake of calories, often limiting their diet to low-calorie and low-fat foods. In contrast, individuals with binge-purge-type anorexia nervosa restrict their food intake but will also periodically binge and purge.[72,73] Some affected individuals will purge after eating only small amounts of food. Anorectics may switch between the two subtypes throughout the course of their disease.

The course of anorexia nervosa varies greatly among individuals. The average age at onset is 14 to 15 years old; however, there appears to be a second peak in incidence at age 18.[74,75] The onset of anorexia nervosa often coincides with stressful life events such as puberty or leaving home for college. [65] About half of the individuals with anorexia nervosa recover fully and about one-third of affected individuals achieve partial recovery.[76] Some, however, will experience chronic debilitating illness that eventually leads to death from starvation, suicide, or cardiac arrest.[66] Mortality rates for anorexia nervosa range from 10% to 22%.[6,66,77]

Figure 5-5

U.S. adolescents in grades 9–12 who reported vomiting or using laxatives to lose weight in the past 30 days by gender and race/ethnicity, 1999

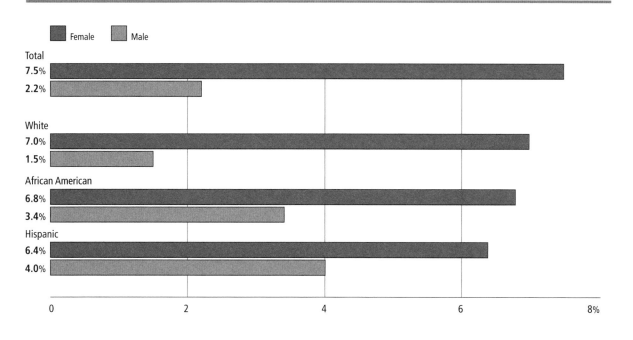

Source: Centers for Disease Control and Prevention. Youth risk behavior surveillance—United States, 1999. June 09, 2000/49(SS05);1–96. Table 38. Atlanta: U.S. Department of Health and Human Services; 1999.

Bulimia Nervosa

Bulimia nervosa affects approximately 1% to 3% of women.[65] The disorder is characterized by binge eating followed by the use of inappropriate compensatory methods at least 2 days per week for 3 months to keep from gaining weight.[6] The diagnosis of bulimia nervosa is only made if the bingeing and purging behaviors occur in the absence of calorie restriction.

Like anorexia, there are two main subtypes of bulimia nervosa: purging and nonpurging.[66] Individuals with purging-type bulimia employ self-induced vomiting or misuse of laxatives, diuretics, or enemas to prevent weight gain. Vomiting is the most common type of purging behavior, seen among 80% to 90% of all purge-type bulimics.[6] In contrast, individuals with nonpurging bulimia nervosa fast or exercise excessively to avoid gaining weight. Despite the

compensatory behaviors, bulimics are often of normal weight.

The course of bulimia nervosa varies in severity and chronicity. The disorder usually starts in late adolescence or early adulthood and typically begins after a period of dieting.[78] Approximately half of bulimics recover fully, whereas about one in five bulimics experience chronic disease.[79] Bulimics who vomit can have severe erosion of their dental enamel and enlarged salivary glands.[64] Up to 3% of bulimics die, usually the result of esophageal tears, gastric rupture, or cardiac arrhythmias.[6,65]

Disordered Eating among Adolescents

Although population-based studies on the prevalence of eating disorders are sparse, each year the YRBS provides information about disordered eating patterns among U.S. adolescents.[48] In the 1999 YRBS, adolescent females (56%) were significantly more likely than adolescent males (25%) to report eating less food, fewer calories, or foods low in fat to lose weight or avoid gaining weight.[48] Female students were also twice as likely as male students to report using diet pills, powders, or liquids to control their weight, (10.9% versus 4.4%, respectively.)[48] Strikingly, female adolescents were three times as likely as males to report fasting, taking laxatives, or vomiting.[48] Figure 5-5 presents the gender- and race-specific prevalence of taking laxatives and vomiting among U.S. adolescents.

References

1. Murray CJL, Lopez AD, editors. The global burden of disease: a comprehensive assessment of mortality and disability from diseases, injuries, and risk factors in 1990 and projected to 2020. Cambridge (MA): Harvard University Press;1996.

2. Kessler RC, McGonagle KA, Zhao S, Nelson CB, Hughes M, Eshleman S, et al. Lifetime and 12-month prevalence of DSM-III-R psychiatric disorders in the United States: results from the National Comorbidity Survey. Arch Gen Psychiatry 1994;51:8–19.

3. Regier DA, Burke JD Jr. Quantitative and experimental methods in psychiatry. In: Sadock BJ, Sadock VA, editors. Kaplan & Sadock's comprehensive textbook of psychiatry. 7th ed. Philadelphia: Lippincott Williams & Wilkins; 2000.

4. McGrath E, Keita GP, Strickland BR, Russ NF. Women and depression: risk factors and treatment issues: final report of the American Psychological Association's National Task Force on Women and Depression. Washington: American Psychological Association; 1990.

5. Kessler RC. Sex differences in DSM-III-R psychiatric disorders in the United States: results from the National Comorbidity Survey. J Am Med Womens Assoc 1998;53:148–157.

6. American Psychiatric Association. Diagnostic and statistical manual of mental disorders: DSM-IV. 4th ed. Washington: American Psychiatric Association; 1994.

7. Regier DA, Boyd JH, Burke JD Jr, Rae DS, Myers JK, Kramer M, et al. One-month prevalence of mental disorders in the United States: based on five epidemiologic catchment area sites. Arch Gen Psychiatry 1988;45:977–986.

8. Greenberg PE, Stiglin L, Finkelstein SN, Berndt ER. The economic burden of depression in 1990. J Clin Psychiatry 1993;54:405–418.

9. Wells KB, Steward A, Hays RD, Burnam MA, Rogers W. Daniels M, et al. The functioning and well-being of depressed patients: results from the Medical Outcomes Study. JAMA 1989;262:914–919.

10. Szewczyk M, Chennault SA. Women's health. Depression and related disorders. Prim Care 1997;24:83–101.

11. Nolen-Hoeksema S. Epidemiology and theories of gender differences in unipolar depression. In: Mary V Seeman, ed. Gender and Psychopathology. 1st ed. Washington: American Psychiatric Press; 1995. p. 63–87.

12. Cross-National Collaborative Group. The changing rate of major depression: cross-national comparisons. JAMA 1992; 268:3098–3105.

13. Kessler RC, McGonagle KA, Nelson CB, Hughes M, Swartz M, Blazer DG. Sex and depression in the National Comorbidity Survey II: cohort effects. J Affect Disord 1994;30:15–26.

14. Kessler RC. Gender and mood disorders. In: Goldman M, Hatch M, editors. Women and health. San Diego: Academic Press; 2000. p. 997–1009.

15. Angold A, Worthman CW. Puberty onset of gender differences in rates of depression: a developmental, epidemiologic, and neuroendocrine perspective. J Affect Disord 1993;29:145–158.

16. Angold A, Costello EJ, Worthman CW. Puberty and depression: the roles of age, pubertal status, and pubertal timing. Psychol Med 1998;28:51–61.

17. Seeman MV. Psychopathology in women and men: focus on female hormones. Am J Psychiatry 1997;154:1641–1647.

18. Gove W. The relationship between sex roles, marital status, and mental illness. Soc Forces 1972;51:34–44.

19. Eaton WW, Kessler LG. Rates of symptoms of depression in a national sample. Am J Epidemiol 1981;114:528–538.

20. Gazmararian JA, James SA, Lepkowski J. Depression in black and white women: the role of marriage and socioeconomic status. Ann Epidemiol 1995;5:455–463.

21. Belle D. Poverty and women's mental health. Am Psychologist 1990;45:385–389.

22. Hirschfeld RM, Klerman GL, Clayton PJ, Keller MB, Andreasen NC. Personality and gender-related differences in depression. J Affect Disord 1984;7:211–221.

23. Bhatia SC, Bhatia SK. Depression in women: diagnostic and treatment considerations. Am Fam Physician 1999;60:225–234, 239–240.

24. Keller MB, McCullough JP, Klein DN, Arnow B, Dunner DL, Gelenberg AJ, et al. A comparison of nefazodone, the cognitive behavioral-analysis system of psychotherapy, and their combination for the treatment of chronic depression. N Engl J Med 2000;342(20):1462–1470.

25. Thase ME, Greenhouse JB, Frank E, Reynolds CF, Pilkonis PA, Hurley K, et al. Treatment of major depression with psychotherapy or psychotherapy-pharmacotherapy combinations. Arch Gen Psychiatry 1997;54:1009–1015.

26. Conte HR, Plutchik R, Wild KV, Karasu TB. Combined psychotherapy and pharmacotherapy for depression. A systematic analysis of the evidence. Arch Gen Psychiatry 1986;43:471–479.

27. Wisner KL, Gelenberg AJ, Leonard H, Zarin D, Frank E. Pharmacologic treatment of depression during pregnancy. JAMA 1999;282:1264–1269.

28. Kapur S, Mann JJ. Role of the dopaminergic system in depression. Biol Psychiatry 1992;32:1–17.

29. Frank E, Thase ME. Natural history and preventative treatment of recurrent mood disorders. Annu Rev Med 1999;50: 453-468.

30. Yalom ID, Lunde DT, Moos RH, Hamburg DA. "Postpartum blues" syndrome: a description and related variables. Arch Gen Psychiatry 1968;18:16–27.

31. Philipps LH, O'Hara MW. Prospective study of post-partum: 4 1/2-year follow-up of women of women and children. J Abnorm Psychol 1991;100:151–155.

32. Spinelli M. Psychiatric disorders during pregnancy and postpartum. J Am Womens Assoc 1998;53:165–169.

33. Epperson CN. Postpartum major depression: detection and treatment. Am Fam Physician 1999;59:2247–2254, 2259–2260.

34. Zuckerman B, Bauchner H, Parker S, Cabral H. Maternal depressive symptoms during pregnancy, and newborn irritability. J Dev Behav Pediatr 1990;11:190–194.

35. Field T. Early interactions between infants and postpartum depressed mothers. Infant Behav Dev 1984;7:517–522.

36. Field T, Healy B, Goldstein S, Perry S, Bendell D, Schanberg S, et al. Infants of depressed mothers show "depressed" behavior even with nondepressed adults. Child Dev 1988;59:1569–1579.

37. Whiffen VE, Gotlib IH. Infants of postpartum depressed mothers: temperament and cognitive status. J Abnorm Psychol 1989; 98:274–279.

38. Cox AD, Puckering C, Pound A, Mills M. The impact of maternal depression in young children. J Child Psychol Psychiatry 1987; 28:917–928.

39. Wisner KL, Wheeler SB. Prevention of recurrent postpartum major depression. Hosp Community Psychiatry 1994;45:1191–1996.

40. Davidson J, Robertson E. A follow-up study of post partum illness, 1946–1978. Acta Psychiatr Scand 1985;71:451–457.

41. Hoyert D, Kochanek K, Murphy S. National Center for Health Statistics, editor. Deaths: final data for 1997. Nat Vital Stat Rep 1999;47(19).

42. Roy A. Psychiatric emergencies. In: Sadock BJ, Sadock VA, editors. Kaplan & Sadock's comprehensive textbook of psychiatry. 7th ed. Philadelphia: Lippincott Williams & Wilkins; 2000.

43. Asnis GM, Friedman TA, Sanderson WC, Kaplan ML, van Praag PH, Harkavy–Friedman JM. Suicidal behaviors in adult psychiatric outpatients, I: description and prevalence. Am J Psychiatry 1993;150:108–112.

44. Remafedi G, French S, Story M, Resnick MD, Blum R. The relationship between suicide risk and sexual orientation: results of a population-based study. Am J Public Health 1998;88:57–60.

45. Cochran SD, Mays VM. Lifetime prevalence of suicide symptoms and affective disorders among men reporting same-sex sexual partners: results from NHANES III. Am J Public Health 2000; 90:573–578.

46. Hirschfeld RM, Russell JM. Assessment and treatment of suicidal patients. N Engl J Med 1997;337:910–915.

47. Moscicki EK. Gender differences in completed and attempted suicides. Ann Epidemiol 1994;4:152–158.

48. Kann L, Kinchen SA, Williams BI, Ross JG, Lowry R, Grunbaum JA, et al. Youth risk behavior surveillance, United States, 1999. State and local YRBS coordinators. J Sch Health 2000;70(7):271–285.

49. National Institute of Mental Health. Facts about anxiety disorders. Publication #0M-99-4152 [1999 Jan]. Available from: URL: www.nimh.nih.gov/anxiety/adfacts.cfm.

50. Schurman RA, Kramer PD, Mitchell JB. The hidden mental health network. Treatment of mental illness by nonpsychiatrist physicians. Arch Gen Psychiatry 1985;42:89–94.

51. Merikangas K, Pollock RA. Anxiety disorders in women. In: Goldman M, Hatch M, editors. Women and health. San Diego: Academic Press; 2000. p. 1010–1023.

52. Regier DA, Narrow WE, Rae DS, Manderscheid RW, Locke BZ, Goodwin FK. The de facto U.S. mental and addictive disorders service system: epidemiologic catchment area prospective 1-year prevalence rates of disorders and services. Arch Gen Psychiatry 1993;50:85–94.

53. Pennington A. Women's health. Anxiety disorders. Prim Care 1997;24:103–111.

54. Horvath E, Weissman M. Anxiety disorders: epidemiology. In: Sadock BJ, Sadock VA, editors. Kaplan & Sadock's comprehensive textbook of psychiatry. 7th ed. Philadelphia: Lippincott Williams & Wilkins; 2000.

55. Kendler KS, Neale MC, Kessler RC, Heath AC, Eaves LJ. The genetic epidemiology of phobias in women: the interrelationship of agoraphobia, social phobia, situational phobia, and simple phobia. Arch Gen Psychiatry 1992;49:273–281.

56. Yonkers K, Gurguis G. Gender differences in the prevalence and expression of anxiety disorders. In: Seeman MV, editor. Gender and psychopathology. 1st ed. Washington: American Psychiatric Press; 1995. p. 113–130.

57. Schneier FR, Johnson J, Hornig CD, Liebowitz MR, Weissman MM. Social phobia: comorbidity and morbidity in an epidemiologic sample. Arch Gen Psychiatry 1992;49:282–288.

58. Fyer AJ, Mannuzza S, Chapman TF, Liebowitz MR, Klein DF. A direct interview family study of social phobia. Arch Gen Psychiatry 1993; 50:286–293.

59. Sable P. Attachment, anxiety and agoraphobia. Women and Therapy 1991;1:55–69.

60. Bourdon KH, Boyd JH, Rae, DS, Burns B, Thompson J, Locke B. Gender differences in phobias: results from the ECA community survey. J Anxiety Disord 1988;2:227–241.

61. Blazer DG, Hughes D, George LK, Swartz M, Boyer R. Generalized anxiety disorders. In: Robins LN, Regier DA, editors. Psychiatric disorders in America: the Epidemiologic Catchment Area Study. New York: Free Press; 1991:181–203.

62. Lucas AR, Beard CM, O'Fallon WM, Kurland LT. 50-year trends in the incidence of anorexia nervosa in Rochester, Minn.: a population-based study. Am J Psychiatry 1991;148:917–922.

63. Kendler KS, MacLean C, Neale M, Kessler R, Heath A, Eaves L. The genetic epidemiology of bulimia nervosa. Am J Psychiatry 1991; 148:1627–1637.

64. Becker AE, Grinspoon SK, Klibanski A, Herzog DB. Eating disorders. N Engl J Med 1999;340:1092–1098.

65. Halmi KA. Eating disorders. In: Goldman M, Hatch M, editors. Women and health. San Diego: Academic Press; 2000.

66. American Psychiatric Association. Practice guideline for the treatment of patients with eating disorders (revision). Am J Psychiatry 2000;157 Suppl:1–39.

67. Johnson WG, Schlundt DG. Eating disorders: assessment and treatment. Clin Obstet Gynecol 1985;28:598–614.

68. Biener L, Heaton A. Women dieters of normal weight: their motives, goals, and risks. Am J Public Health 1995;85:714–717.

69. Halmi KA. Eating disorders. In: Sadock BJ, Sadock VA, editors. Kaplan & Sadock's comprehensive textbook of psychiatry. 7th ed. Philadelphia: Lippincott Williams & Wilkins; 2000.

70. Garner DM, Garfinkel PE. Handbook of treatment for eating disorders. 2nd ed. New York: Guilford Press; 1997.

71. Walters EE, Kendler KS. Anorexia nervosa and anorexic-like syndromes in a population-based female twin sample. Am J Psychiatry 1995;152:64–71.

72. Garfinkel PE, Moldofsky H, Garner DM. The heterogeneity of anorexia nervosa: bulimia as a distinct subgroup. Arch Gen Psychiatry 1980;37:1036–1040.

73. Strober M, Salkin B, Burroughs J, Morrell W. Validity of the bulimia-restricter distinction in anorexia nervosa: parental personality characteristics and family psychiatric morbidity. J Nerv Ment Dis 1982;170:345–351.

74. Halmi KA, Eckert E, Marchi P, Sampugnaro V, Apple R, Cohen J. Comorbidity of psychiatric diagnoses in anorexia nervosa. Arch Gen Psychiatry 1991;48:712–718.

75. Halmi KA, Casper RC, Eckert ED, Goldberg SC, Davis JM. Unique features associated with age of onset of anorexia nervosa. Psychiatry Res 1979;1:209–215.

76. Steinhausen HC. Treatment and outcome of adolescent anorexia nervosa. Horm Res 1995;43:168–170.

77. Theander S. Outcome and prognosis in anorexia nervosa and bulimia: some results of previous investigations, compared with those of a Swedish long-term study. J Psychiatr Res 1985; 19:493–508.

78. Warren MP. Anorexia nervosa and related eating disorders. Clin Obstet Gynecol 1985;28:588–597.

79. Keel PK, Mitchell JE. Outcome in bulimia nervosa. Am J Psychiatry 1997;154:313–321.

Chapter 6

Health Behaviors

Contents

Introduction

This chapter focuses on behaviors that can influence a woman's health. Recently, public health efforts have focused on increasing awareness of how healthy behaviors can reduce avoidable mortality. Many of these behaviors were discussed briefly in the preceding chapters in descriptions of the risk factors for particular diseases (e.g., smoking and lung cancer). It is important to note that although the adoption of healthy behaviors (e.g., beginning an exercise program) or cessation of unhealthy ones (e.g., smoking) may improve health, this does not imply that women themselves are solely responsible for their health. Other individual-level factors, such as health insurance coverage, certainly play critical roles (see chapter 8), as do the social, economic, and political forces that shape women's health (see chapter 1).

Smoking

Cigarette smoking is a major preventable cause of morbidity and mortality among women. Approximately 22 million women 18 years and older and 1.5 million adolescent girls in the United States currently smoke cigarettes.[1] Moreover, women are beginning to smoke at younger ages, which increases their risk of developing smoking-related diseases.[2]

Slightly more than one in five adult women are current smokers (22.1% in 1997, Table 6-1).[3] The percentage of women who smoke as well as the number of cigarettes smoked per day increases with the age of the woman through the childbearing years. After the childbearing years, the percentage of women who are current smokers begins to decline as more women quit smoking and few begin. Figure 6-1 shows the smoking status of women after age 55. Among older women, declines in current smoking are a function both of quitting and differential mortality rates. (Death rates are higher among smokers as they age.) By age 75, just 7.8% of women were current smokers based on National Health Interview Survey (NHIS) 1993–1995 data.[4]

There are racial and ethnic differences in smoking rates. The 1997 NHIS reported that Asian American women have the lowest rates of smoking, and the highest rates are found among white and Native American women.[3] However, because the number of Native Americans studied is so small, averages over a 2-year period are considered more representative of smoking rates for Native American women. Based on 1994–1995 aggregate NHIS age-adjusted rates of smoking, Native American women remain much more likely to be smokers (32.9%, nearly identical to the rate of 31.3% in Table 6-1) than are whites (25.0%) or African Americans (22.2%).[5] While smoking prevalence among Asian American women has risen from 4.3% in 1995 to 12.4% in 1997, changes in design and content of questions on the NHIS for Asian American women may be responsible.[3] Data from the Commonwealth Fund 1998 Survey of Women's Health are generally consistent with the NHIS data, with Asian American women having the lowest rate (4%) and white women the highest rate (25%).[6]

Women from low-income families or with low levels of education are more likely to smoke than their higher socioeconomic counterparts. Results from the 1997 NHIS show that women with 9–11 years of education are 3 times more likely to smoke than women who are college graduates. The differential by poverty status is not as marked.[3] In contrast, data from the Commonwealth Fund 1998 Survey of Women's Health suggest substantial differences by income with low-income women ($16,000 or less annually) more than twice as likely to be smokers compared to other women.[6]

Overall, the prevalence of smoking among women has been declining in the United States since the mid-1960s (Figures 6-2 and 6-3).[7] This is a function both of smoking cessation efforts and declines in initiation of smoking. These declines, however, vary by race/ethnicity and age with some groups even experiencing increases.[7] Recent trends show plateauing rates of smoking among young adult women.[8] The

Table 6-1

Cigarette smoking among women* by selected characteristics, 1997

Characteristic	Percent of women ≥18 years of age currently smoking
Total	**22.1**
Race/ethnicity	
White, non-Hispanic	23.3
Black, non-Hispanic	22.4
Hispanic	14.3
American Indian/Alaskan Native	31.3
Asian/Pacific Islander	12.4
Education (years)**	
≤8	15.1
9–11	30.5
12	25.7
13–15	23.1
≥16	10.1
Age group (years)	
18–24	25.7
25–44	26.1
45–64	21.5
≥65	11.5
Poverty status***	
Below 100% poverty level	29.8
At or above 100% poverty level	21.8
Unknown	18.2

*Persons who reported having smoked ≥ 100 cigarettes during their lifetime and who reported now smoking every day or some days.

**Limited to persons aged ≥ 25 years.

***Published 1996 poverty thresholds from the Bureau of the Census are used in these calculations.

Source: Centers for Disease Control and Prevention. Cigarette smoking among adults, United States, 1997. MMWR Morb Mortal Wkly Rep 1999;48:993–996.

Figure 6-1

Smoking among women aged 55 years and older, 1993–1995

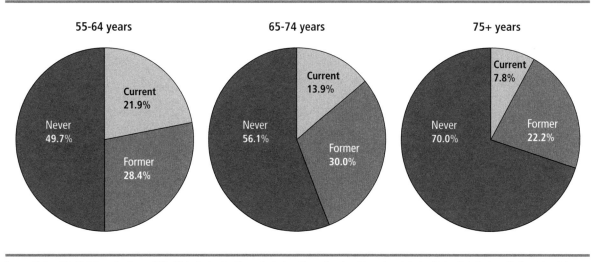

Source: National Health Information Survey,1993–95. In: Centers for Disease Control and Prevention. Surveillance for selected public health indicators affecting older adults, United States. MMWR Morb Mortal Wkly Rep 1999;48:116–118.

rate of decline in smoking since 1965 has been greatest among African American women aged 18 to 24 years. This decline is being accelerated by declines in African American adolescents.[9]

The vast majority of smokers begin tobacco use between the sixth and ninth grades (ages 11–15 years) and few adopt smoking after age 20.[10] Based on 1992 NHIS data, it is estimated that approximately 8% of female smokers began by age 10 or younger. In the 1999 National Youth Tobacco Survey (NYTS), 11.3% of middle school girls reported currently using tobacco products. In the 1999 Youth Risk Behavior Survey (YRBS), approximately 60% of ninth graders reported ever trying cigarettes with the prevalence reaching 75% by twelfth grade. Overall, approximately 70% of adolescent females in grades 9–12 reported ever trying cigarettes and 35% reported currently smoking.[11] Current smoking rates in adolescent females vary by race/ethnicity with patterns similar to adult women. Based on 1999 YRBS data, white adolescent females are the most likely to be current and frequent smokers and blacks are the least likely (Figure 6-4), with Hispanics having

rates closer to whites.[11] Recent data show a rise in the adoption of smoking by female students overall in grades 8–12.[8] Among black female high school seniors, however, rates have dropped dramatically, falling from 24.7% in 1976–1977 to 3.5% in 1991–1992.[12] These declines in adolescent smoking among blacks have meant dramatic declines are now being reported for young black women, along with an increasing divergence of smoking rates for young black and white women.[9]

Based on 1996 Behavioral Risk Factor Surveillance System (BRFSS) data, 11.8% of pregnant women smoke. This represents a substantial decline from a rate of 16.3% in 1986.[13] Women of lower socioeconomic status and unmarried women have higher than average rates of smoking during pregnancy.[14] Smoking during pregnancy is less frequent among young black women than among young white and older black women, but the lowest rates have been noted for Asian American and Hispanic women. Women who drink or use illicit substances during pregnancy are also more likely to smoke during pregnancy than women

Figure 6-2

Current cigarette smoking among white women by age, 1965–1995

Prevalence of smoking (white women)

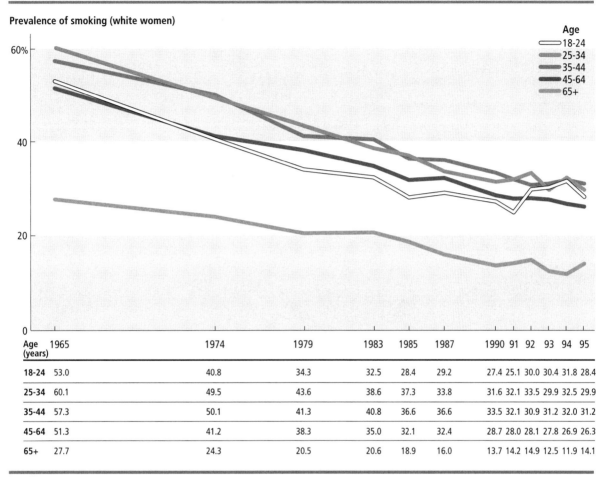

Age (years)	1965	1974	1979	1983	1985	1987	1990	91	92	93	94	95
18-24	53.0	40.8	34.3	32.5	28.4	29.2	27.4	25.1	30.0	30.4	31.8	28.4
25-34	60.1	49.5	43.6	38.6	37.3	33.8	31.6	32.1	33.5	29.9	32.5	29.9
35-44	57.3	50.1	41.3	40.8	36.6	36.6	33.5	32.1	30.9	31.2	32.0	31.2
45-64	51.3	41.2	38.3	35.0	32.1	32.4	28.7	28.0	28.1	27.8	26.9	26.3
65+	27.7	24.3	20.5	20.6	18.9	16.0	13.7	14.2	14.9	12.5	11.9	14.1

Source: National Center for Health Statistics. Health, United States, 1998. Table 62. (PHS)98–1232. Hyattsville (MD): U.S. Department of Health and Human Services; 1998.

who do not use these substances.[15] Rates of smoking are higher among young pregnant women (ages 18–24) than rates for the general population of women in this age group.[14] Women continue to smoke during pregnancy for most of the same reasons that they do when they are not pregnant.[16] Most women who smoke are aware of the risks to developing fetuses. As a result, pregnant women are less likely to smoke than women who are not pregnant because they are more likely to spontaneously quit or reduce smoking during pregnancy.[17,18,19,20] Many women resume smoking after delivery,[18,21] but women who quit during pregnancy are somewhat less

likely to relapse within 1 year than nonpregnant women who have quit.[18]

As illustrated by the higher smoking rates among low-income women, socioeconomic status appears to influence adoption and maintenance of this habit. The reason for these high rates appears to be related in part to the use of smoking for stress management.[22,23] Among female teenagers, smoking is related to other risk-taking behaviors including use of marijuana, binge drinking, and multiple sex partners.[24] Other risk factors among teenagers include access to substances in the home, working more

Figure 6-3

Current cigarette smoking among black women by age, 1965–1995

Prevalence of smoking (black women)

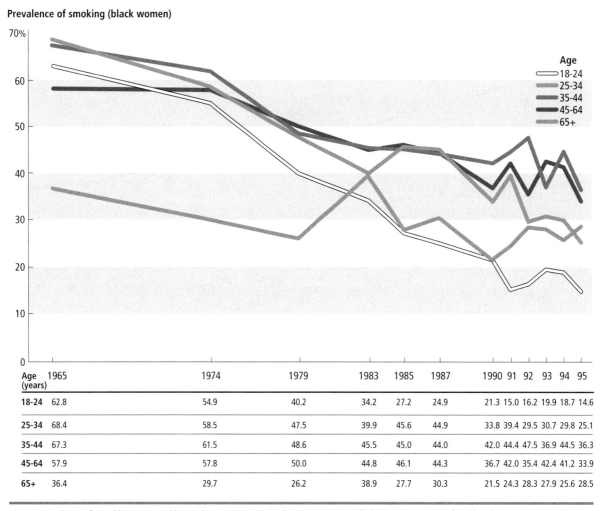

Age (years)	1965	1974	1979	1983	1985	1987	1990	91	92	93	94	95
18-24	62.8	54.9	40.2	34.2	27.2	24.9	21.3	15.0	16.2	19.9	18.7	14.6
25-34	68.4	58.5	47.5	39.9	45.6	44.9	33.8	39.4	29.5	30.7	29.8	25.1
35-44	67.3	61.5	48.6	45.5	45.0	44.0	42.0	44.4	47.5	36.9	44.5	36.3
45-64	57.9	57.8	50.0	44.8	46.1	44.3	36.7	42.0	35.4	42.4	41.2	33.9
65+	36.4	29.7	26.2	38.9	27.7	30.3	21.5	24.3	28.3	27.9	25.6	28.5

Source: National Center for Health Statistics. Health, United States, 1998. Table 62. (PHS)98–1232. Hyattsville (MD): U.S. Department of Health and Human Services; 1998.

than 20 hours per week, and repeating a grade in school.[25]

Once they start, women continue to smoke for a number of reasons, most often because of nicotine addiction but also to manage stress and to combat depression. Women appear to respond more than men to non-nicotine effects of smoking, such as smoking in social groups, adding to their difficulty in quitting.[26] Among

adult women, heavy smoking is related to having friends who smoke, being overweight, smoking within 30 minutes of waking, smoking similar amounts at work and home, and smoking for more than 10 years.[27] They also may fear weight gain following quitting and continue to smoke as a form of weight management.[28,29] Although women may gain some weight after quitting, it may be more of a symptom of nicotine withdrawal, which can be minimized

Figure 6-4

Cigarette smoking among adolescent female students in grades 9–12 by race/ethnicity, 1999

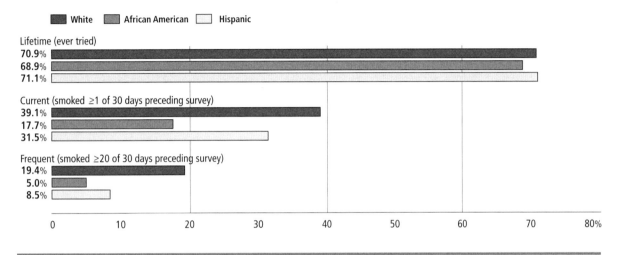

Source: Kann L, Kinchen S, Williams B, Ross J, Lowry R, Grunbaum JA, et al. Youth risk behavior surveillance—United States, 1999. MMWR Morb Mortal Wkly Rep 2000;49(SS05):1–96.

through changes in dietary habits.[30] On average, women tend to gain more weight than men after quitting.[29]

The most well-known smoking-related health problem is lung cancer. Men experienced higher rates of lung cancer during most of the twentieth century, but the rates for women and men have converged in recent years[31] due to the increasing numbers of women who took up smoking during the second half of the century.[29] In fact, lung cancer surpassed breast cancer in 1987 as the leading cause of cancer death in women[32] (see chapter 4).

Cigarette smoking is also strongly associated with cancers of the mouth, pharynx, larynx, esophagus, pancreas, uterine cervix, kidney, and bladder. It accounts for at least 30% of all cancer deaths and is associated with diseases such as chronic bronchitis, chronic obstructive pulmonary disease, and emphysema.[29,33] Cigarette smoking is also a major preventable cause of heart disease as well as a risk factor in the devel-

opment of cerebrovascular diseases and atherosclerotic peripheral vascular disease. An adverse effect of smoking unique to women is an increased risk of cardiovascular disease among smokers who use oral contraceptives; this risk increases with age and amount smoked.[34]

Cigarette smoking may complicate pre-existing chronic illnesses such as diabetes. Smokers miss more days of work, make more visits to the doctor, and have greater average lifetime medical costs than nonsmokers.[35] Women who smoke also appear to experience accelerated aging, including a greater risk of osteoporosis, early menopause, and skin wrinkling.[36] In addition, smoking has been shown to be detrimental to healing following periodontal treatment, as well as to the severity of periodontal disease in postmenopausal women.[37]

Finally, smoking is an important health behavior for women because of its effects on pregnancy. An increased risk of infertility has been reported for women who smoke.[38] One study reported

Table 6-2

Alcohol use among females by age and race/ethnicity, 1998

	Percent	
	Used during past year	Used during past month
Total	60.0	45.1
Age (years)		
12–17	32.7	18.7
18–25	68.9	51.7
26–34	71.5	54.2
35+	59.7	45.8
Race/ethnicity		
White, non-Hispanic	65.0	49.7
Black, non-Hispanic	45.1	32.3
Hispanic	48.4	33.6

Source: Substance Abuse and Mental Health Services Administration (SAMSHA). National Household Survey on Drug Abuse Population Estimates, 1998. Rockville (MD): U.S. Department of Health and Human Services; 1999.

Table 6-3

Alcohol use among adolescent female students in grades 9–12 by race/ethnicity, 1999

	Percent		
	Current use*	Episodic heavy drinking**	Before age 13***
Total	42.7	28.1	26.8
Race/ethnicity			
White, non-Hispanic	49.8	32.2	25.2
Black, non-Hispanic	40.7	14.7	26.5
Hispanic	49.3	26.8	30.7

*Current use is defined as ≥1 drink on 3 days of the 30 days preceding the interview.

**Episodic heavy drinking is defined as five or more drinks on the same occasion on more than one day in the past month.

*** Use before age 13 represents more than "a few sips."

Source: Kann L, Kinchen S, Williams B, Ross J, Lowry R, Grunbaum JA, et al. Youth risk behavior surveillance, United States, 1999. MMWR Morb Mortal Wkly Rep 2000;49(SS05):1–96.

fertility rates of smokers to be only about 70% of those for nonsmokers, and smokers were more than three times more likely to take longer than 1 year to conceive.[39] Women who smoke during pregnancy are twice as likely to give birth to a low-birth-weight (LBW) baby (weighing less than 2,500 grams at birth) as women who do not smoke; their babies weigh on average 200 grams less than nonsmokers' babies.[40,41,42,43]

Alcohol and Drug Use

Although the awareness among the general public of the ill effects of alcohol and drug abuse has increased over the past decade, substance abuse still remains a pervasive problem among women in the United States.

Alcohol Use

In 1998, nearly 10% of current drinkers (about 8 million people) met the diagnostic criteria for alcohol dependence and an additional 7% (more than 5.6 million people) met the diagnostic criteria for alcohol abuse. Similar to illicit drug use, data on alcohol use is collected as part of the National Household Survey on Drug Abuse (NHSDA).[44] Rates among women are lower than among men. Table 6-2 provides estimates on use of alcohol by women in the past year and in the past month. Among women who used alcohol in the past year, 17.5% reported drinking at least 51 days or more.[44] The peak age for use of alcohol is between the ages of 26–34 years.[44] Alcohol use tends to be less prevalent among blacks than among other racial and ethnic groups. In 1998, non-Hispanic white women reported the highest prevalence of lifetime use and past year use, followed by non-Hispanic black and Hispanic women. Estimates are not available for rates of use among Asian American or Native American women in this survey.

Among those who initiate alcohol use prior to age 15, more than 40% will become dependent on alcohol in their lifetime compared to less than 10% who wait until age 20 years or later.[45] Hispanic female students had the highest rates of ever use (ever had at least one drink) and use before age 13. Current use and episodic heavy drinking (five or more drinks on at least one occasion on one or more days in the past month) were much less common among black female students relative to either white or Hispanic female students (Table 6-3).[11] Although rates of ever use and current use (on at least 1 day of past month) of alcohol among male students were similar to those of female students, males were more likely than females to try alcohol before 13 years of age (37.4% versus 26.8%).[11]

The percentage of pregnant women reporting alcohol use in the BRFSS surveys is considerably lower than for all women of childbearing age. While 50.6% of all women reported use in the past month in 1995, only 16.3% of pregnant women did so. Strikingly, more than four times as many pregnant women reported frequent use in the past month in 1995 than in 1991 (3.5% versus 0.8%).[46]

The percentages of women reporting use of alcohol during pregnancy in the BRFSS surveys are somewhat lower than other estimates because they are estimates of prevalence at one point in time rather than throughout pregnancy. Moreover, the number of pregnant women in the samples is sufficiently small to be concerned about random variability and possible systematic errors.[46] In the 1992 National Pregnancy and Health Survey (NPHS), 18.8% of women reported using alcohol during pregnancy, but use dropped markedly as pregnancy progressed. Young women (under the age of 25 years) in the NPHS

Table 6-4

Alcoholism-related mortality* rates in women, 1992–1994

| Age (years) | Mortality rates per 100,000 population** | |
	American Indian/ Alaskan Native women (1992–94)	U.S. all races women (1993)
15–24	2.1	0.1
25–34	26.1	1.4
35–44	64.2	4.9
45–54	87.6	6.3
55–64	61.5	9.9
65–74	49.3	8.3
75–84	20.1	4.9
85+	***	1.6

*Includes ICD-9 codes 291, 303, 305.0, 357.5, 425.5, 535.3,571.0-571.3, 790.3, E860.

** Rates adjusted to compensate for miscoding of Indian race on death certificates.
***Not available.

Source: U.S. Indian Health Service. Trends in Indian health, 1997. Rockville (MD): U.S. Department of Health and Human Services; 1998. Available from: URL: www.ihs.gov/publicinfo/publications/trends97/tds97pt1.pdf.

were least likely to report using alcohol in pregnancy. Rates also varied by race/ethnicity, with the highest rates for Native American and white women. Trends by age were similar for white, black, and Hispanic pregnant women.[47]

The major risk period for initiation of alcohol use is over by the age of 20, and almost no individuals initiate use after age 29.[48] Studies of twin and family histories support the inherited susceptibility of alcoholism.[49,50] Other risk factors for heavy drinking include drinking by a woman's partner or spouse, drinking by friends, depression, marital distress and/or sexual dysfunction, and the amount of time spent in drinking situations or social events.[50,51] Additionally, women who are heavy drinkers are more likely to report having had behavioral or emotional problems in childhood and adolescence, particularly in response to early painful experiences, and a history of sexual abuse and childhood victimization.[52,53]

Liver disease is the most frequently reported direct effect of heavy alcohol use, particularly cirrhosis of the liver. Women who use alcohol have higher rates of liver disease and related mortality than men and at earlier ages.[54,55] Additionally, the incidence of breast cancer also appears to increase directly with alcohol intake.[56] Light-to-moderate drinking can have beneficial effects on the heart, particularly after menopause.[57] Long-term heavy drinking, however, increases risk for high blood pressure and heart disease.[58] The all-cause death rates for women who are chronic heavy users of alcohol are higher than rates for male alcoholics.[49] Because of biological differences, alcohol has different effects on the health of women than it does on men; women's susceptibility to the physiological consequences of alcohol abuse is considered higher than males. That is, women reach higher blood alcohol concentrations from the same weight-adjusted levels of consumption and may develop liver disorders after lower levels of regular alcohol consumption compared to men.[59]

Alcohol abuse is reported to be rare among Asian American women, but Native American women appear to be particularly vulnerable to problem drinking, although they drink less than Native American men do.[49,60] Table 6-4 shows the toll of alcoholism on Native American women; rates of alcoholism-related mortality are at least 10 times higher for Native American women compared to other women.

Illicit Drug Use

As discussed here, illicit drug use refers to use of marijuana, cocaine, inhalants, hallucinogens, heroin, or use of any prescription-type psychotherapeutic (e.g., benzodiazepines such as Valium) for nonprescribed purposes. Overall, the current use (past month) of illicit drugs in the

Table 6-5

Past month illicit drug use among respondents aged 12 years and older by gender, 1979–1998

| Year | Percent | | | | | |
| | Any illicit drugs | | Marijuana | | Cocaine | |
	Women	Men	Women	Men	Women	Men
1979	9.4	19.2	8.7	18.1	1.8	3.5
1985	9.5	14.9	7.1	12.6	2.1	3.9
1990	5.3	8.2	4.2	6.8	0.6	1.2
1992	4.2	7.6	3.1	6.4	0.4	1.0
1995	4.5	7.8	3.3	6.2	0.4	1.1
1997	4.5	8.5	3.5	7.0	0.5	0.9
1998	4.5	8.1	3.5	6.7	0.5	1.1

Source: Substance Abuse and Mental Health Services Administration (SAMSHA). National Household Survey on Drug Abuse Population Estimates, 1998. Rockville (MD): U.S. Department of Health and Human Services; 1999.

United States over the past two decades has decreased sharply (Table 6-5). Reported drug use has declined by almost half since 1979 among both men and women.[44] The rates of current illicit drug use were lower among women than those among men with 4.5% of women reporting use within the past month as compared to 8.1% of men. Despite this general decline, based on data from the 1998 NHSDA, it is estimated that there were 13.6 million current users of an illicit drug in the total population aged 12 years and older. In 1998, 30.3% of women aged 12 and older reported ever using any illicit drug.[44]

The peak age for use of illicit drugs among women coincides with the peak childbearing ages, 18–34 years, while the lowest lifetime, past year, and past month use rates for adults are found among women aged 35 or older (Table 6-6).[44] Age

Table 6-6

Illicit drug use among women by age and race/ethnicity,* 1998

	Percent		
	Ever used during lifetime	Used past year	Used past month
Age (years)			
12–17	20.5	16.0	9.5
18–25	41.9	22.1	11.7
26–34	44.9	9.3	4.3
35+	26.0	4.0	2.4
Race/ethnicity			
White, non-Hispanic	33.1	8.4	4.5
Black, non-Hispanic	26.4	9.0	5.2
Hispanic	20.3	7.9	4.5

*Data not reported for Native American and Asian/Pacific Islander women. See text for estimates.

Source: Substance Abuse and Mental Health Services Administration (SAMSHA). National Household Survey on Drug Abuse Population Estimates, 1998. Rockville (MD): U.S. Department of Health and Human Services; 1999.

Table 6-7

Illicit drug use among women by type of drug and race/ethnicity, 1998

	Percent		
	Ever used during lifetime	Used past year	Used past month
Marijuana	**27.9**	**6.5**	**3.5**
White, non-Hispanic	30.9	6.7	3.6
Black, non-Hispanic	23.5	7.2	3.8
Hispanic	16.9	5.8	3.2
Cocaine	**8.2**	**1.2**	**0.5**
White, non-Hispanic	9.2	1.3	0.5
Black, non-Hispanic	5.6	1.3	0.9
Hispanic	5.8	1.3	0.8
Crack cocaine	**1.4**	**0.3**	**0.2**
White, non-Hispanic	1.2	0.3	0.1
Black, non-Hispanic	2.7	0.8	0.4
Hispanic	1.2	0.4	0.2
Heroin	**0.8**	**0.1**	**0.1**
White, non-Hispanic	*	*	*
Black, non-Hispanic	*	*	*
Hispanic	*	*	*
Inhalant	**3.7**	**0.6**	**0.2**
White, non-Hispanic	4.3	0.7	0.2
Black, non-Hispanic	1.3	0.3	0.1
Hispanic	2.5	0.7	0.3
Hallucinogen	**7.4**	**1.3**	**0.6**
White, non-Hispanic	8.8	1.6	0.7
Black, non-Hispanic	2.6	0.2	**
Hispanic	3.7	1.0	0.3
Psychotherapeutic	**7.6**	**2.1**	**0.9**
White, non-Hispanic	8.3	2.2	0.9
Black, non-Hispanic	5.5	1.7	0.9
Hispanic	5.4	2.6	1.1
Stimulant	**3.2**	**0.5**	**0.2**
White, non-Hispanic	3.7	0.5	0.2
Black, non-Hispanic	1.8	0.5	0.2
Hispanic	2.1	0.7	0.3

*Not available.

**Low precision, no estimate reported.

Source: Substance Abuse and Mental Health Services Administration (SAMSHA). National Household Survey on Drug Abuse Population Estimates, 1998. Rockville (MD): U.S. Department of Health and Human Services; 1999.

Table 6-8

Illicit drug use among adolescent female students in grades 9–12 by type of drug and race/ethnicity, 1999

	Percent					
	Marijuana		Cocaine		Inhalants	
	Ever-use	Current use	Ever-use*	Current use	Ever-use**	Current use***
Total	47.2	26.7	9.5	4.0	14.6	4.2
Female	43.4	22.6	8.4	2.9	14.6	3.9
Male	51.0	30.8	10.7	5.2	14.7	4.4
White, non-Hispanic						
Female	42.3	22.9	8.7	2.8	16.5	4.3
Male	49.2	29.6	11.0	5.3	16.2	4.4
Black, non-Hispanic						
Female	42.7	21.9	1.5	1.1	5.5	3.1
Male	54.8	31.2	2.8	1.0	3.4	1.4
Hispanic						
Female	46.4	21.8	12.3	5.4	16.6	5.0
Male	55.8	34.8	18.3	8.0	15.6	4.7

*Ever-use of cocaine includes ever trying any form of cocaine (e.g., power, "crack", freebase).

**Ever-use of inhalants is defined as ever sniffed glue or breathed contents of aerosol spray cans or inhaled any paints or sprays to become intoxicated.

***Current use of inhalants is defined as use on at least one occasion in the 30 days preceding the interview.

Source: Kann L, Kinchen S, Williams B, Ross, Lowry R, Grunbaum JA, et al. J. Youth risk behavior surveillance, United States, 1999. MMWR Morb Mortal Wkly Rep 2000;49(SS05):1–96.

patterns are similar for each specific drug (e.g., cocaine) although the peak age for use is 18–25 years in some instances.[44] Rates of substance use and the choice of substances also vary by a woman's race and ethnicity. In 1998, non-Hispanic white women aged 12 or older reported more lifetime use of any illicit drug, as well as more lifetime use of most of the specific drugs (marijuana, cocaine, hallucinogens, inhalants, stimulants, and psychotherapeutics) than non-Hispanic black or Hispanic women (Table 6-7). However, rates of ever-use of crack cocaine were highest for non-Hispanic black women. Rates of illicit drug use in 1995, the most recent year for which data for other racial or ethnic groups are available, were lowest for women of Asian or Pacific Island descent. Native Americans reported the highest use of illicit drugs, marijuana, and other drugs.[44]

Looking at drug use among women by specific type of drug categorized by ever-use, use in past year, and use in past month, marijuana was the most commonly reported illicit drug among women in 1998. Use of cocaine among women has remained relatively stable over the past decade after peaking in 1985. Heroin use among women is infrequent. Needle use (not included in the table) is also rare with 0.1% of women reporting use of a needle to inject drugs (heroin, cocaine, or a stimulant) in the past year, representing nearly 120,000 women in 1998. Approximately 2.1% of women reported using psychotherapeutic drugs in the past year for nonmedical reasons, making them the second most commonly used illicit drug.[44]

Table 6-8 provides estimates of drug use among adolescent students based on the 1999 YRBS.[11] Like adult women, the most commonly used illicit drug among high-school girls in grades 9-12 is marijuana but it is followed by inhalants, a drug used much more frequently by adolescents than adults. The use of marijuana did not vary by race/ethnicity, but rates of ever-use of cocaine were much higher for Hispanic and white female students than for black female students. Rates of marijuana use are higher among adolescent boys than girls across all categories of use (e.g., 30.8% of boys reported currently using versus 22.6% of girls). Likewise, overall rates of cocaine use are higher for male students than female students with nearly twice the proportion of male students currently using (5.2% versus 2.9%). Interestingly, there was almost no difference in the current use of inhalants by gender (4.4% of boys versus 3.9% of girls).[11]

Drug use among women is also influenced by pregnancy. In the 1992 NPHS, an estimated 5.5% of women had used an illicit substance during pregnancy, with the most commonly reported substance being marijuana (2.9%). An estimated

1.1% of women used cocaine and 1.5% nonprescription psychotherapeutic drugs, with much lower levels of use of other substances. Crack cocaine use was reported by three-fourths of cocaine users.[47] The choice of substances and their frequency of use varied in the NPHS by age and race/ethnicity. Women 25 years of age and younger were less likely to report using crack cocaine than women 25 years or older. In contrast to rates among nonpregnant women, pregnant black women had higher rates of use of any illicit drug than pregnant white or Hispanic women. Among white and black women, rates of use of any substances dropped from 3 months prior to pregnancy through the second trimester, after which they stabilized. For Hispanic women, they continued to drop throughout pregnancy although to a lesser extent in the third trimester.[47]

The most important predictor of drug use in women more than 17 years old is initiation of alcohol or drug use at a young age. Risk factors include appearing older than schoolmates, having a low grade point average, working 20 hours or more per week, living in a family without two biological parents, moving frequently, receiving welfare (through a family member), and having emotional or behavioral problems.[61] Protective factors against marijuana use for adolescents include high levels of parent and family connectedness, school connectedness, and self-esteem, as well as the importance of religion in student's lives.[61]

Risk factors for illicit substance use among women include a history of sexual abuse as a child, of violence as an adult, and of drug or alcohol abuse in the family.[62,63] Women who abuse substances also have been found to have fewer social supports, fewer members in their social networks, and lower social esteem; they are also more likely to experience depression than nonusers.[64]

Like substance-using women in general, women who use drugs during pregnancy are more likely to have a partner who uses drugs, to have been introduced to drugs by their partner, to have a family history of drug or alcohol abuse, to be depressed, and to have fewer social supports and less stable living situations.[62,65,66,67] They are more likely to move several times or be homeless and to drink alcohol and smoke cigarettes during their pregnancy.[47,62,66,67,68,69]

Women who use illicit substances are more likely to have poor nutrition, to be below average weight for their height, and to have serious medical and infectious disease, including elevated blood pressure, increased heart rate, and/or sexually transmitted diseases (STDs).[70,71] Substance-using women are also more likely to die from drug overdose, suicide, and violence, with black women having slightly higher death rates from drug-induced causes than white women.[71] Furthermore, substance abuse often co-occurs with mental disorders, and women tend to have higher rates of co-occurring disorders compared to men.[72,73]

The specific effects of substance use during pregnancy depend upon the type and amount of drug used, the mother's overall health, the gestational age of the fetus at the time of use, and the functional state of the placenta.[59,60,74] Moreover, when there is multiple drug use, it is often difficult to isolate the effect of any single drug.[59,75] Many other factors in the lives of women who use drugs are also related to poor pregnancy outcomes.

Women who are substance users often face barriers, including social and health care access, when they attempt to seek help for their addiction. These barriers contribute to problems of women entering and remaining in treatment[76] (see chapter 8).

Physical Activity

The risks of many chronic diseases are lower among women who exercise regularly, and exercise can ameliorate symptoms or improve functioning for women with particular chronic diseases (e.g., arthritis). Exercise is also an important component in weight control and obesity

Table 6-9

Frequent exercise* among women by race/ethnicity, income, and education, 1998

	Percent reporting frequent exercise
Total	39
Race/ethnicity	
White	42
African American	32
Hispanic	32
Asian American	16
Income	
$16,000 or less	32
$16,001–$35,000	38
$35,001–$50,000	40
$50,001 or more	48
Education	
Less than high school	26
High school/ some college	41
College or more	47

*Exercise is defined as physical activity that entails heavy breathing and acceleration of the heart and pulse rates for at least 20 minutes three or more days per week.

Source: Collins K, Schoen C, Joseph S, Duchon L, Simantov E, Yellowitz M. Health concerns across a woman's lifespan: The Commonwealth Fund 1998 Survey of Women's Health. New York: The Commonwealth Fund; 1999.

prevention. Despite these benefits, however, overall rates of exercise among women continue to be low.

Data from the 1998 BRFSS illustrate the generally low levels of physical activity among women.[77] Only 19.5% of adult women participated in regular, sustained physical activity (≥5 sessions per week, ≥30 minutes per session, regardless of intensity) and 13.6% in regular, vigorous physical activity (≥3 sessions per week, ≥20 minutes per session, at 50% or more capacity). In the

Table 6-10

Physical activity among adolescent students in grades 9–12 by gender and race/ethnicity, 1999

	Percent							
	Female				Male			
Type of activity	Total	White, non-Hispanic	Black, non-Hispanic	Hispanic	Total	White, non-Hispanic	Black, non-Hispanic	Hispanic
Vigorous*	57.1	59.7	47.2	49.5	72.3	74.6	64.6	71.6
Moderate**	24.4	25.8	17.8	16.7	29.0	31.7	24.3	26.1
Strengthening***	43.6	45.9	33.1	38.8	63.5	64.8	57.9	66.4

*Activities that caused sweating and hard breathing for ≥20 minutes on ≥3 of the 7 days preceding the survey.

**Activities that did not cause sweating and hard breathing for ≥20 minutes on ≥3 of the 7 days preceding the survey.

***For example, push-ups, sit-ups, or weight lifting on ≥3 of the 7 days preceding the survey.

Source: Kann L, Kinchen S, Williams B, Ross J, Lowry R, Grunbaum JA, et al. Youth risk behavior surveillance, United States, 1999. MMWR Morb Mortal Wkly Rep 2000;49(SS05):1–96.

Commonwealth Fund's 1998 Survey of Women's Health, almost four in 10 women (39%) reported frequent exercise defined as physical activity that entails heavy breathing and acceleration of the heart and pulse rates for at least 20 minutes on 3 or more days per week (Table 6-9). This figure represents an increase compared to the 31% reported in the 1993 survey.[6]

Physical activity participation differs by a number of individual characteristics. These issues have been explored in more detail in the National Health and Nutrition Examination Survey III (NHANES III), which contains somewhat older data than the data available from the BRFSS. In NHANES III, non-Hispanic black women and Mexican American (other Hispanic groups not studied) women reported a higher rate of inactivity compared with non-Hispanic white women.[78] Rates of inactivity also increase with age in NHANES III.[78] Due to small numbers, most surveys cannot estimate the prevalence of inactivity and activity for American Indian/Native Alaskan women.

Patterns were more complex with regard to vigorous physical activity three or more days per week in NHANES III, although rates were very low for all groups.[78] Among women 20–39 years of age, the rate of participation in vigorous activity was similar for each of the ethnic groups, at about 4%. But among women aged 40–59, non-Hispanic white women (4%) were twice as likely to participate in vigorous activity compared to either non-Hispanic black women (2%) or Mexican American women (2%). For women 60 years and older, non-Hispanic white women (5%) were most likely to participate in vigorous activity followed by non-Hispanic black women (3%) and then Mexican American women (2%).

In The Commonwealth Fund survey, rates also varied by race/ethnicity, with Asian American women the least likely and whites the most likely to report exercising frequently. Additionally, there were marked differences according to education level and income, with the lowest rates found for women with less than a high school education and those with lower incomes.[6]

The four most frequently reported leisure-time physical activities for adult women aged 20 years and older, based on NHANES III, are walking, gardening/yard work, calisthenics, and cycling. Among Mexican American and non-Hispanic black women, however, dancing (not including aerobic dance or aerobics classes) is one of the four most frequent activities, rather than cycling.[78]

Estimates of physical activity among young people have shown that girls, like their adult female counterparts, are less likely than males of the same age to participate in physical activity. In the 1999 YRBS,[11] male high school students were more likely to exercise than female students in each racial/ethnic group (Table 6-10). The gender gap is largest for vigorous activity. Of those who exercised, females (65.4%) were more likely to exercise to lose weight or control weight gain than males (39.9%). As with adult women, rates vary by race and ethnicity with rates of vigorous physical activity among non-Hispanic white females greater than those of non-Hispanic black and Hispanic females. Boys and girls both tend to decrease levels of physical activity as they become older.[11]

Strikingly, in the NHANES III data, 29.9% of the adult women reported no leisure time physical activity.[77] Little change has been seen overall (men and women combined) in these proportions since 1991, suggesting that increases in obesity cannot be explained by declines in physical activity.[79]

In a cross-sectional national survey of older women (the U.S. Women's Determinants Study) minority women were oversampled to estimate physical inactivity and activity in these groups. The highest prevalence of leisure time physical inactivity was found among American Indian/Alaskan Native women (48.7%) and the lowest among white women (30.7%).[80]

As described above, factors that may be related to regular physical activity include gender, age, race/ethnicity, education, and income level. According to the U.S. Surgeon General's Report, social support for exercise from family and friends is positively related to regular physical activity.[81] Other correlates related to physical activity include self-efficacy, self-esteem, and perceived benefits and barriers.[82] Based on 1996 BRFSS data from five states, a Centers for Disease Control and Prevention (CDC) analysis concluded that physical inactivity was more common among people who perceived their neighborhood to be unsafe. Nearly half of women who rated their neighborhood as "not at all safe" reported physical inactivity as compared with one-third of women who rated their neighborhood as "extremely safe." This association with safety was much stronger for women than for men.[83] Creating opportunities for physical activity, reinforcing physical activity habits, and ensuring that neighborhoods are safe for outdoor activity may promote exercise among women.[81]

Physical activity is an important health behavior that can substantially reduce a woman's risk of cardiovascular disease[84,85,86,87] and osteoporosis,[88] and there is emerging evidence that physical activity may decrease the risk of breast cancer [89,90] and colon cancer (see chapter 4).[91] Physical activity also prevents obesity, which indirectly improves health because several conditions are linked to or exacerbated by obesity. Finally, physical activity may improve overall health-related quality of life and mood.[81]

Nutrition

Dietary factors have been found to be associated with four of the 10 leading causes of death (coronary heart disease, some forms of cancer, stroke, and type II diabetes[92]), as well as osteoporosis, the leading cause of bone fractures in postmenopausal women.[93] Nutritional concerns include nutrient deficiencies as well as excesses and imbalances in diet composition. The Food and Drug Administration (FDA) developed recommended dietary allowances (RDAs) in 1943 to serve as a goal for nutritional well-being.[94] Now in its tenth edition, *Recommended Dietary Allowances* can be used as a benchmark to judge adequacy of nutrient intake. Few women have diets that meet the RDAs

Table 6-11

Women's body mass index (BMI)* by race/ethnicity, 1988–1994

	Percent of women					
	Underweight	Normal	Overweight	Obesity class I	Obesity class II	Obesity class III
BMI	<18.5	18.5–24.9	25–29.9	30–34.9	35–39.9	≥40.0
White, non-Hispanic	3.49	46.78	25.96	13.73	6.50	3.55
Black, non-Hispanic	2.47	28.59	29.99	19.77	11.01	8.57
Mexican American	1.35	30.04	32.29	22.36	3.57	5.38
Other	2.45	44.11	25.50	19.33	5.74	2.86

*BMI is body weight in kilograms divided by height in meters squared: kg/m².

Source: Must A, Spadano J, Coakley E, Field A, Colditz G, Dietz W. The disease burden associated with overweight and obesity. JAMA 1999;282:1523–1529.

for key nutrients. This is not suprising given the overall composition of most women's diets.

The 1998 BRFSS reported that less than one-third of women meet the recommendation to consume at least five servings of fruits and vegetables per day.[77] In the 1994–1996 U.S. Department of Agriculture (USDA) Continuing Survey of Food Intakes by Individuals (CSFII), more than half of women aged 20 years and older reported that at least one food item was obtained and eaten away from home, with the highest proportions reported by the youngest women. Although nutritious foods are available, approximately 30% of women more than 20 years old who ate out obtained at least some of their food from a fast food restaurant.[95] The poor quality of women's diets does not appear to be entirely the result of a lack of knowledge as the majority of the women in the CSFII perceived dietary guidance (e.g., recommendations to choose a diet low in saturated fat) as very important.[95] Interestingly, the majority of women more than 20 years old in the USDA 1994–96 CSFII reported taking vitamin or mineral supplements.[95]

Table 6-12

Overweight among adolescent female students in grades 9–12 by race/ethnicity, 1999

	Percent			
	At risk for over-weight*	Over-weight**	Thought they were over-weight	Attempting weight loss
Total	14.4	7.9	36.4	59.4
White, non-Hispanic	12.4	6.8	35.7	61.4
Black, non-Hispanic	22.6	12.8	32.3	48.3
Hispanic	18.3	9.7	42.3	63.6

*≥85th percentile but <95th percentile BMI age and sex based on reference data from NHANES I.

**≥95th percentile BMI age and sex based on reference data from NHANES I.

Source: Kann L, Kinchen S, Williams B, Ross J, Lowry R. Grunbaum JA, et al. Youth Risk Behavior Surveillance, United States, 1999. MMWR Morb Mortal Wkly Rep 2000;49(SS05):1–96.

Obesity

Obesity and overweight have been increasing over the past two decades among U.S. women (see Figure 4-4 in chapter 4). Next to tobacco, obesity has been identified as the most significant health problem facing American women.[96]

Data from the NHANES III indicate that in 1988–1994, 35% of women aged 20 to 74 years of age were overweight (including being obese).[98] Overweight and obesity among women in the NHANES III sample can also be examined in more detail by body mass index (BMI, measured as kilograms body weight divided by height in meters squared; Table 6-11). Although Mexican American women are the most likely to be either overweight or in obesity class I, non-Hispanic black women are the most likely to be classified in obesity classes II and III. Data on obesity are also available from the USDA 1995 CSFII. In this survey, limited to adults 20 years

and older, approximately 31% of women were determined to be overweight with the highest rates among women 40–59 years of age (approximately 39%).[97]

The percentage of women who are overweight or obese has been increasing over the past 25 years. Based on NHANES data, the percentage of obese persons has risen from 14.5% from 1976–1980 to 22.5% from 1988–1994.[99] From 1991 to 1998, increases were seen for men and women alike, but the highest increases in prevalence of obesity were among the youngest and most educated. The BRFSS data, which rely on self-reported body weight and height to compute BMI, also show an increase in the prevalence of obesity. The prevalence of obesity among women increased from 12.2% in 1991 to 18.1% in 1998.[79] (BRFSS data likely underestimate obesity due to reliance on self-reporting.)

Reports from the 1999 YRBS provide information about the problem of overweight among adolescents (defined differently than for adults, see Table 6-12). Many adolescents are at risk or already have become overweight, but even more perceive themselves to be overweight and report attempting to lose weight. It is unclear whether those who perceive themselves to be overweight are accurate in their perceptions. Female students were significantly more likely than male students to believe that they were overweight and were trying to lose weight. Among female students, blacks are approximately two times more likely to be overweight or at risk for being overweight.[11]

Essentially, obesity and overweight are problems resulting from an energy intake imbalance, meaning that obesity and overweight occur when an individual consumes too many calories relative to their calorie expenditure through activity.

Obesity is associated with increased mortality and morbidity related to several chronic health problems in women, including diabetes, cardiovascular disease, osteoarthritis, and some forms of cancer.[100,101,102,103,104,105,106,107] Data from the

Table 6-13

U.S. adolescents and women with nutrient intake below 100% of the RDA by age, 1994–1996			
Age (years)	**Percent of women with diets containing less than 100% RDA**		
	Calcium	**Folate**	**Iron**
12–19	86.6	41.8	72.5
20–29	83.1	47.6	74.1
30–39	74.7	48.0	73.4
40–49	76.1	48.1	77.9
50–59	76.7	45.4	44.8
60–69	79.3	44.7	40.7
70+	79.2	41.1	40.8

Source: U.S. Department of Agriculture. Agricultural Research Service. Data tables: results from USDA's 1994-1996 Continuing Survey of Food Intakes by Individuals. Beltsville (MD): U.S. Department of Agriculture, Agricultural Research Service, Beltsville Human Nutrition Research Center; 1997.

Table 6-14

Calcium supplement use among women by age, race/ethnicity, income, and education, 1998

	Percent taking calcium supplements
Total	39
Age (years)	
18–44	26
45–64	52
65+	57
Race/ethnicity	
White	44
African American	21
Hispanic	29
Asian American	38
Income	
$16,000 or less	29
$16,001–$35,000	37
$35,001–$50,000	42
$50,001 or more	46
Education	
Less than high school	31
High school/some college	38
College or more	49

Source: Collins K, Schoen C, Joseph S, Duchon L, Simantov E, Yellowitz M. Health concerns across a woman's lifespan: The Commonwealth Fund 1998 Survey of Women's Health. New York: The Commonwealth Fund; 1999.

NHANES III have been used to estimate the overall disease burden associated with overweight and obesity. For all but one of the conditions examined, the prevalence of morbidity increases with increasing severity of overweight and obesity.[108] Some studies, however, do not report a relationship between obesity and increased mortality.[109,110]

Calcium

Peak bone mass is attained between the ages of 20 and 30 years. From this point onward, calcium is lost from bones at a very slow rate until menopause, when bone loss increases rapidly. Diet and exercise can decelerate this process. Calcium stored in bones can compensate for short-term deprivation, but chronic shortages are associated with loss of bone mass and bone structure that may be irreversible (see chapter 4). The *Third Report on Nutrition Monitoring in the United States* (1995) reported that median calcium intakes from dietary sources were below recommended levels among adolescents and adult females.[111] Table 6-13 describes the proportion of adolescents and women whose diets contain less than 100% of the RDA for calcium and other nutrients. Among adult women (older than 20 years of age), just 22% of women had diets that achieved 100% of the RDA for calcium.[95]

The Commonwealth Fund 1998 Survey of Women's Health examined the use of calcium supplements, a critical behavior given the generally low levels of dietary calcium consumed by women. The proportion of women using calcium supplements rose from 28% in 1993 to 39% in 1998. The increase was more pronounced for older women.[6] Rates of supplementation also varied by race/ethnicity, income, and education (Table 6-14). Even in the groups most likely to report supplement use, less than half of the women are taking calcium supplements. Many women not taking supplements (77%), however, reported consuming calcium-rich dietary sources to ensure adequate calcium intake.[6]

Folate

Folate can be found in whole grain breads, various meats and eggs, green leafy vegetables, lentils, beans, and citrus juices.[112] Inadequate folate intake very early in pregnancy is a well-established risk factor for neural tube defects.[113,114,115] It is recommended that all women of childbearing age consume 400 micrograms per day as a preventive measure, because it is too late to increase intake by the time most women discover they are pregnant.[94] Nevertheless, a 1998 national telephone survey by the March of Dimes Birth Defects Foundation revealed that 68% of women reported ever having heard of or read about folic acid, a 31% increase from 52% in 1995.[116] The CDC reports that folic acid supplementation prior to pregnancy has only risen to 29%, an increase of 4% over 3 years. In addition, disparities exist, as older, college-educated women of higher socioeconomic status are the most likely to take folic acid supplements.[116]

According to the USDA 1995 CSFII, nearly half of adult women consume diets containing less than 100% of the RDA for folate with little variation by age.[97] Fortification of cereals and grains with folic acid began shortly after 1996 in an effort to decrease the incidence of neural tube defects in pregnancy. One study revealed that adult serum folate values rose from 12.6 to 18.7 micrograms per liter from 1994 to 1998. This change is likely attributable to folic acid food fortification.[117] A woman may experience folate deficiency as a result of inadequate intake or poor absorption of folate. The most important external factor that reduces folate absorption is alcohol. Many medications influence absorption of folate. Of particular importance for women, oral contraceptives appear to decrease folate absorption.[118] Folate deficiency can also result in anemia, leading to lethargy and weakness.[112,118]

Iron

Anemia resulting from iron deficiency is the most common micronutrient deficiency in developing and developed countries. The RDA for iron among women aged 12–49 years is 15 milligrams per day and drops to 10 milligrams per day for women aged 50 years and older.[94]

Among persons aged 12 years and older, iron deficiency and iron deficiency anemia are more common in women than in men.[119]

Approximately 7.8 million adolescent girls and women of childbearing age are iron deficient.[120] Iron deficiency rates are highest for women aged 16–19 and 20–49 years (11%). The prevalence of anemia associated with iron deficiency was highest for the women aged 20–49 years. The prevalence is higher in African American women and women in some Hispanic ethnic groups than in non-Hispanic white women.[120,121]

Data from the USDA 1994–1996 CSFII show that women 40–49 years old are the least likely and women over 50 years the most likely to achieve the RDA for iron.[95] Menstruation, particularly if blood loss is heavy, increases the risk of iron deficiency anemia for girls and women.[119] Use of an intrauterine device, high parity, and low iron intake all increase the risk for iron deficiency anemia in women.[120,122] Oral contraceptives are associated with a reduced risk because they tend to reduce menstrual blood losses.[123,124] Women may experience anemia, weakness, and headaches if iron deficient.[94] In adults, iron-deficiency anemia may have an effect on cognitive function but this has not yet been clearly established.[125]

Hormone Replacement Therapy (HRT)

Hormone replacement therapy, consisting of estrogen or a combination of estrogen and progestin, is the most often prescribed medication for women in the United States with an estimated 6 million users in 1992.[126,127] Menopausal women experience a decrease in estrogen during and after menopause that is associated with symptoms such as hot flashes and decreased vaginal lubrication and chronic diseases such as coronary heart disease (CHD) and osteoporosis. Hormone replacement therapy alleviates the symptoms of menopause and may reduce the risk of CHD and

Figure 6-5

Women using hormone replacement therapy by year and type of menopause, 1925–1992

Percent

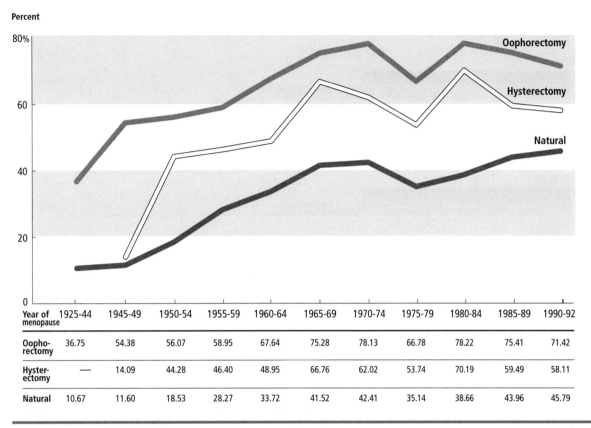

Year of menopause	1925-44	1945-49	1950-54	1955-59	1960-64	1965-69	1970-74	1975-79	1980-84	1985-89	1990-92
Oopho-rectomy	36.75	54.38	56.07	58.95	67.64	75.28	78.13	66.78	78.22	75.41	71.42
Hyster-ectomy	—	14.09	44.28	46.40	48.95	66.76	62.02	53.74	70.19	59.49	58.11
Natural	10.67	11.60	18.53	28.27	33.72	41.52	42.41	35.14	38.66	43.96	45.79

Source: Brett KM, Madans JH. Use of postmenopausal hormone replacement therapy: estimates from a nationally representative cohort study. Am J Epidemiol 1997 Mar 15;145(6):536–545.

osteoporosis after menopause.[128] There may also be risks associated with use of HRT, such as increased rates of endometrial[129] and breast cancers.[130]

Using data from the NHANES I Epidemiologic Followup Study (NHEFS), the overall use of HRT was estimated to be 45% among women who were menopausal by 1992.[126] Among women who became menopausal between 1970–1992, the odds of HRT use were 4.2 times greater among women who experienced menopause after surgical removal of their ovaries (oophorectomy) than for those women who experienced natural menopause. Similarly, women who experienced menopause after hysterectomy were 2.4 times more likely to use HRT than women with natural menopause.[126] Furthermore, women who under-

went oophorectomy were 1.9 times more likely to continue hormone replacement therapy for at least 5 years. Trends in the use of HRT by year of menopause and by type of menopause (i.e. natural, oophorectomy, hysterectomy) are shown in Figure 6-5. In general, use is higher for later cohorts. However, HRT use after hysterectomy and oophorectomy is more common among women who became menopausal in the early 1980s compared to later years.

Data from the Commonwealth Fund's 1993 and 1998 Surveys of Women's Health can be used to examine more recent trends in HRT use as well as variability by sociodemographic characteristics. From 1993 to 1998, the percentage of women aged 50 years or older using HRT increased overall (from 23% to 34%) and in all

Figure 6-6

Hormone replacement therapy use among women aged 50 years and older by income,
1993 and 1998

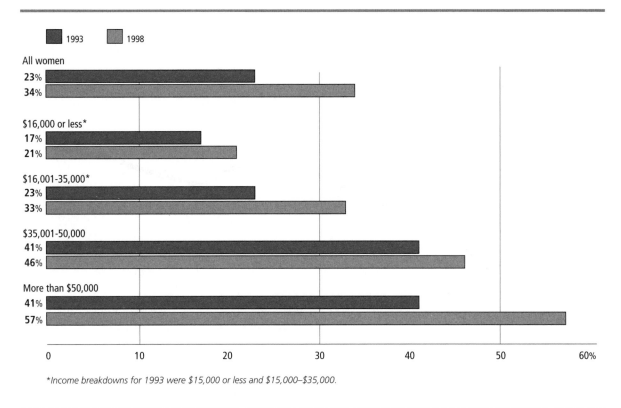

*Income breakdowns for 1993 were $15,000 or less and $15,000–$35,000.

Source: Collins K, Schoen C, Joseph S, Duchon L, Simantov E, Yellowitz M. Health concerns across a woman's lifespan: the Commonwealth Fund 1998 Survey of Women's Health. New York: The Commonwealth Fund; 1999.

categories of income (Figure 6-6) and education (Figure 6-7).[6] Higher income and educational levels were associated with higher rates of HRT. Education was also positively related to HRT use among black women enrolled in the Black Women's Health Study.[131]

Based on the NHEFS, black women were much less likely to be users of HRT (prevalence of 32.7%) compared to white women (51.4%).[126] Similarly, results from a study of ambulatory physician office visits demonstrated that menopausal black women are two times less likely to receive a prescription for HRT than white women of similar age.[132] Data from the Commonwealth Fund's 1998 Survey of Women's Health echo these findings.[6] Prevalence of HRT use for Hispanic women has been infrequently

reported. The 1998 Commonwealth Fund Survey found a 23% prevalence of HRT use among Hispanic women aged 50 years and older, making them somewhat more likely than African American women (16%) and less likely than white women (37%) to use HRT.[6]

As with other health behaviors, the decision to initiate HRT must be an informed one, taking into account both the risks and potential benefits of therapy. Data from the NHIS demonstrate that 43% of women aged 40 to 60 years and 62.4% of women aged 50 to 54 years received HRT counseling from a healthcare provider.[133] Black women were 0.6 times less likely to receive counseling as compared with women who were white. Women who had received a college education were 2.5 times more likely to receive

Figure 6-7

Hormone replacement therapy use among women aged 50 years and older by education, 1993 and 1998

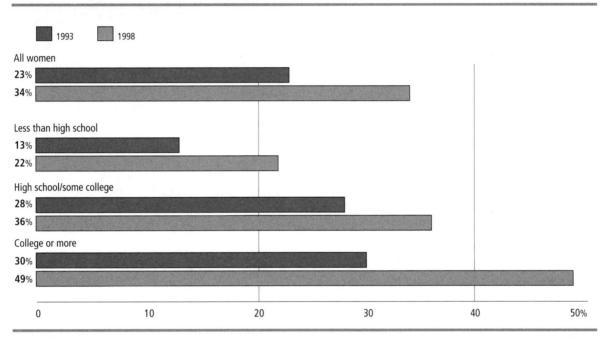

Source: Collins K, Schoen C, Joseph S, Duchon L, Simantov E, Yellowitz M. Health concerns across a woman's lifespan: the Commonwealth Fund 1998 Survey of Women's Health. New York: The Commonwealth Fund; 1999.

counseling compared to women who had not completed college. [133]

There are regional differences in the use of HRT among women in the United States. Based on the NHEFS data, when they are compared with women in the Northeast, women in the West are two times more likely to use HRT therapy, women in the South are 1.9 times more likely, and women in the Midwest are 1.6 times more likely.[126] Other studies corroborate these findings.[6,131]

Data from large randomized controlled trials are not yet available from which to estimate the risks and benefits of HRT. However, there are several observational studies that have examined the effects of HRT use. Based on these studies, the use of postmenopausal HRT appears to carry both the benefit of a reduced risk of CHD[134] and osteoporosis[136] and a potential for an increased risk of breast and endometrial cancer[137,138,139] (see

chapter 4). Data from the Nurses' Health Study demonstrate that women who take estrogen HRT without progestin have a 40% reduction in the risk of developing CHD compared to women who do not take any HRT. Additionally, women who use combined estrogen and progestin HRT have a 60% reduction in risk. However, the risk of stroke increased by 27% for women who take estrogen alone.[134] The only published, randomized, controlled trial of HRT confined to a group of women who already had heart disease did not find any reduction of new episodes of heart disease.[135]

The declining levels of estrogen that accompany menopause also lead to increasing bone loss in postmenopausal women. Hormone replacement therapy with estrogen has been shown to reduce the risk of hip fracture among menopausal women. In a pooled analysis based upon several studies, a 25% reduction in risk of hip fractures was achieved.[136]

The risk of endometrial cancer with long-term use of estrogen alone among menopausal women is 8.2 times greater than for those who do not use therapy. However, this risk is reduced to 3.1 with the use of combined estrogen and progestin therapy with less than 10 days of progestin a month.[129] Another study reported no increase from baseline incidence with estrogen and progestin for at least 12 days a month.[140]

The relationship between breast cancer and HRT is less clear than that of endometrial cancer. Pooled results of 39 studies revealed that long-term use of estrogen increased the risk of breast cancer by 25%. However, there appears to be no increased risk among short-term users.[136] A recent study on the risk of breast cancer associated with combined estrogen and progestin reported a 1.4 times greater risk in thin women currently taking estrogen and progestin but did not find an increased risk with estrogen alone.[130] An analysis of the NHEFS data found no increase in breast cancer in women using estrogen replacement therapy or combined estrogen/progestin HRT even with more than 10 years of use.[141]

Overall, HRT appears to reduce mortality. In the Nurses' Health Study, the risk of all-cause mortality among current hormone users was 37% lower than among women who never used hormones. However, the long-term benefit over a period of 10 or more years of HRT use was not quite as large (a 20% reduction in overall mortality) due to the increased breast cancer mortality.[142] Based on data from a large cohort of women in a retirement community, there is an estimated 41% reduction in all-cause mortality for women between the ages of 50 and 75 taking estrogen.[143] A study in San Francisco reported a 46% reduction in mortality for women taking estrogen for 5 or more years.[144] (See chapter 4 discussion of breast cancer.)

Table 6-15

Douching practices among women aged 15–44 years by age, education, and region, 1995

| | Percent who douche regularly | | | |
	Total	White, non-Hispanic	Black, non-Hispanic	Hispanic
All women 15–44 years	26.9	20.8	55.3	33.4
Age (years)				
15–19	15.5	10.8	36.8	16.4
20–24	27.8	20.4	60.4	32.5
25–29	30.0	23.9	58.7	38.0
30–34	30.6	24.5	60.4	35.1
35–39	28.9	21.9	62.5	41.2
40–44	26.9	21.1	53.1	38.5
Education				
No high school diploma or GED	52.9	52.5	69.7	44.1
High school diploma or GED	36.5	30.2	64.5	43.6
Some college, no bachelor's degree	25.0	18.6	54.6	31.9
Bachelor's degree or higher	11.5	8.6	40.3	16.7
Region of residence				
Northeast	23.3	17.7	47.4	41.0
Midwest	24.4	18.8	60.3	39.5
South	35.0	28.3	57.0	33.0
West	20.5	15.2	49.3	30.1

Source: Abma J, Chandra A, Mosher W, Peterson L, Piccinino L. Fertility, family planning, and women's health: new data from the 1995 National Survey of Family Growth. Vital Health Stat 1997;23:1–114.

Vaginal Douching

Vaginal douching is a widespread practice among American women that may be hazardous to their reproductive health. According to recent industry figures, 200 million disposable douche preparations are sold in the U.S. annually.

Based on the 1995 National Survey of Family Growth (NSFG), it is estimated that about one quarter (27%) of U.S. women aged 15–44 years practice vaginal douching.[145] This represents a decline from the 1988 NSFG when 37% of women reported douching.[146] Although the overall prevalence has declined, douching is still more common among minority women (black and Hispanic) and less educated women (Table 6-15).[145] Among non-Hispanic black women without a high school diploma or GED, most women (approximately 70%) reported douching regularly. Rates are lowest for teenagers and vary little among women over 20 years of age. However, due to the cross-sectional nature of these data, it is not known if the low rates of douching among teenagers will continue as they age or whether they will initiate this behavior in their twenties.

Recent studies suggest that douching is associated with a number of adverse health outcomes, particularly pregnancy outcomes. Studies have directly linked douching to an increased risk of ectopic pregnancy,[147,148,149,150] preterm delivery,[151,152] and LBW babies.[153] Many studies have also documented an increased risk of infection and related conditions among women who douche. These include HIV,[154] pelvic infammatory disease (PID),[147] and bacterial vaginosis.[155,156] These infections can have far-reaching consequences even years after being acquired. Infections increase the risk of infertility through an increased risk of an ectopic pregnancy,[157,158,159,160,161] as well as through the development of PID subsequent to infection.[162,163,164] A variety of specific douching practices, such as frequency of douching, type of douching solution, timing (e.g., near ovulation, around intercourse), presence of infection, and douching technique, may influence degree of exposure and therefore the effect of douching on health outcomes. Prior studies examining these practices in detail have not made any effort to link them to adverse health outcomes. Consequently, it is not known which aspects of vaginal douching are most important in causing its untoward health effects.

References

1. Centers for Disease Control and Prevention. Cigarette smoking among adults—United States, 1995. MMWR Morb Mortal Wkly Rep 1997;46:1217–1220.

2. U.S. Public Health Service. Preventing tobacco use among young people: a report of the Surgeon General. Atlanta: U.S. Department of Health and Human Services, Public Health Service, Centers for Disease Control and Prevention, National Center for Chronic Disease Prevention and Health Promotion, Office on Smoking and Health; 1994. Available from: URL: www.cdc.gov/tobacco/sgryth2.htm.

3. Centers for Disease Control and Prevention. Cigarette smoking among adults—United States, 1997. MMWR Morb Mortal Wkly Rep 1999;48:993–996.

4. Blackman DK, Kamimoto LA, Smith SM. Overview: surveillance for selected public health indicators affecting older adults—United States. MMWR Morb Mortal Wkly Rep 1999;48:1–6.

5. U.S. Public Health Service. Tobacco use among U.S. racial/ethnic minority groups: African-Americans, American Indians and Alaska Natives, Asian Americans and Pacific Islanders: a report of the Surgeon General. Washington: U.S. Department of Health and Human Services, Centers for Disease Control, National Center for Chronic Disease Prevention and Health Promotion, Office on Smoking and Health; 1998. Available from: URL: www.cdc.gov/tobacco/sgr-minorities.htm.

6. Collins K, Schoen C, Joseph S, Duchon L, Simantov E, Yellowitz M. Health concerns across a woman's lifespan: The Commonwealth Fund 1998 Survey of Women's Health. New York: The Commonwealth Fund; 1999.

7. National Center for Health Statistics. Health, United States, 1998. Hyattsville (MD): U.S. Department of Health and Human Services; 1998.

8. Husten CG. Cigarette smoking among girls and women in the United States, 1965–1994. J Med Assoc Ga 1997;86:213–216.

9. Husten CG, Chrismon JH, Reddy MN. Trends and effects of cigarette smoking among girls and women in the United States, 1965–1993. J Am Med Womens Assoc 1996;51:11–18.

10. Healton C, Messeri P, Reynolds J, Wolfe C, Stokes C, Ross J, et al. Tobacco use among middle and high school students—United States, 1999. MMWR Morb Mortal Wkly Rep 2000;49:49–53.

11. Kann L, Kinchen S, Williams B, Ross J, Lowry R, Grunbaum JA, et al. Youth Risk Behavior Surveillance—United States, 1999. MMWR Morb Mortal Wkly Rep 2000;49(SS05):1–96.

12. Tobacco Use and Ethnicity. Washington: Campaign for Tobacco-Free Kids; 1997.

13. Ebrahim SH, Floyd RL, Merritt RK, Decoufle P, Holtzman D. Trends in pregnancy-related smoking rates in the United States, 1987–1996. JAMA. 2000;283:361–366.

14. Tollestrup K, Frost FJ, Starzyk P. Smoking prevalence of pregnant women compared to women in the general population of Washington State. Am J Prev Med 1992;8:215–220.

15. Day N, Richardson G. Comparative teratogenicity of alcohol and other drugs. Alcohol Health Res World 1994;18:42–48.

16. McCormick MC, Brooks-Gunn J, Shorter T, Holmes JH, Wallace CY, Heagarty MC. Factors associated with smoking in low-income pregnant women: relationship to birth weight, stressful life events, social support, health behaviors and mental distress. J Clin Epidemiol 1990;43:441–448.

17. Albrecht SA, Rosella JD, Patrick T. Smoking among low-income, pregnant women: prevalence rates, cessation interventions, and clinical implications. Birth 1994;21:155–162.

18. Fingerhut LA, Kleinman JC, Knedrick JS. Smoking before, during, and after pregnancy. Am J Public Health 1990;80:541–544.

19. O'Campo P, Davis MV, Gielen AC. Smoking cessation interventions for pregnant women: review and future directions. Semin Perinatol 1995;19:279–285.

20. Williamson DF, Serdula MK, Kendrick JS, Binkin NJ. Comparing the prevalence of smoking in pregnant and nonpregnant women, 1985 to 1986. JAMA 1989;261:70–74.

21. O'Campo P, Faden RR, Brown H, Gielen A. The impact of pregnancy on women's prenatal and postpartum smoking behavior. Am J Prev Med 1992;8:1–13.

22. Manfredi C, Lacey L, Warnecke R, Buis M. Smoking-related behavior, beliefs, and social environment of young black women in subsidized public housing in Chicago. Am J Public Health 1992;82:267–272.

23. Shervington DO. Attitudes and practices of African-American women regarding cigarette smoking: implications for interventions. J Natl Med Assoc 1994;86:337–343.

24. Escobedo LG, Reddy M, DuRant RH. Relationship between cigarette smoking and health risk and problem behaviors among U.S. adolescents. Arch Pediatr Adolesc Med 1997;151:66–71.

25. Resnick MD, Bearman PS, Blum RW, Bauman KE, Harris KM, Jones J, et al. Protecting adolescents from harm: findings from the National Longitudinal Study on Adolescent Health. JAMA 1997;278:823–832.

26. Perkins KA, Sexton JE, DiMarco A. Acute thermogenic effects of nicotine and alcohol in healthy male and female smokers. Physiol Behav 1996;60:305–309.

27. Wilson D, Taylor A, Roberts L. Can we target smoking groups more effectively? A study of male and female heavy smokers. Prev Med 1995;24:363–368.

28. Crisp A, Sedgwick P, Halek C, Joughin N, Humphrey H. Why may teenage girls persist in smoking. J Adolesc 1999;22:657–672.

29. Kristeller J, Johnson T. Smoking effects and cessation. In: Rosenfeld J, editor. Women's Health in Primary Care. Baltimore: Williams & Wilkins; 1997. p. 93–116.

30. Vierola H. Tobacco and women's health. Helsinki: Hakapaino Oy; 1998. p. 324.

31. Devesa SS, Blot WJ, Stone BJ, Miller BA, Tarone RE, Fraumeni JF Jr. Recent cancer trends in the United States. J Natl Cancer Inst 1995;87:175–182.

32. Centers for Disease Control and Prevention. Mortality trends for selected smoking-related cancers and breast-cancer—United States, 1950–1990. MMWR Morb Mortal Wkly Rep 1993;42:857, 863–866.

33. American Cancer Society. Cancer Facts & Figures—2000. Atlanta: American Cancer Society; 2000.

34. Association of Reproductive Health Professionals. Clinical proceedings: implications of smoking and oral contraceptive use. ARHP Clin Proc 1996 Mar:1–12.

35. MacKenzie TD, Bartecchi CE, Schrier RW. The human costs of tobacco use. N Engl J Med 1994;330:975–980.

36. Baron J, Weiderpass E. Birth control, hormones, and reproduction. ARHP Clin Proc 1996 Oct:3–8.

37. Qandil R, Sandhu HS, Matthews DC. Tobacco smoking and periodontal diseases. J Can Dent Assoc 1997;63:187–192.

38. American College of Obstetricians and Gynecologists. Smoking and reproductive health: ACOG Technical Bulletin Number 180—May 1993. Int J Gynaecol Obstet 1993;43:75–81.

39. Baird DD, Wilcox AJ. Cigarette smoking associated with delayed conception. JAMA 1985;253:2979–2983.

40. Cigarette smoking and the risk of low birth weight: a comparison in black and white women. Alameda County Low Birth Weight Study Group. Epidemiology 1990;1:201–205.

41. Hellerstedt WL, Himes JH, Story M, Alton IR, Edwards LE. The effects of cigarette smoking and gestational weight change on birth outcomes in obese and normal-weight women. Am J Public Health 1997;87:591–596.

42. Li CQ, Windsor RA, Perkins L, Goldenberg RL, Lowe JB. The impact of infant birth weight and gestational age of cotine-validated smoking reduction during pregnancy. JAMA 1993;269:1519–1524.

43. Walsh RA. Effects of maternal smoking on adverse pregnancy outcomes: examination of the criteria of causation. Hum Biol 1994;66:1059–1092.

44. Substance Abuse and Mental Health Services Administration (SAMSHA). National Household Survey on Drug Abuse: population estimates, 1998. Rockville (MD): U.S. Department of Health and Human Services, Office of Applied Statistics; 1999. Available from: URL: www.samhsa.gov/statistics/statistics.html.

45. Grant BF, Dawson DA. Age at onset of alcohol use and its association with DSM-IV alcohol abuse and dependence: results from the National Longitudinal Alcohol Epidemiologic Survey. J Subst Abuse 1997;9:103–110.

46. Centers for Disease Control and Prevention. Alcohol consumption among pregnant and childbearing-aged women—United States, 1991 and 1995. MMWR Morb Mortal Wkly Rep 1997; 46:346–350.

47. National Institute on Drug Abuse. National pregnancy & health survey: Drug use among women delivering live births: 1992. Rockville (MD): U.S. Department of Health and Human Services; 1996.

48. Chen K, Kandel DB. The natural history of drug use from adolescence to the mid-thirties in a general population sample. Am J Public Health 1995;85:41–47.

49. Allen K, Feeney E. Alcohol and other drug use, abuse, and dependence. In: Allen K, Phillips J, editors. Women's health across the lifespan: a comprehensive perspective. Philadelphia: Lippincott; 1997. p. 256–288.

50. Kendler KS, Heath AC, Neale MC, Kessler RC, Eaves LJ. A population-based twin study of alcoholism in women. JAMA 1992;268:1877–1882.

51. Howard JM, editor. Women and alcohol: issues for prevention research. Bethesda (MD): National Institutes of Health, National Institute on Alcohol Abuse and Alcoholism; 1996.

52. Gomberg ES. Alcoholic women in treatment: early histories and early problem behaviors. Adv Alcohol Subst Abuse 1989;8:133–147.

53. Miller BA, Downs WR, Testa M. Interrelationships between victimization experiences and women's alcohol use. J Stud Alcohol 1993;11 Suppl:109–117.

54. Hall P. Factors affecting individual susceptibility to alcoholic liver disease. In: Hall P, editor. Alcoholic liver disease: pathology and pathogenesis. 2nd ed. Boston: Edward Arnold; 1995. p. 299–316.

55. Gavaler J, Arria A. Increased susceptibility of women to alcohol liver disease: artifactual or real? In: Hall P, editor. Alcoholic liver disease: pathology and pathogenesis. 2nd ed. Boston: Edward Arnold; 1995. p. 123–133.

56. Mishra L, Sharma S, Potter JJ, Mezey E. More rapid elimination of alcohol in women as compared to their male siblings. Alcohol Clin Exp Res 1989;13:752–754.

57. Kannel WB, Ellison RC. Alcohol and coronary heart disease: the evidence for a protective effect. Clin Chim Acta 1996;246:59–76.

58. Fraser G. Preventive cardiology. New York: Oxford University Press; 1986.

59. Wilsnack S, Wilsnack R, Hiller-Sturmhofel S. How women drink: epidemiology of women's drinking and problem drinking. Alcohol Health Res World 1994;18.

60. U.S. Indian Health Service. Trends in Indian health. Washington: U.S. Department of Health and Human Services, U.S. Indian Health Service, Office of Planning, Evaluation, and Legislation; 1994.

61. Resnick MD, Bearman PS, Blum RW, Bauman KE, Harris KM, Hones J, et al. Protecting adolescents from harm. Findings from the National Longitudinal Study on Adolescent Health. JAMA 1997;278:823–832.

62. Hutchins E, DiPietro J. Psychosocial risk factors associated with cocaine use during preganancy: a case-control study. Obstet Gynecol 1997;90:142–147.

63. Paltrow L. Perspective of a reproductive rights attorney. The Future of Children 1991;1(1):85–86.

64. Lindenberg CS, Gendrop SC, Reiskin HK. Empirical evidence for the social stress model of substance abuse. Res Nurs Health 1993;16:351–362.

65. Chavkin W. Psychiatric histories of drug-using mothers: treatment implications. J Subst Abuse Treat 1993;10:445–448.

66. Robins L, Mills J. Effects of in utero exposure to street drugs. Am J Public Health 1993;83 Suppl:1–32.

67. Lindenberg CS, Alexander EM, Gendrop SC, Nencioli M, Williams DG. A review of the literature on cocaine abuse in pregnancy. Nurs Res 1991;40:69–75.

68. Bendersky M, Alessandri S, Gilbert P, Lewis M. Characteristics of pregnant substance abusers in two cities in the northeast. Am J Drug Alcohol Abuse 1996;22:349–362.

69. Lutiger B, Graham K, Einarson T, Koren G. Relationship between gestational cocaine use and pregnancy outcome: a meta-analysis. Teratology 1991;44:405–414.

70. Beebe D. Addictive behaviors. In: Rosenfeld J, editor. Women's health in primary care. Baltimore: Williams & Wilkins; 1997. p. 227–240.

71. Lex B. Alcohol and other drug abuse among women. Alcohol Health Res World 1994;18:212–220.

72. Rach-Beisel J, Dixon L, Gearon J. Awareness of substance abuse problems among dually diagnosed psychiatric inpatients. J Psychoactive Drugs 1999;31:53–57.

73. Regier DA, Farmer ME, Rae DS, Locke BZ, Keith SJ, Judd LL. Comorbidity of mental disorders with alcohol and other drug abuse. Results from the Epidemiologic Catchment Area Study. JAMA 1990;264:2511–2518.

74. Dattel BJ. Substance abuse in pregnancy. Semin Perinatol 1990;14:179–187.

75. Mayes LC, Granger RH, Bornstein MH, Zuckerman B. The problem of prenatal cocaine exposure. A rush to judgement. JAMA 1992;267:406–408.

76. Substance Abuse and Mental Health Services Administration (SAMHSA). Summary of findings from the 1999 National Household Survey on Drug Abuse. Rockville (MD): U.S. Department of Health and Human Services, SAMHSA, Office of Applied Studies; 2000. Available from: URL: www.samhsa.gov/statistics/statistics.html.

77. Centers for Disease Control and Prevention. Behavioral risk factor surveillance system: 1998 summary prevalence report; 1998. Available from: URL: www.cdc.gov/hccdphp/brfss/pdf/98prvrpt.pdf.

78. Crespo CJ, Keteyian SJ, Heath GW, Sempos CJ. Leisure-time physical activity among U.S. adults. Results from the Third National Health and Nutrition Examination Study. Arch Intern Med 1996;156:93–98.

79. Mokdad AH, Serdula MK, Dietz WH, Bowman BA, Marks JS, Koplan JP. The spread of the obesity epidemic in the United States, 1991–1998. JAMA 1999;282:1519–1522.

80. Brownson RC, Eyler AA, King AC, Brown DR, Shyu Y-L, Sallis JF. Patterns and correlates of physical activity among U.S. women 40 years and older. Am J Public Health 2000;90:264–270.

81. U.S. Public Health Service. Physical activity and health: a report of the Surgeon General. S/N 017–023–00196–5. Atlanta: U.S. Department of Health and Human Services, Centers for Disease Control and Prevention, National Center for Chronic Disease Prevention and Health Promotion; 1996.

82. Sallis JF, Prochaska JJ, Taylor WC. A review of correlates of physical activity among children and adolescents. Med Sci Sport Exerc 2000;32:963–975.

83. Centers for Disease Control and Prevention. Neighborhood safety and the prevalence of physical inactivity—selected states, 1996. MMWR Morb Mortal Wkly Rep 1999;48:143–146.

84. Sesso HD, Paffenbarger RS, Ha T, Lee I-M. Physical activity and cardiovascular disease risk in middle-aged and older women. Am J Epidemiol 1999;150:408–416.

85. Rockhill B, Willett WC, Hunter DJ, Manson JE, Hankinson SE, Colditz GA. A prospective study of recreational physical activity and breast cancer risk. Arch Intern Med 1999;159:2290–2296.

86. Hu FB, Stampfer MJ, Colditz GA, Ascherio A, Rexrode KM, Willett WC, et al. Physical activity and risk of stroke in women. JAMA 2000;283:2961–2967.

87. Hu FB, Sigal RJ, Rich-Edwards JW, Colditz GA, Solomon CG, Willett WC, et al. Walking compared with vigorous physical activity and risk of type 2 dibetes in women: a prospective study. JAMA 1999;282:1433–1439.

88. Kelley GA. Exercise and regional bone mineral density in post-menopausal women: a meta-analytic review of randomized trials. Am J Phys Med Rehabil. 1998;77:76–87.

89. Brinton LA, Bernstein L, Colditz GA. Summary of the workshop: workshop on physical activity and breast cancer, November 13–14, 1997. Cancer 1998;83 Suppl:595–599.

90. Friedenreich CM, Thune I, Brinton LA, Albanes D. Epidemiologic issues related to the association between physical activity and breast cancer. Cancer 1998;83(3 Suppl):600–610.

91. Giovannucci E, Colditz GA, Stampfer MJ, Willett WC. Physical activity, obesity, and risk of colorectal adenoma in women (United States). Cancer Causes Control 1996;7:253–263.

92. National Center for Health Statistics. Report of final mortality statistics, 1995. Mon Vital Stat Rep 1997;45 Suppl 2.

93. Fox B, Cameron A. Food science, nutrition and health. 6th ed. Boston: Edward Arnold; 1995. p. 388.

94. National Research Council, National Institutes of Health, Food and Nutrition Board NRC. Recommended dietary allowances. Subcommittee on the Tenth Edition of the RDAs. 10th ed. Washington: National Academy Press; 1989. p. 285.

95. U.S. Department of Agriculture ARS. Data tables: results from USDA's 1994–96 Continuing Survey of Food Intakes by Individuals. U.S. Department of Agriculture, Agricultural Research Service, Beltsville Human Nutrition Research Center; 1997. Available from: URL: nps.ars.usda.gov/publications/publications.htm.

96. Albu J, Allison D, Boozer CN, Heymsfield S, Kissileff H, Kretsser A, et al. Obesity solutions: report of a meeting. Nutr Rev 1997; 55:150–156.

97. U.S. Department of Agriculture ARS. Data tables: results from USDA's 1995 Continuing Survey of Food Intakes by Individuals and 1995 Diet and Health Knowledge Survey. U.S. Department of Agriculture, Agricultural Research Service, Beltsville Human Nutrition Center; 1995.

98. Centers for Disease Control and Prevention. Update: prevalence of overweight among children, adolescents, and adults—United States, 1988–1994. MMWR Morb Mortal Wkly Rep 1997;46: 198–202.

99. Flegal KM, Carroll MD, Kuczmarski RJ, Johnson CI. Overweight and obesity trends in the United States: prevalence and trends, 1960–1994. Int J Obes Relat Metab Disord 1998;22:39–47.

100. Manson JE, Stampfer MJ, Hennekens CH, Willett WC. Body weight and longevity. A reassessment. JAMA 1987;257:353–358.

101. Manson JE, Willett WC, Stampfer MJ, Colditz GA, Hunter DJ, Hankinson SE, et al. Body weight and mortality among women. N Engl J Med 1995;333:677–685.

102. National Research Council. Committee on Diet and Health. Diet and health: implications for reducing chronic disease risk. Washington: National Academy Press; 1989.

103. Colditz GA, Willett WC, Stampfer MJ, Manson JE, Hennekens CH, Arky RA, et al. Weight as a risk factor for clinical diabetes in women. Am J Epidemiol 1990;132:501–513.

104. Kannel WB, D'Agostino RB, Cobb JL. Effect of weight on cardiovascular disease. Am J Clin Nutr 1996;63(3 Suppl):419S–422S.

105. Felson DT. Weight and osteoarthritis. Am J Clin Nutr 1996;63(3 Suppl):430S–432S.

106. Ballard-Barbash R, Swanson C. Body weight: estimation of risk for breast and endometrial cancers. Am J Clin Nutr 1996;63(3 Suppl):437S–431S.

107. Pi-Sunyer F. Weight and non-insulin-dependent diabetes mellitus. Am J Clin Nutr 1996;63(3 Suppl):426S–429S.

108. Must A, Spadano J, Coakley EH, Field AE, Colditz G, Dietz WH. The disease burden associated with overweight and obesity. JAMA 1999;282:1523–1529.

109. Rissanen A, Heliovaara M, Knekt P, Reunanen A, Aromaa A, Maatela J. Risk of disability and mortality due to overweight in a Finnish population. BMJ 1990;301:835–837.

110. Seidell JC, Verschuren WM, Van Leer EM, Kromhout D. Overweight, underweight, and mortality. A prospective study of 48,287 men and women. Arch Intern Med 1996;156:958–963.

111. Federation of American Societies for Experimental Biology LSRO. Third report on nutrition monitoring in the United States: executive summary. Washington: Interagency Board for Nutrition Monitoring and Related Research; 1995. p. 51.

112. Winick M. The Columbia encyclopedia of nutrition. New York: Putnam's; 1987:349.

113. Mills JL, Scott JM, Kirke PN, McPartlin JM, Conley MR, Weir DG, et al. Homocysteine and neural tube defects. J Nutr 1996;126:756S–760S.

114. Smithells RW, Sheppard S, Schorah CT, Seller MJ, Nevin NC, Harris R, et al. Apparent prevention of neural tube defects by periconceptional vitamin supplementation. Arch Dis Child 1981;56:911–918.

115. Wald N. Folic acid and the prevention of neural tube defects. BMJ 1995;310:1019–1020.

116. Centers for Disease Control and Prevention. Knowledge and use of folic acid by women of childbearing age—United States, 1995 and 1998. MMWR Morb Mortal Wkly Rep 1999;48:325–327.

117. Lawrence JM, Petitti DB, Watkins M, Umekubo MA. Trends in serum folate after food fortification. Lancet 1999;354:915–916.

118. Winick M. Nutrition in health and disease. New York: Wiley; 1980. p. 261.

119. Centers for Disease Control and Prevention. Recommendations to prevent and control iron deficiency in the United States. MMWR Morb Mortal Wkly Rep 1998;47:1–29.

120. Looker AC, Dallman PR, Carroll MD, Gunter EW, Johnson CL. Prevalence of iron deficiency in the United States. JAMA 1997;277:973–976.

121. Earl RO, Woteki CE, editors. Institute of Medicine. Iron deficiency anemia: recommended guidelines for the prevention, detection, and management among U.S. children and women of childbearing age. Washington: National Academy Press; 1993.

122. Yip R, Dallman P. Iron. In: Ziegler E, Filer LJ, editors. Present knowledge in nutrition. 7th ed. Washington: International Life Sciences Institute Press; 1996. p. 277–292.

123. Mooij PN, Thomas CM, Doesburg WH, Eskes TK. The effects of oral contraceptives and multivitamin supplementation on serum ferritin and hematological parameters. Int J Clin Pharmacol Ther Toxicol 1992;30:57–62.

124. Bothwell T, Charlton R. Iron deficiency in women. Washington: The Nutrition Foundation; 1981.

125. Lee G. Iron deficiency and iron-deficiency anemia. In: Wintrobe MM, Lee GR, editors. Wintrobe's clinical hematology. 10th ed. Baltimore: Williams & Wilkins; 1999:979–1010.

126. Brett KM, Madans JH. Use of postmenopausal hormone replacement therapy: estimates from a nationally representative cohort study. Am J Epidemiol 1997;145:536–545.

127. Wysowski DK, Golden L, Burke L. Use of menopausal estrogens and medroxyprogesterone in the United States, 1982–1992. Obstet Gynecol 1995;85:6–10.

128. Belchetz PE. Hormonal treatment of postmenopausal women. N Engl J Med 1994;330:1062-1071.

129. Beresford SA, Weiss NS, Voigt LF, McKnight B. Risk of endometrial cancer in relation to use of oestrogen combined with cyclic progestagen therapy in postmenopausal women. Lancet 1997;349:458–461.

130. Schairer C, Lubin J, Troisi R, Sturgeon S, Brinton L, Hoover R. Menopausal estrogen and estrogen-progestin replacement therapy and breast cancer risk. JAMA 2000;283:485–491.

131. Rosenberg L, Plamer JR, Rao RS, Adams-Campbell L. Correlates of postmenopausal female hormone use among black women in the United States. Obstet Gynecol 1998;91:454–458.

132. Marsh JV, Brett KM, Miller LC. Racial differences in hormone replacement therapy prescriptions. Obstet Gynecol 1999; 93:999–1003.

133. Zhang P, Tao G, Anderson LA. Prevalence of and factors associated with hormone replacement therapy counseling: results from the 1994 National Health Interview Survey. Am J Public Health. 1999;89:1575–1577.

134. Grodstein F, Stampfer MJ, Manson JE, Colditz GA, Willett WC, Rosner B, et al. Postmenopausal estrogen and progestin use and the risk of cardiovascular disease. N Engl J Med 1996; 335:453–460.

135. Hulley S, Grady D, Bush T, furberg C, HerringtonD, Riggs B, et al. Randomized trial of estrogen plus progestin for secondary prevention of coronary heart disease in postmenopausal women. Heart and Estrogen/Progestin Replacement Study (HERS) Research Group. JAMA 1998;280:605–613.

136. Grady D, Rubin SM, Pettiti DB, Fox CS, Black D, Ettinger B, et al. Hormone therapy to prevent disease and prolong life in postmenopausal women. Ann Intern Med 1992;117:1016–1037.

137. Bush TL, Whiteman MK. Hormone replacement therapy and risk of breast cancer. JAMA 1999;281:2140–2141.

138. Colditz GA. Hormones and breast cancer: evidence and implications for consideration of risks and benefits of hormone replacement therapy. J Womens Health 1999;8:347–357.

139. Gapstur S, Morrow M, Sellers T. Hormone replacement therapy and risk of breast cancer with a favorable histology: results of the Iowa Women's Health Study. JAMA 1999;281:2091–2097.

140. Persson I, Yuen J, Bergkvist L, Schairer C. Cancer incidence and mortality in women receiving estrogen and estrogen-progestin replacement therapy—long-term follow up of a Swedish cohort. Int J Cancer 1996;67:327–332.

141. Lando JF, Heck KE, Brett KM. Hormone replacement therapy and breast cancer risk in a nationally representative cohort. Am J Prev Med 1999;17:176–180.

142. Grodstein F, Stampfer MJ, Colditz GA, Willet WC, Manson JE, Joffe M, et al. Postmenopausal hormone therapy and mortality. N Engl J Med 1997;336:1769–1775.

143. Henderson BE, Ross RK, Pagini-Hill A, Mack TM. Estrogen use and cardiovascular disease. Am J Obstet Gynecol 1986; 154:1181–1186.

144. Ettinger B, Friedman GD, Bush T, Quesenberry CP. Reduced mortality associated with long-term postmenopausal estrogen therapy. Obstet Gynecol 1996;87:6–12.

145. Abma JC, Chandra A, Mosher WD, Peterson LS, Piccinino LJ. Fertility, family planning, and women's health: new data from the 1995 National Survey of Family Growth. Vital Health Stat 1997;23:1–114.

146. Aral SO, Mosher WD, Cates W. Vaginal douching among women of reproductive age in the United States: 1988. Am J Public Health 1992;82:210–214.

147. Zhang J, Thomas G, Leybovich E. Vaginal douching and adverse health effects: a meta-analysis. Am J Public Health 1997;87:1207–1211.

148. Kendrick JS, Atrash HK, Strauss LT, Gargiullo PM, Ahn YW. Vaginal douching and the risk of ectopic pregnancy among black women. Am J Obstet Gynecol 1997;176:991–997.

149. Daling JR, Weiss NS, Schwartz SM, Stergachis A, Wang SP, Foy H, et al. Vaginal douching and the risk of tubal pregnancy. Epidemiology 1991;2:40–48.

150. Chow WH, Daling JR, Weiss NS, Moore DE, Soderstrom R. Vaginal douching as a potential risk factor for ectopic pregnancy. Am J Obstet Gynecol 1985;153:727–729.

151. Bruce FC, Kendrick JS, Strauss LT, Gargiullo PM, Atrash HK. Does vaginal douching increase the risk of preterm delivery? Baltimore: Society for Pediatric Epidemiologic Research; 1999.

152. Bruce FC, Fiscella K, Kendrick JS. Vaginal douching and preterm birth: an intriguing hypothesis. Med Hypotheses 2000;54:448–452.

153. Fiscella K, Franks P, Kendrick JS, Bruce FC. The risk of low birth weight associated with vaginal douching. Obstet Gynecol 1998;92:913–917.

154. Gresenguet G, Kreiss JK, Chapko MK, Hillier SL, Weiss NS. HIV infection and vaginal douching in central Africa. AIDS 1997; 11:101–106.

155. Hawes SE, Hillier SL, Benedetti J, Stevens CE, Koutsky LA, Wolner-Hanssen P, et al. Hydrogen peroxide-producing lactobacilli and acquisition of vaginal infections. J Infect Dis 1996;174:1058–1063.

156. Onderdonk AB, Delaney ML, Hinkson PL, DuBois AM. Quantitative and qualitative effects of douche preparations on vaginal microflora. Obstet Gynecol 1992;80(3 Pt 1):333–338.

157. Brunham RC, Binns B, McDowell J, Paraskevas M. Chlamydia trachomatis infection in women with ectopic pregnancy. Obstet Gynecol 1986;67:722–726.

158. Cates W, Wasserheit JN. Genital chlamydial infections: epidemiology and reproductive sequelae. Am J Obstet Gynecol 1991;164(6 Pt 2):1771–1781.

159. Chow JM, Yonekura ML, Richwald GA, Greenland S, Sweet RL, Schacter J. The association between Chlamydia trachomatis and ectopic pregnancy. A matched-pair, case control study. JAMA 1990;263:3164–3167.

160. Chrysostomou M, Karafyllidi P, Papadimitriou V, Bassiotou V, Mayakos G. Serum antibodies to Chlamydia trachomatis in women with ectopic pregnancy, normal pregnancy, or salpingitis. Eur J Obstet Gynecol Reprod Biol 1992;44:101–115.

161. Phillips RS, Tuomala RE, Feldblum PJ, Schachter J, Rosenberg MJ, Aronson MD. The effect of cigarette smoking, Chlamydia trachomatis infection, and vaginal douching on ectopic pregnancy. Obstet Gynecol 1992;79:85–90.

162. Westrom L. Effect of pelvic inflammatory disease on fertility. Venereology 1995;8:219–222.

163. Coste J, Job-Spira N, Fernandez H, Papiernik E, Spira A. Risk factors for ectopic pregnancy: a case-control study in France with special focus on infectious factors. Am J Epidemiol 1991;133:839–849.

164. Brunham RC, Binns B, Guijon F, Danforth D, Kosseim ML, Rand F, et al. Etiology and outcome of acute pelvic inflammatory disease. J Infect Dis 1988;158:510–517.

Chapter 7

Violence Against Women

Contents

Introduction

Violence against women is a significant public health problem in the United States. Its consequences pervade all ethnic, racial, and socioeconomic groups. Although violent victimization rates for both men and women have declined in recent years, rates remain high. Based on 1998 National Crime Victimization Survey (NCVS) data, women experienced approximately 3.5 million nonlethal, violent victimizations—rapes, sexual assaults, robberies, aggravated assaults, and simple assaults—compared with 4.6 million experienced by men (Table 7-1).[1] It should be noted, however, that routine data sources likely underestimate violence, particularly violence against women by intimate partners. Over the past decade, recognition of violence against women has increased among health care providers. Currently, all U.S.-accredited medical schools include domestic violence training in their curricula.[2]

The rates of violent victimization are higher for some women than others. Table 7-2 describes rates of nonlethal violence for men and women by characteristics of the victim based on 1998 NCVS data.[1] Rates are higher for African American women and adolescent and young women. Married and widowed women experienced the lowest rates of nonlethal violence. Marital status is interesting to examine as those who are divorced or separated are the only group in which women experience higher rates of victimization than men.[1] In an analysis of older (1994) NCVS data, investigators compared men and women across these and other characteristics to determine whether differences were statistically significant. Statistically higher rates were found for males across race, ethnicity, household income, place of residence (urban/rural/suburban), age, education, and marital status. In a few groups, male rates were higher, but the difference was not statistically significant (African Americans, household income $7,500–$14,999, 25–34 years old). In one group (marital status of separated), women had higher rates than men (127.8 versus 79.1 per 1,000).[3]

Table 7-1

Nonlethal violent victimization by sex, race, and ethnicity of victim, 1998

	Rates per 1,000 persons aged 12 years or older							
	Women				Men			
	Race/Ethnicity				Race/Ethnicity			
	Total	White	Black	Hispanic	Total	White	Black	Hispanic
All violent crimes	30.4	29.7	37.5	26.8	43.1	43.1	46.6	38.9
Rape/sexual assault	2.7	2.7	3.3	1.7	0.2	0.2	0.5	0
Robbery	3.5	3.1	5.6	4.9	4.6	4.3	6.2	7.8
Aggravated assault	4.7	4.3	7.1	4.1	10.5	9.7	17.6	8.2
Simple assault	19.5	19.6	21.5	16.1	27.8	29.0	22.2	22.9

Note: "White" and "Black" categories include Hispanic and non-Hispanic persons.

Source: U.S. Department of Justice, Bureau of Justice Statistics. Criminal victimization in the United States, 1998 statistical tables. Data tables 2, 6, 7. NCJ-181585. 2000 May 25. Available from: URL: www.ojp.usdoj.gov/bjs/abstract/cvusst.htm.

Although less likely than males to experience violent crime, women are five times more likely to be victimized by an intimate partner (at rates of 767 versus 146 per 100,000 persons, respectively).[4] From 1992 to 1998, violent victimization by an intimate partner accounted for 22% of the violence experienced by women, amounting to an estimated 876,340 victimizations each year.[4] An additional one-third of these crimes were committed by a friend or acquaintance. Three million of the 5 million violent crimes against women in 1994 were committed by someone known to the victim.[3] These proportions vary greatly depending on the crime committed (e.g., rape, murder). The term intimate partner violence (IPV) is used to describe actual or threatened physical, sexual, or psychological abuse. Many terms have been commonly used to describe IPV, including domestic violence, domestic abuse, spouse abuse, battering, marital rape, and date rape. Intimate partners include current or former spouses, boyfriends, or girlfriends and encompass both heterosexual and homosexual relationships.

Consequences of Violence

The consequences of violence are both physical and psychological. They may be severe and long term. Short-term physical consequences include broken bones, bruises, and cuts.[5] Medical problems include miscarriage, preterm labor, fetal injury, sexually transmitted diseases (STDs), hearing or vision loss, chronic headaches, and chronic pain.[5] Psychological effects can include depression, anxiety, suicide attempts, substance abuse, post-traumatic stress disorder, and revictimization.[6] The medical consequences of abuse are likely to be underreported, as most women do not disclose their abuse history to their health care providers nor are providers comfortable asking. There are also many social consequences to abuse; these include but are not limited to job loss, diminished work productivity, and social isolation.[5]

Injuries and Medical Care

Reports of injuries and subsequent health care seeking behavior depend upon whether the

Table 7-2

Violence victimization rates by characteristics of victims, 1998*		
	Rates per 1,000 persons aged 12 years or older	
Victim characteristic	**Women**	**Men**
Crimes of violence**	30.4	43.1
Race		
White	29.7	43.1
Black	37.5	46.6
Ethnicity		
Hispanic	26.8	38.9
Non-Hispanic	30.8	43.2
Age (years)		
12–15	62.3	101.7
16–19	72.6	108.6
20–24	59.9	75.6
25–34	35.2	47.9
35–49	28.9	31.0
50–64	13.1	17.9
65 and over	2.1	3.8
Marital Status		
Never married	55.7	75.9
Married	13.3	22.0
Widowed	6.9	5.8
Divorced or separated	61.3	51.8

*These rates do not include homicide.

**Includes verbal threats of rape and sexual assault.

Source: U.S. Department of Justice, Bureau of Justice Statistics. Criminal victimization in the United States, 1998 statistical tables. Data tables 2, 4, 6, 8, 12. NCJ-181585. 2000 May 25. Available from: URL: www.ojp.usdoj.gov/bjs/abstract/cvusst.htm.

perpetrator is a stranger or someone who is a partner.[4] Slightly more than half of female victims of violence by an intimate partner are physically injured in the attack; however, only four in 10 of these women seek professional medical treatment.[4] Hospital emergency department data demonstrate that women account for 39% of hospital emergency department visits for violence-related injuries. However, 84% of the women who did visit the hospital were treated for injuries inflicted by an intimate partner.[7]

Economic Costs of Violence

Few studies have examined the direct and indirect costs of violence against women. Those that have suggest that the costs to both the victims and society are considerable. These include the costs of health care, child welfare, foster care, emergency shelter, criminal arrests, and incarceration. Estimates based on medical treatment, lost worker productivity, and quality of life have indicated that costs to the nation may be as high as $67 billion annually.[8] Recent findings from the NCVS have yielded lower estimates, concluding that victims lost $150 million a year in medical expenses, cash loss, property damage or loss, and lost pay (Table 7-3).[7] Cost of medical and psychological services to victims of violence is estimated to range between $1,075 and $1,633 per woman each year.[7,9]

Causes of Violence

Research has unveiled a number of theories regarding the causes of violence against women. Most emphasize the importance of social context. Issues include poverty and economic deprivation; exposure to racism and classism for the perpetrators and sexism for the victim; women having more economic or human capital resources than their partners; patriarchal traditions permitting men to exercise their will over female partners; pathological personality characteristics of the perpetrators; poor coping skills in response to stress by the perpetrators; and social learning by the perpetrators in the home during childhood, experiences in young adulthood and through media influences.[5]

Table 7-3

Expenses for women victims of nonlethal intimate violence, 1992–1996

	Women victims of intimate violence		
	Percent of victims experiencing an expense or loss	Average expense or loss per victim reporting a loss	Estimated total loss annually (in millions of dollars)
Medical expenses	6.0	$1,075	$61.8
Cash loss	1.1	455	4.9
Property			
Loss	4.3	734	30.3
Repair	5.8	189	10.5
Replacement	5.3	478	24.3
Lost pay from			
Injury	4.3	261	10.8
Other cause	2.8	255	6.9

Note: These are the most recent figures available that estimate total dollar costs of nonlethal intimate partner violence.

Source: Greenfeld LA, Rand MR, Rand D, Craven PA, Klaus CA, Perkins C, et al. Violence by intimates: analysis of data on crimes by current or former spouses, boyfriends, and girlfriends. Bureau of Justice statistics factbook. NCJ–167237. Washington: Bureau of Justice Statistics, U.S. Department of Justice; 1998.

Risk factors for victims include young age; social isolation; higher educational or occupational status than the male partner; pregnancy, early postpartum period; substance use on the part of the partners and/or victims; economic strain and unemployment of the partner; exposure to other stressors such as economic, occupational, or race discrimination; and previous violent relationships.[10]

Data Collection and Reporting

How researchers define different types of violence against women plays an important role in determining the scope of the problem. Reporting of violence is likely to be underestimated by routine sources such as police reports, crime surveys, and medical records.[11] Such routine sources are likely to underestimate victimization rates because approximately half of women who have been victimized do not report their experiences to anyone.[6] In-person interviews and telephone surveys tend to yield higher estimates of violence because of women's greater willingness to disclose sensitive information when asked directly. In addition, reports to law enforcement entities of physical and sexual abuse by intimate partners are underestimated because some women may not view such acts as abusive.[10] Reports of abuse may not be documented in medical records because of the victim's fear that documentation will lead to denial of health insurance.[10]

Physical Assault

Physical assault encompasses a range of attacks, including being pushed, hit, slapped, kicked, bitten, choked, attacked, or threatened with a gun or knife. According to the 1998 NCVS, there were approximately 2.8 million aggravated and simple assaults against women ages 12 and older.[1] The 1995–1996 National Violence Against Women Survey (NVAW) found that 52% of women reported being physically assaulted either as a child or as an adult.[11] Based on these reports, an estimated 52 million women have been assaulted during their lifetimes.[11]

Women are significantly more likely to be assaulted by an intimate partner than men.[3] A 1996 review of the literature reported that 8% to 17% of women in the past year have experienced acts of violence inflicted by current or former partners.[12] One study suggests that an estimated 4.4 million women are physically assaulted by intimate partners, and 1.7 million of these women suffer severe abuse each year.[13]

Women who are physically assaulted are more likely to be younger, separated or divorced, of lower socioeconomic status, and unemployed.[12]

Studies of possible associations between violence and race or ethnic background have been less conclusive.[12]

Physical injuries inflicted on women include cuts, scratches, bruises, sprains, broken bones, knife wounds, broken teeth, burns, bites, and broken eardrums.[14] Psychological consequences for victims of physical assault include depression, anxiety, lowered self-esteem, suicidal thoughts, substance abuse, and post-traumatic stress disorder.[10]

Violence Against Pregnant Women

Intimate partner violence does not end when a woman becomes pregnant. On the contrary, pregnancy is a period of increased risk for violence perpetrated by intimate partners. Population-based data from the Pregnancy Risk Assessment Monitoring System (PRAMS) indicate that between 3.8% and 6.9% of women reported being physically hurt by their husband or partner in the 12 months preceding childbirth.[15] One study, however, found no difference in reports of violence between pregnant and nonpregnant women, after controlling for the ages of the women and their partners.[16]

A number of studies have attempted to identify the risk factors for violence during pregnancy. Rates of physical violence have been found to be higher for women who are young, have fewer than 12 years of education, are unmarried, are of low socio-economic status, participated in the WIC program during pregnancy, had delayed or no prenatal care, and have had an unintended pregnancy.[15,17]

Research into the effects of physical violence during pregnancy on birth outcomes has reached mixed conclusions. Some studies have demonstrated effects on birthweight, preterm labor, medical complications, spontaneous abortion and use of health care, yet other studies find no such differences.[18,19,20,21] Others have hypothesized that adverse pregnancy outcomes could be a result of either the direct trauma from physical violence or the stress associated with physical and emotional abuse.[22]

Rape and Sexual Assault

National rates of rape and sexual assault vary substantially by the source of data. The Uniform Crime Reporting (UCR) program of the Federal Bureau of Investigation (FBI) reported that in 1999 there were 89,107 attempted or completed forcible rapes against women reported to law enforcement agencies, the seventh consecutive annual decrease. Figure 7-1 depicts these data but excludes cases of statutory rape without force or other sexual assaults.[23] It has been estimated that more than two-thirds of rapes and sexual assaults against women are not reported to law enforcement agencies and, therefore, are not included in the UCR data.[3,24] The proportion of women who report the rape drops even further when the crime was committed by someone they knew.[23] The 1998 NCVS concluded that women aged 12 years and older experienced 307,110 rapes and sexual assaults in that year alone. The 1998 annual incidence of rape and sexual assault was estimated to be about 2.7 per 1,000 for women, more than 10 times the rate for men.[3] Using a definition of rape that includes forced vaginal, oral, or anal sex, the 1995–1996 NVAW survey yielded higher estimates of sexual violence than even those generated by the NCVS. The NVAW results indicate that one in six women (18%) aged 18 years and older had experienced an attempted or completed rape at some time in their lives.[11]

Multiple studies have indicated that women are more likely to be the victim of a rape or sexual assault committed by an intimate partner or acquaintance (64%) than by a stranger (32%).[3] The intimate offender is more likely to be a boyfriend or ex-boyfriend than a spouse, a finding that may reflect some reluctance to report violence by a spouse or to consider the act criminal.

The majority of rapes and sexual assaults are committed against children and adolescents. The highest incidence of rape occurs among older adolescents.[11] Age at *first* rape also shows the preponderance of young women as victims of

Figure 7-1

Forcible rapes against women recorded by law enforcement, 1976–1999

Number of rapes* per 1,000 females

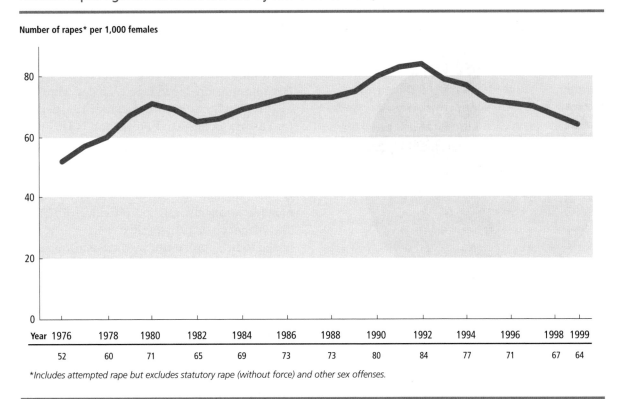

Year	1976	1978	1980	1982	1984	1986	1988	1990	1992	1994	1996	1998	1999
	52	60	71	65	69	73	73	80	84	77	71	67	64

*Includes attempted rape but excludes statutory rape (without force) and other sex offenses.

Source: Federal Bureau of Investigation. Crime in the United States: uniform crime reports for the United States; 1976–1999. Available from: URL: www.fbi.gov/ucr/ucr.htm.

this crime (Figure 7-2).[11] A survey of high-school students determined that one in five had already experienced forced sex; however, only half had told someone about the event.[25] Several studies have concluded that women who were sexually assaulted as children and adolescents are at greater risk of being sexually assaulted as adults. The 1995–1996 NVAW survey found that 18% of women raped before age 18 were also raped after age 18, twice the rate of those who had not been raped before age 18.[11] Findings from the NVAW survey indicate that nonwhite women are more frequent victims of rape than white women. In addition, Hispanic women are less likely to report being raped to law enforcement agencies than non-Hispanic women.[11]

Most studies indicate that people with disabilities are at greater risk for sexual violence than people without disabilities.[26] Estimated rates of sexual

assault range from 51% to 79% among women with disabilities[27] and approximately 24% among adolescent girls.[28] Most perpetrators are male (88% to 98%) and are known to the victim, including family members, acquaintances, other people with disabilities, and health care providers.[27]

Physical and Psychological Consequences

Additional physical injuries occur in as many as 65% of attempted and completed cases of rape and sexual assault against women.[3] Fatalities occur in 0.1% of rape cases.[29] The NVAW survey found that 31.5% of female rape victims sustained injuries. Most of these injuries were minor, including scratches, bruises, and welts (72.6%), although a few women reported broken bones and dislocations (14.1%), head and spinal cord

Figure 7-2

Women victims' age at first rape, 1995–1996

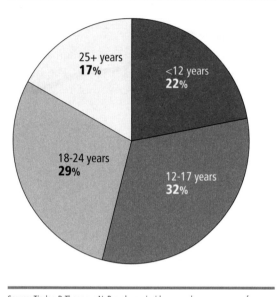

Source: Tjaden P, Thoennes N. Prevalence, incidence, and consequences of violence against women: findings from the National Violence Against Women Survey. Washington: National Institute of Justice, U.S. Department of Justice; Centers for Disease Control and Prevention, U.S. Department of Health and Human Services; 1998.

injuries (6.6%), lacerations (6.2%), and internal injuries (5.8%).[11] If a woman suffers injuries other than the rape or sexual assault itself, it is more likely that the police are notified of the crime. Women who sustained additional injuries reported 37% of the crimes, a rate that is significantly higher than the 22% of rapes and sexual assaults that did not include other injuries.[3] The long-term physical and psychological consequences of sexual assault may be extensive. These may include chronic headaches, insomnia, fatigue, recurrent nausea, eating disorders, menstrual pain, sexual dysfunction, suicide attempts, and substance abuse.[29,30]

Research shows a range of responses from women about contracting STDs from sexual assaults. From 3.6% to 30% of women are reported to contract STDs as a result of sexual assault.[29] Most research, however, has concluded

that bacterial and viral infections in adult and adolescent women were likely to have been present at the time of assault.[31] These conclusions are based on the assumption that most STDs diagnosed within days of the rape are not related to the rape; however, these findings have met with much controversy.[31] Data on the risk of HIV transmission due to rape is limited, although case reports have been presented. The Centers for Disease Control and Prevention (CDC) have estimated the HIV transmission rate in cases of rape is 1 in 500.[29] The risk of HIV transmission may be higher in certain situations, such as genital trauma, repeated abuse over time, multiple assailants, and the presence of STDs.[32] The pregnancy rate associated with rape is estimated to be approximately 5% among women of reproductive age. Therefore, rape accounts for an estimated 32,101 pregnancies each year.[33] Research on rape-related pregnancies found that most often the perpetrator was a boyfriend (29.4%), husband (17.6%), or friend (14.7%).[33]

Homicide

According to the FBI's UCR program, there were 15,533 murders and non-negligent manslaughters in 1998 (referred to as murders or homicides hereafter; excludes justifiable homicides).[23] Among the 12,658 murders for which data were available, 3,085 females ages 12 and older were victims of murder in 1998 as compared with 9,558 men.[23] Although men are nearly four times more likely to be murdered than women in the United States, women are significantly more likely than men to be killed by someone they know (Table 7-4). Close to one-third of murdered women are killed by an intimate partner, compared to approximately 4% of men.[4] This difference is greatest for those aged 18 to 24 years.[7]

Over recent decades, the number of homicides involving spouses, ex-spouses, and other intimate partners has been declining (Figure 7-3).[4] This decline, however, has been more pronounced for male victims than female victims.

Table 7-4

Homicides of persons aged 12 years or older by victim-offender relationship, 1994

	Percent of homicides		
	---	---	---
Offenders	Total victims	Women victims	Men victims
Intimates	9.4	31.0	3.8
Spouse	5.1	17.2	2.0
Ex-spouse	0.4	1.6	0.1
Boy/girlfriend	3.9	12.3	1.7
Other relatives	4.5	7.0	3.9
Friend/acquaintance	32.3	23.9	34.3
Stranger	13.6	7.9	15.0
Unknown	40.2	30.1	42.9

Note: Although more recent data are available on overall rates of homicide by intimate partners (see Figure 7-3), these are the most recent figures on the proportions of homicides according to relationship of the perpetrator to the victim.

Source: Craven D. Sex differences in violence victimization, 1994. NCJ–164508. Washington: Bureau of Justice Statistics, U.S. Department of Justice; 1997.

On average, the number of male victims of intimate homicide fell 4% each year, in contrast to a 1% decline among female victims.[4] This differential has resulted in an increasing female-to-male ratio for victims of intimate homicide. By the mid-1990s, there were more than three white females for every white male killed by an intimate partner and 1.5 African American females for every African American male killed by an intimate partner.[7]

The decline in intimate murder rates over the past two decades (1976 to 1996) also varied by race. During that time, African American women experienced a 5% decline and white women a 1% decline each year in murder rates by intimates. Therefore, although African American women were still much more likely to be murdered by an intimate partner than white women, the gap in rates had declined from a sevenfold difference in 1976 to just a threefold difference in 1996.[7]

Weapon Type

In 1996, 65% of all homicides by intimate partners were committed with a firearm.[7] The type of weapon used varied by the type of relationship. Over the past two decades, there has been a pronounced decline in the number of intimate homicides committed using a gun, with an average decrease of 3% per year. The number of intimate homicides committed by other methods has remained constant. Consequently, the decrease in the total number of intimate murders between 1976 and 1996 has been primarily attributed to the substantial decline in the number of crimes committed with a firearm.[7]

Many women believe that owning a firearm protects them against assault by both strangers and violent intimates. Rather than conferring protection for women, one study determined that having a gun in the home was associated with an increased risk of domestic homicide.[34] Another concluded that assaults by an intimate partner with a gun are 12 times more likely to end in death than assaults involving other types of weapons.[35]

Homicide in the Workplace

Homicide is the leading cause of occupational injury death for women and accounts for 42% of all deaths of women in the workplace.[36] Nonetheless, female workers are at much lower risk of homicide than their male counterparts, with rates of 0.32 and 1.01 deaths per 100,000 workers, respectively. An analysis by the National Institute for Occupational Safety and Health found that more than 2,000 women were victims of homicide at their place of work from 1980 to 1992. The majority of these victims were employed in the retail trade (46%) and service (22%) sectors, industries that are predicted to see substantial growth in the years to come.[36]

Figure 7-3

Homicides of intimates by gender of victim, 1976–1998

Number of homicides by intimates

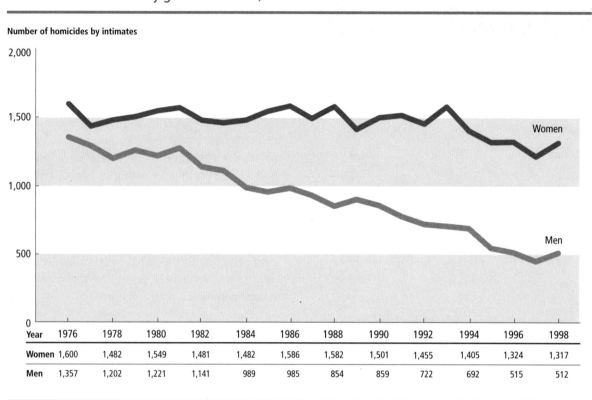

Year	1976	1978	1980	1982	1984	1986	1988	1990	1992	1994	1996	1998
Women	1,600	1,482	1,549	1,481	1,482	1,586	1,582	1,501	1,455	1,405	1,324	1,317
Men	1,357	1,202	1,221	1,141	989	985	854	859	722	692	515	512

Source: Rennison CM, Welchans S. Intimate partner violence. NCJ–178247. Washington: Bureau of Justice Statistics, U.S. Department of Justice; 2000.

Stalking

Stalking refers to a range of harassing and threatening behaviors that occur repeatedly and may be accompanied by a threat of serious harm.[43] Stalkers may follow or spy on a victim at home or at work, make unsolicited phone calls, send unwanted letters, or vandalize property. The legal definition of stalking varies from state to state, and the prevalence of stalking depends greatly on the definition being used.

Although stalking has gained national media attention over the past decade, little scientific research has focused on the prevalence of this form of violence. Most research on stalking has been limited to case studies on the characteristics of perpetrators, small unrepresentative clin-ical studies on known stalkers, and law journal reviews on the constitutionality of state anti-stalking statutes.[37,43] The NVAW survey, the first national survey to measure the impact of stalking in the United States, found annual rates of stalking five times higher than projected. At this time, data on stalking are not collected through the NCV survey or the UCR program, the two primary sources of violent victimization data within the Department of Justice.

The NVAW survey, using a definition that requires victims to feel fear of bodily harm, found that one of every 12 (8%), or a total of 8.2 million women, have been stalked at some point in their lifetimes.[43] One percent of women in the NVAW survey reported being stalked in the previous 12 months, providing an estimate

Figure 7-4

Women victims' age when first stalked, 1995–1996

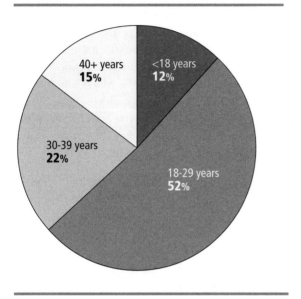

40+ years
15%

<18 years
12%

30-39 years
22%

18-29 years
52%

Source: Tjaden P, Thoennes N. Stalking in America: findings from the National Violence Against Women Survey. Washington: National Institute of Justice, U.S. Department of Justice; Centers for Disease Control and Prevention, U.S. Department of Health and Human Services; 1998.

that more than 1 million women are stalked annually in the United States. Using a less stringent definition of stalking, one that requires victims only to feel frightened by the behavior of their perpetrator, substantially raises the estimates of the number of women who experience stalking in their lifetimes (12%) or during the previous 12 months (6%).[43] In a study on a college campus, 30% of female students reported having been stalked at some time in their lives.[38] It has been estimated that stalkers are violent to their victims between 25% and 35% of the time; most of these crimes are committed by intimates.[37]

Although both men and women may experience stalking, women are significantly more likely to be stalked than men. In the NVAW survey, 78% of those who reported a history of being stalked

were female. Eighty-seven percent of the perpetrators, however, were male.[43]

Risk of stalking tends to vary by the age of the victim, with young adults being the principal targets (Figure 7-4).[43] Stalking rates for women also differ by racial and ethnic background. The NVAW survey found that American Indian/Alaskan Native women are the most likely and Asian and Pacific Islander women the least likely to be victims of stalking. However, this finding must be interpreted cautiously due to the small sample size for these groups and possible underreporting. Overall, Hispanic women were more than twice as likely as non-Hispanic women to report ever having been stalked.[43]

In the majority of stalking cases, the victim knew the stalker, either as an intimate partner or an acquaintance. The 1995–1996 NVAW survey concluded that only 23% of female victims had been stalked by strangers, whereas 59% were stalked by a current or former husband, cohabiting partner, boyfriend, or date.[43] A college-based study found similar results: 80% knew their stalkers, and 40% had seriously dated their stalkers.[38] Some research has found that stalking tends to occur after the woman attempts to leave the relationship, but the NVAW survey concluded that more than half of stalking by intimate partners begins while the relationship is still intact.[43]

The NVAW survey also found a significant association between stalking and other forms of violence between intimate partners. Of the women who reported being stalked by a current or former spouse or cohabiting partner, four of five were also physically assaulted and one of three was sexually assaulted by that partner. Former husbands who stalk their female partners were found to be significantly more likely to engage in emotionally abusive or controlling behavior in their relationship than husbands who do not stalk.[43]

Elder Mistreatment

Elder mistreatment includes physical, psychological, sexual, or financial abuse, and intentional or unintentional neglect. The aging of the U.S. population and new definitions of what constitutes abuse and neglect, have resulted in increased public attention and research on this topic. However, comprehensive data on this issue are not yet routinely reported and available.

Using aggregate data from the states, it was reported that there were 227,000 cases of elder mistreatment in 1991, an increase of 94% since 1986.[39] A large community-based study in Boston found that 3.2% of adults had experienced some form of abuse or neglect since reaching age 65. Forms of abuse included physical violence (2.0%), chronic verbal aggression (1.1%), and neglect (0.4%). These rates are considered to be underestimates, due to both underreporting and the narrow definitions used by the study. It was found that 58% of the abusers were spouses and 24% were adult children.[40]

Elder mistreatment is a particularly important health problem for women. The majority of studies have concluded that women are more likely to be victims of elder abuse than men.[39,40] This finding may reflect the fact that women outnumber men among the elderly at a rate of three to two. Thus, women are disproportionately affected by the increasing incidence of elder mistreatment. Because women live longer, they may be more likely to experience chronic illness that may require them to be dependent on others for care. There is also evidence that some elder abuse is spousal, including wife abuse continued from earlier years.[39] Also, women are more likely to be physically abused by their children, which is more likely to be reported than spousal abuse. Men are more likely to be neglected by their spouse, a crime which is less likely to be reported.[40]

Little is known about the association between homicide, assault, and elder abuse at this time. From 1987 to 1996, 50% of older homicide victims were killed by someone they knew: 25% by a family member and 25% by an acquaintance. This is in part because older adults tend to spend less time outside the home, thus limiting their exposure to strangers.[41]

Factors that may increase the risk of being a victim of elder abuse or neglect include poor health, functional impairment, cognitive impairment, substance abuse or mental illness of the abuser, greater dependence, shared living arrangement, external factors causing stress, social isolation, and a history of violence between the perpetrator and the abused.[39,42]

References

1. Office of Justice Programs, Bureau of Justice Statistics. Criminal victimization in United States, 1998 statistical tables. Washington: U.S. Department of Justice; 2000. Available from: URL: www.ojp.usdoj.gov/bjs/abstract/cvusst.htm.

2. American Association of Medical Colleges. AAMC curriculum directory 2000. 2nd ed. Washington: The Association; 2000. p. 9.

3. Craven D. Sex differences in violence victimization, 1994. NCJ–164508. Washington: Bureau of Justice Statistics, U.S. Department of Justice; 1997.

4. Rennison CM, Welchans S. Intimate partner violence. NCJ–178247. Washington: Bureau of Justice Statistics, U.S. Department of Justice; 2000.

5. O'Campo P, Baldwin K. Abuse against women by their intimate partners. In: Grason H, Hutchins J, Silver G, editors. Charting a course for the future of women's and perinatal health. Baltimore: Women's and Children's Health Policy Center, Johns Hopkins University School of Public Health; 1999. p. 168–181.

6. Bell RN, Duncan MM, Eilenberg J, Fullilove M, Hein D, Innes L, et al. Violence against women in the United States: a comprehensive background paper. 1st ed. New York: The Commonwealth Fund; 1995.

7. Greenfeld LA, Rand MR, Rand D, Craven PA, Klaus CA, Perkins C, et al. Violence by intimates: analysis of data on crimes by current or former spouses, boyfriends, and girlfriends. Bureau of Justice statistics factbook. NJS-167237. Washington: Bureau of Justice Statistics, U.S. Department of Justice; 1998.

8. Laurence L, Spalter-Roth R. Measuring the costs of domestic violence against women and the cost-effectiveness of interventions. Washington: Institute for Women's Policy Research; 1996.

9. Meyer H. The billion-dollar epidemic. Am Med News 1992 Jan 6.

10. Crowell NA, Burgess A. Understanding violence against women. Washington: National Academy Press; 1996.

11. Tjaden P, Thoennes N. Prevalence, incidence, and consequences of violence against women: findings from the National Violence Against Women Survey. Washington: National Institute of Justice, U.S. Department of Justice; Centers for Disease Control and Prevention, U.S. Department of Health and Human Services; 1998.

12. Wilt S, Olson S. Prevalence of domestic violence in the United States. J Am Womens Assoc 1996;51:77–82.

13. Plichta S. Violence and abuse: implications for women's health. In: Falik M, Collins K, editors. Women's health: the Commonwealth Fund Survey. Baltimore: The Johns Hopkins University Press; 1996. p. 237–270.

14. Centers for Disease Control and Prevention. Lifetime and annual incidence of intimate partner violence and resulting injuries, Georgia, 1995. MMWR Morb Mortal Wkly Rep 1998;47:849–853.

15. Centers for Disease Control and Prevention. Physical violence during the 12 months preceding childbirth: Alaska, Maine, Oklahoma, and West Virginia, 1990–1991. MMWR Morb Mortal Wkly Rep 1994;43:132–137.

16. Gelles R. Violence in pregnancy: are pregnant women at greater risk of abuse? J Marriage Fam 1988;50:841–847.

17. Gazmararian JA, Adams MM, Salzman LE, Johnson CH, Bruce FC, Marks JS, et al. The relationship between pregnancy intendedness and physical violence in mothers of newborns. Obstet Gynecol 1995;85:1031–1038.

18. Amaro H, Fried LE, Cabral H, Zuckerman B. Violence during pregnancy and substance use. Am J Public Health 1990;80:575–579.

19. Berenson AB, Wiemann CM, Wilkinson GS, Jones WA, Anderson GD. Prenatal morbidity associated with violence experienced by pregnant women. Am J Obstet Gynecol 1994;170:1766–1769.

20. Helton AS, McFarlane J, Anderson ET. Battered and pregnant: a prevalence study. Am J Public Health 1987;77:1337–1339.

21. Hillard PJA. Physical abuse in pregnancy. Obstet Gynecol 1985;66:185–190.

22. Petersen R, Gazmararian JA, Spitz A, Rowley DL, Goodwin MM, Saltzman LE, et al. Violence and adverse pregnancy outcomes: a review of the literature and directions for future research. Am J Prev Med 1997;13:366–373.

23. Federal Bureau of Investigation. Crime in the United States: uniform crime reports for the United States. Washington: U.S. Department of Justice; 1998. Available from: URL: www.fbi.gov/ucr.htm.

24. Greenfeld LA. Sex offenses and offenders: an analysis of data on rape and sexual assault. NCJ–163392. Washington: Bureau of Justice Statistics, U.S. Department of Justice; 1997.

25. Davis TC, Peck GQ, Storment JM. Acquaintance rape and the high school student. J Adolesc Health 1993;14:220–224.

26. Bachman R, Saltzman LE. Violence against women: estimates from the redesigned survey. Bureau of Justice Statistics: special report. NCJ-154348. Washington: U.S. Department of Justice; 1995 Aug.

27. National Center for Injury Prevention and Control. Sexual violence against people with disabilities. Atlanta: Centers for Disease Control and Prevention, U.S. Department of Health and Human Services; 1998. Available from: URL: www.cdc.gov/ncipc/factsheets/disabvi.htm.

28. Surís J-C, Resnick MD, Cassuto N, Blum RW. Sexual behavior of adolescents with chronic disease and disability. J Adolesc Health 1996;19:124–131.

29. National Center for Injury Prevention and Control. Rape fact sheet. http://www.cdc.gov/ncipc/factsheets/rape.htm. Atlanta: Centers for Disease Control and Prevention, U.S. Department of Health and Human Services; 1999.

30. Laws A, Golding J. Sexual assault history and eating disorder symptoms among White, Hispanic, and African American Women and Men. Am J Public Health 1996;86:579–582.

31. Jenny C, Hooton TM, Bowers A, Copass MK, Krieger JN, Hillier SL, et al. Sexually transmitted diseases in victims of rape. N Engl J Med 1990;322:713–716.

32. Beck-Sague CM, Solomon F. Sexually transmitted diseases in abused children and adolescent and adult victims of rape: review of selected literature. Clin Infect Dis 1999;28 Suppl 1:S74–S83.

33. Holmes MM, Resnick HS, Kilpatrick DG, Best CL. Rape-related pregnancy: estimates and descriptive characteristics from a national sample of women. Am J Obstet Gynecol 1996;175:320–324.

34. Bailey JE, Kellermann AL, Somes GW, Banton J, Rivara FP, Rushforth NP. Risk factors for violent death of women in the home. Arch Intern Med 1997;157:777–782.

35. Saltzman LE, Mercy JA, O'Carroll PW, Rosenberg ML, Rhodes PH. Weapon involvement and injury outcomes in family and intimate assaults. JAMA 1992;267:3043–3047.

36. Jenkins EL. Homicide against women in the workplace. J Am Womens Assoc 1996;51:118–119, 122.

37. Violence Against Women Office. Stalking and domestic violence: the third annual report to Congress under the Violence Against Women Act. NCJ–1772204. Washington: U.S. Department of Justice; 1998.

38. Fremouw WJ, Westrup D, Pennypacker J. Stalking on campus: the prevalence and strategies for coping with stalking. J Forensic Science 1997;42:666–669.

39. Hudson MF. Elder mistreatment: its relevance to older women. J Am Womens Assoc 1997;52:142–146, 158.

40. Pillemer K, Finkelhor D. The prevalence of elder abuse: a random sample survey. Gerontologist. 1988;28:51–57.

41. Stevens JA, Hasbrouck LM, Durant TM, Dellinger AM, Batabyal PK, Crosby AE, et al. Surveillance for injuries and violence among older adults. MMWR Morb Mortal Wkly Rep 1999;48:27–50.

42. Lachs MS, Pillemer K. Abuse and neglect of elderly persons. N Engl J Med 1995;332:437–443.

43. Tjaden P, Thoennes N. Stalking in America: findings from the National Violence Against Women Survey. Washington: National Institute of Justice, U.S. Department of Justice; Centers for Disease Control and Prevention, U.S. Department of Health and Human Services; 1998.

Chapter 8

Access, Utilization, and Quality of Health Care

Contents

Introduction

Women have a large stake in how health care services are financed and delivered. Often, they coordinate health care for their families and have primary responsibility for family health care decisions, and they use more health care services than men do.[1,2] Access to affordable, high-quality care is an important issue for women's health. Over the past decade, changes in health care policies, financing, and delivery in both the private and public health care sectors have affected health care access for women. The growth of managed care has changed the way health care services are organized, financed, and delivered. Changes in public policies related to Medicaid, welfare, and immigration have also affected health care coverage and access. This chapter addresses three broad areas: access to health insurance coverage and services, utilization of health care services, and quality of health care services.

Federal agencies and other research institutions routinely collect data on women's health care coverage and utilization through several surveys. The March supplement of the Current Population Survey, conducted by the U.S. Bureau of the Census, provides national estimates of health insurance coverage of the civilian noninstitutionalized population living in the United States. Other major, federally sponsored sources of data on health service utilization and costs are the Medical Expenditure Panel Survey (MEPS), conducted by the Agency for Healthcare Research and Quality, and the National Health Interview Survey (NHIS), conducted by the National Center for Health Statistics. Although aggregate data are routinely published, national estimates of coverage and access to care for adult women are either not often readily available, do not include the broad range of access concerns that are specific to women, or are not released in a timely fashion. The Commonwealth Fund Survey of Women's Health was developed and fielded in 1993 and 1998 to fill these gaps, and, although the sample size of the survey is not as robust as its federally funded counterparts, it does provide up-to-date, self-reported information on many access issues that are important to women.

Coverage and access to health care services are also strongly influenced by policies at the state and federal levels, including public program funding levels, Medicaid eligibility rules, and private insurance mandates. In addition, coverage and access are affected by private sector decisions regarding the cost and scope of coverage and care. Information on public and private sector policies is not routinely collected or published by state or federal agencies. Therefore, this information is not readily available or included in the peer-reviewed medical literature upon which this data book relies. Instead, such information provided in this chapter is based upon the most accurate and reliable data available from other sources.

Access to Health Care Services

Access to health care services is influenced by a wide of range of factors, both financial and nonfinancial. Financial factors include availability of health insurance, the type and scope of coverage, and ability to afford out-of-pocket costs for health care. Nonfinancial factors include the availability of needed health services in communities, of enabling factors such as transportation and child care, and of culturally appropriate services.

Health Insurance Coverage for Women Aged 18–64 Years

One important factor that is amenable to policy change is health insurance coverage. The mechanisms for obtaining health insurance coverage are embedded in complex social and economic situations, which have important implications for women. Factors, such as income, marital status, employment, and age, all affect women's access

to coverage. Among women 18 to 64 years of age, 68% are covered by private health insurance, obtained through their own employment or the employment of a spouse or parent (Figure 8-1). Private coverage can also be purchased directly from an insurer, but this is typically a more costly option. Medicaid, a state- and federally financed entitlement program, provides coverage for eligible low-income and disabled individuals. Disabled women may be eligible for health coverage through Medicare, a federal entitlement program. Other forms of government coverage, such as the Civilian Health and Medical Program for the Uniformed Services (CHAMPUS) and the Veterans Health Administration (VHA) system, cover a very small portion of women.

Figure 8-1

Health insurance coverage of adults aged 18–64 years by gender, United States, 1999

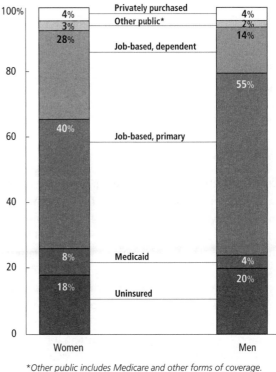

*Other public includes Medicare and other forms of coverage.
Note: Totals may not equal 100% due to rounding.

Source: University of California, Center for Health Policy Research analyses of the March 2000 Current Population Survey, U.S. Bureau of Census.

Figure 8-2

Women's health insurance trends, 1987–1998

Percent of women aged 18–64 years

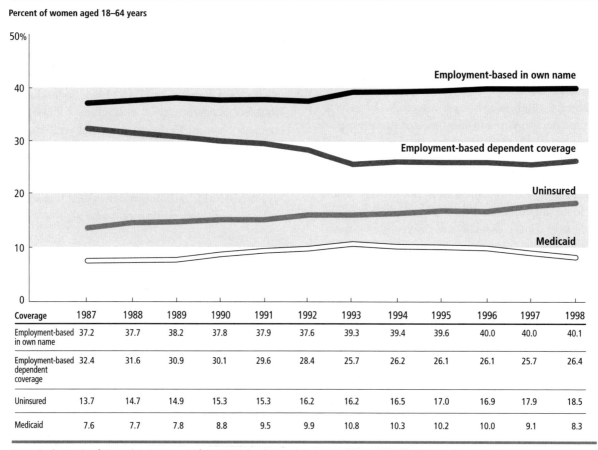

Coverage	1987	1988	1989	1990	1991	1992	1993	1994	1995	1996	1997	1998
Employment-based in own name	37.2	37.7	38.2	37.8	37.9	37.6	39.3	39.4	39.6	40.0	40.0	40.1
Employment-based dependent coverage	32.4	31.6	30.9	30.1	29.6	28.4	25.7	26.2	26.1	26.1	25.7	26.4
Uninsured	13.7	14.7	14.9	15.3	15.3	16.2	16.2	16.5	17.0	16.9	17.9	18.5
Medicaid	7.6	7.7	7.8	8.8	9.5	9.9	10.8	10.3	10.2	10.0	9.1	8.3

Source: Employment Benefit Research Institute Issue Briefs 1997-2000, based on March Current Population Surveys,1988–1999, U.S. Bureau of the Census.

Employment-Based Coverage. Coverage rates through employment are similar for women and men; however, women are more likely than men to have coverage as a dependent and less likely than men to have coverage in their own name. Over time, women have become more likely to have insurance coverage in their own name and less likely to be covered as a dependent (Figure 8-2). This is attributable to a combination of women's growing workforce participation and rising costs for dependent coverage, which may lead workers to drop dependent coverage. In 2000, according to a national survey of private employers, the average worker's contribution for family coverage was $138 per month, which represented 27% of the total premium costs (with the remaining share borne by the employer), compared to $28 per month for individuals, accounting for 14% of the total premium costs.[3]

Individually purchased coverage, separate from employment, plays a small role in insuring women, covering 4% of women aged 18–64 years. Premiums in the individual market vary significantly based on the age of the applicant. Such coverage is often denied to people with health problems or offered only at very high cost for their coverage. Insurers often raise premiums or add riders for people in the individual market to waive coverage for pre-existing health conditions or risk factors.[4]

Figure 8-3

Health plans with contraceptive coverage by type of plan, 2000

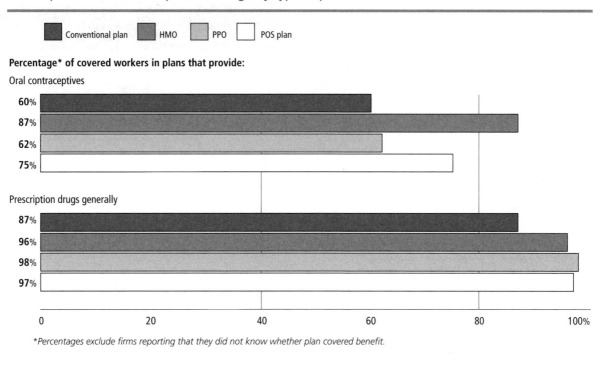

Conventional plan   HMO   PPO   POS plan

Percentage* of covered workers in plans that provide:

Oral contraceptives

60%	
87%	
62%	
75%	

Prescription drugs generally

87%	
96%	
98%	
97%	

0   20   40   60   80   100%

*Percentages exclude firms reporting that they did not know whether plan covered benefit.

Source: Henry J. Kaiser Family Foundation and Health Research and Educational Trust. Survey of Employer Health Benefits. Menlo Park (CA): The Foundation; 2000.

Benefits and scope of coverage often depend on the type of care arrangement in which an employee or their dependent is enrolled. On average, those enrolled in managed care arrangements, such as health maintenance organizations (HMOs) and point-of-service (POS) plans, are more likely than those in conventional fee-for-service or indemnity plans to have coverage for a broad range of preventive services. For example, according to employers responding to a national survey, adult physical examinations are a covered benefit for 97% of covered workers in HMO plans, compared to 71% of covered workers in conventional plans.[3] Insurance coverage of alternative treatments also varies significantly depending on the type of plan and the type of services. Coverage of chiropractic care, for example, ranged from 74% of workers enrolled in HMO plans to 88% of those enrolled

in preferred provider organizations (PPOs). Coverage of acupuncture, however, was more limited; 28% to 35% of workers had coverage for this treatment.[3]

Although nearly all women with employer-based coverage have prescription drug benefits and prenatal care coverage, far fewer have specific coverage for oral contraceptives, and fewer still are covered for a broad range of reversible contraceptives. Coverage varies considerably across health plan type, with HMOs more likely than other types of health plans to cover oral contraceptives (Figure 8-3).[3] As of October 2000, 13 states had enacted legislation that requires coverage for contraceptive services and supplies under the same terms and conditions as coverage for other prescription medication. An additional nine states have more limited provisions.[5] Of the

13 states with comprehensive coverage, nine include some form of a conscience clause, which applies to either the employer, the insurer, or both, that provides an exemption to providing birth control based on religious belief.[5]

Most workers with insurance have coverage for both inpatient and outpatient mental health services, but many plans place annual limits on either the number of visits permitted or days covered. For example, on average, according to a survey of employers, 26% of insured workers have coverage for 20 or fewer outpatient mental health visits, and only 11% had coverage for unlimited outpatient visits. Similar restrictions exist with inpatient mental health benefits, with those in managed care arrangements experiencing the greatest degree of limits on days covered.[3]

Medicaid. Medicaid is an important safety net for women who do not have access to or cannot afford employment-based or other forms of coverage.[6] Medicaid is the nation's health insurance program for the poor and provides millions of low-income women with comprehensive health coverage. Authorized under Title XIX of the Social Security Act and enacted in 1965, Medicaid is a means-tested entitlement program financed by state and federal governments and administered by the states. Overall, women are twice as likely to have Medicaid coverage as men (8% versus 4%), because women are more likely to meet Medicaid's restrictive income and categorical eligibility criteria. Nevertheless, being poor does not automatically qualify women for Medicaid. Generally, unless a woman is pregnant, disabled, or more than 65 years old, she is not eligible for Medicaid assistance, no matter how poor she is (unless she has one or more children). Because states establish eligibility criteria under broad federal guidelines, there is considerable variation in income eligibility levels across states. Data from the Current Population Survey show that nationwide, 33% of nonelderly women with incomes less than 100% of the federal poverty level (FPL) had Medicaid coverage in 1999 (Table 8-1). Medicaid plays an

Table 8-1

Health insurance coverage of women by age, family structure, poverty level, and race/ethnicity, 1999

	Percent			
	Medicaid	Employ-ment-based coverage	Other coverage	Un-insured
Age (years)				
18–29	12	59	5	25
30–44	7	72	6	16
45–54	5	74	6	14
55–64	7	63	14	16
Family structure				
Single, children	25	45	4	25
Single, no children	8	61	7	24
Married, children	4	77	6	12
Married, no children	3	75	9	14
Poverty level				
<100% of FPL*	33	19	8	40
100%–199% of FPL	14	46	10	31
200% of FPL and higher	2	81	6	11
Race/Ethnicity				
Hispanic	13	46	5	37
White, non-Hispanic	5	74	7	13
Black, non-Hispanic	16	56	5	23
Asian/Pacific Islander	6	64	7	24

Note: Due to rounding, the rows may not equal 100%.

*FPL is the federal poverty level, which was $13,290 for a family of three in 1999.

Source: University of California, Los Angeles, Center for Health Policy Research analysis of the March 2000 Current Population Survey, U.S. Bureau of the Census.

important role for low-income women who are young, women of color, and single mothers.

Medicaid pays for a broad range of health services for women, including inpatient and outpatient hospital care; services of a physician, midwife, or certified nurse practitioner; laboratory and X-ray testing; and, in almost all states, outpatient prescription drugs with nominal or no copayments.[7] Medicaid also covers prenatal visits, delivery, other pregnancy-related care, and postpartum care. Screening services, such as mammograms and Pap tests, sexually transmitted disease (STD) testing and treatment, and preventive services are all mandatory Medicaid benefits.[7]

Medicaid covers "family planning services and supplies," for low-income women, but, as with other services, it is up to the states to define the scope, amount, and duration of these benefits. States have used Medicaid to expand family planning services to uninsured women. The federal government matches the cost of family planning services at a higher rate than it does for other health services—90 cents for every dime a state spends.[8] By mid-2000, 12 states had Section 1115 Research and Demonstration waivers needed to expand family planning services coverage to low-income, uninsured women.[9] Six additional states were awaiting approval to expand services to women.

In the absence of Medicaid or private insurance coverage, many low-income women turn to Title X clinics for their gynecologic care. The federal Title X program funds family planning and reproductive health clinics to provide health services to clients regardless of their age, income, or insurance status.[10] States administer their Title X funds in different ways, but all clinics use sliding-fee scales for services and subsidize visits for women whose income is 250% or less of the FPL.[9]

An important new optional Medicaid eligibility category expands coverage to uninsured women with breast or cervical cancer. The Breast and Cervical Cancer Prevention and Treatment Act, passed in 2000, enables states to use Medicaid funding to provide full Medicaid benefits to unin-

sured women under age 65 who are in need of treatment for breast or cervical cancer.[11] Women diagnosed through the National Breast and Cervical Cancer Early Detection Program, or an eligible equivalent, may qualify for this program regardless of income so long as they meet general Medicaid requirements.

Abortion coverage is restricted under Medicaid. Federal Medicaid funds for abortions can only be used in cases of rape, incest, or if the woman's life is in danger. Sixteen states choose to fund through the use of state or local funds other "medically necessary" abortions sought by women.[12]

Today, Medicaid finances over one-third of all U.S. births,[7] largely due to federal and state expansions in eligibility for pregnant women that occurred in the late 1980s and 1990s. These laws broadened Medicaid eligibility and established a nationwide floor of eligibility for all pregnant women with incomes under 133% of the FPL. States can also choose to cover pregnant women with incomes up to 185% of the FPL or higher. Coverage is, however, limited to pregnancy-related care and ends 60 days after a woman gives birth unless she meets other eligibility requirements.[5]

Although Medicaid expansions resulted in broadened eligibility for low-income women, significant numbers of pregnant women are uninsured. One study estimated that in 1997, 13.7% of pregnant women (465,000 women) lacked coverage, of whom 77% were likely eligible for Medicaid.[13]

Uninsured Rates and the Risk of Being Uninsured. The current insurance system, with its reliance on employment-based coverage and Medicaid as a safety net, leaves many women uninsured. Data from the Current Population Survey show that in 1999, even with a strong economy and low unemployment, 18% of women between the ages of 18 and 64 years—approximately 15.1 million women—were uninsured. Women are slightly less likely to be uninsured than men (20%), because some women are eligible for Medicaid.[14]

There are considerable differences in patterns of coverage among women. Younger women aged 18–29 years are the most likely to be uninsured (25%); uninsured rates drop in each successive age group and then start to rise again among women in the 55–64 age group. Poorer women are also less likely to have coverage. Forty percent of women with family incomes below the FPL and approximately one-third of near-poor women (family income 100% to 199% of the FPL) are uninsured. Women with lower incomes have much less access to employment-based coverage, even when working full time for the full year.[15] Among uninsured women, 82% are in working families, with nearly one-half in families with a full-time, full-year worker.[15]

Family structure also has important implications for women's coverage. Eligibility for Medicaid is based mainly on income and family composition, whereas employment-based insurance for many women is based on access to spousal coverage. Women who are married are more likely to have employment-based coverage and are less likely to be uninsured than women who are single because of access to coverage through a spouse. Approximately one of four single women is uninsured, a rate nearly twice that of their married counterparts. Medicaid buffers single, poor mothers from even higher uninsured rates. Yet, Medicaid rates have been declining rapidly for this population, going from 66% in 1994 to 52% in 1998 while the rate of uninsurance continues to rise.[15]

Women of color have higher uninsurance rates and lower rates of employment-based coverage than do white women. Uninsurance rates are especially high for Hispanics, with nearly four of 10 lacking coverage in 1999. Medicaid is a particularly important source of coverage for many women of color, filling in the gaps in the current health insurance system.

Coverage Trends. During the past decade, the number and proportion of the U.S. population without health insurance coverage has grown.[16]

Table 8-2

Health insurance coverage of low-income women* aged 18–64 years by source of coverge and poverty level,** 1994 and 1998		
	Percent	
	1994	**1998**
Uninsured		
Low-income (<200% of FPL)	**32**	**35**
Less than 100% of FPL	34	39
100%–199% of FPL	30	32
Medicaid		
Low-income (<200% of FPL)	**26**	**23**
Less than 100% of FPL	42	34
100%–199% of FPL	14	14
Job-based coverage		
Low-income (<200% of FPL)	**32**	**33**
Less than 100% of FPL	16	19
100%–199% of FPL	45	45
Other government		
Low-income (<200% of FPL)	**5**	**4**
Less than 100% of FPL	4	4
100%–199% of FPL	5	4
Privately purchased		
Low-income (<200% of FPL)	**6**	**4**
Less than 100% of FPL	5	4
100%–199% of FPL	6	5

*<200% of the FPL.

**FPL is the federal poverty level, which was $13,003 for a family of three in 1998.

Source: Wyn R, Solis B, Ojeda V, Pourat N. Falling through the cracks: low-income women and their health insurance coverage. Menlo Park (CA): Henry J. Kaiser Family Foundation; 2001.

Among women, the uninsured rate has steadily increased, going from 13.7% in 1987 to 18.5% in 1998. This increase in uninsured rates is partly attributable to a decrease in dependent coverage, which declined steadily between 1987 (32.4%) and the mid-1990s when it leveled off, to a level of 26.4% in 1998. During this time, employment-based coverage in one's own name increased for women, from 37.2% to 40.1%. The Commonwealth Fund Surveys of 1993 and 1998 also found an overall increase in the proportion of women without coverage, notably among poor women and Hispanics.[2]

Recent years have seen a decrease in the proportion of women covered through Medicaid. Between 1994 and 1998, Medicaid coverage decreased for low-income women, increasing their uninsured rate[15] (Table 8-2). This trend was most pronounced among poor women, the group disproportionately affected by changes in welfare law which severed the automatic link between cash welfare and Medicaid benefits.[17] This law, the 1996 Personal Responsibility and Work Opportunities Act, uncoupled the historical link between public assistance (welfare) and Medicaid. Prior to the passage of welfare reform, families eligible for assistance were automatically enrolled in Medicaid.[18] The legislation also imposed new time limits on receipt of benefits and work requirements on recipients. Although women leaving welfare are often eligible to receive transitional Medicaid as they begin to work, many may not know of this option or may have difficulties following through.[19] Only 35% of former welfare recipients had Medicaid 6 to 11 months after leaving welfare, and nearly half of women were uninsured 12 or more months later.[17]

Health Insurance Coverage for Women Aged 65 Years and Older

Health insurance coverage issues differ for women aged 65 years and over. The vast majority have coverage through Medicare and often a supplemental form of coverage, yet the increasing need for health care and gaps in coverage create access problems for these women.

Medicare. Medicare functions as a partner program to Social Security and provides health care coverage to nearly all the U.S population 65 years of age and older and for many with disabilities who are younger than 65. Medicare coverage has two components: Part A, which is hospital insurance and is financed primarily through a payroll tax paid for by workers and employers, and Part B, or supplementary medical insurance, financed by beneficiary premiums ($50 per month in 2001) and general revenue. Medicare plays a critical role for older women for several reasons. Compared to men, women rely on Medicare for more years because they live longer, they are more likely to experience multiple health problems, and they have higher rates of poverty and, therefore, less income to pay for out-of-pocket health care needs.[20]

Women outnumber men in the U.S. population and, by age 85, they outnumber men two to one.[21] According to data from the Medicare Current Beneficiary Survey, women also outnumber men in the Medicare population. Of the 34.5 million Medicare beneficiaries aged 65 years and older, 19.4 million (56%) are women, and among those 85 and older, approximately 70% of beneficiaries are women.[22] Within each beneficiary age group, the proportion of female beneficiaries is higher than males (Figure 8-4). As the baby boomers age, the number of women on Medicare will continue to increase.

Given women's longer life spans (79 years versus 72 years for men),[23] women on Medicare are more likely than men to have multiple health problems and functional limitations. They rely more on long-term care services and constitute the majority of users of home health care and nursing home services.[24] Exacerbating their poorer health status is their worse financial situation. Women are at greater risk of poverty than men are at every age, disparities that are marked in old age[21] and that

Figure 8-4

Gender of Medicare beneficiaries by age, 1996

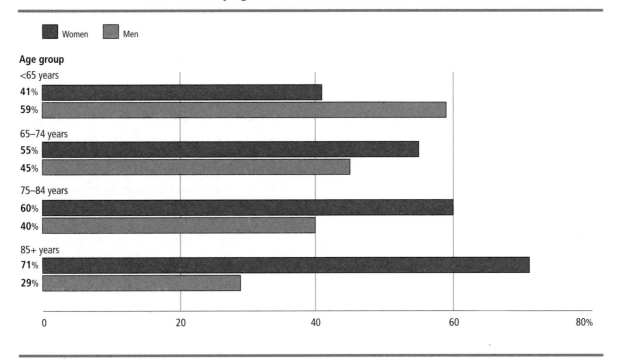

Source: Henry J. Kaiser Family Foundation. Medicare and women. Menlo Park (CA): Henry J. Kaiser Family Foundation, Kaiser Medicare Policy Project; 1999.

affect the affordability of health care. Data from the Current Population Survey show that older women are twice as likely as older men to have incomes below $10,000[25] and that nearly 70% of Medicare beneficiaries of all ages with incomes below poverty are female.[24]

Private and Public Supplements. Although Medicare provides access to basic insurance coverage for a full range of health care services, it does have cost-sharing requirements and gaps in the benefits package, such as a lack of coverage for prescription drugs and certain specialized care. Consequently, many beneficiaries also have private or public supplemental insurance or must pay out-of-pocket to fill the gaps in Medicare's benefit package. In 1997, 60% of female Medicare beneficiaries had private supplemental coverage, either as a retiree benefit (33%) or a privately purchased Medigap policy (27%). An additional 14% were enrolled in

Medicare HMOs and 15% had Medicaid in addition to Medicare. Just 10% relied solely on Medicare benefits without any form of supplemental coverage.[26] The Balanced Budget Act of 1997 created the Medicare+Choice program to increase Medicare enrollees' participation in private HMO plans as a way of reducing out-of-pocket spending, but results thus far have been inconclusive.[27]

Medicare does not pay for most long-term care. It covers only limited amounts of skilled nursing care and some home health services, usually following a hospitalization. Medicaid serves as an important complement to Medicare for the poor elderly, especially in providing coverage for long-term care services. The extent of coverage provided to Medicare beneficiaries varies by income eligibility, but most dually eligible beneficiaries receive coverage for Medicare Part B premiums, cost-sharing, prescription drugs, and long-term care. Medicaid is the largest payor of

Figure 8-5

Out-of-pocket spending on medical care as a percent of income for Medicare beneficiaries* by gender and other characteristics, 1998

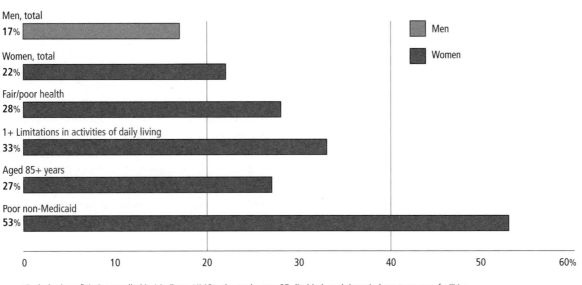

*Excludes beneficiaries enrolled in Medicare HMOs, the under-age-65 disabled, and those in long-term care facilities.

Source: Gibson MJ, Brangan N. Out-of-pocket spending on health care by women aged 65 years and over in fee-for-service Medicare: 1998 projections. Washington; AARP Public Policy Institute; 1998.

long-term care services for Medicare beneficiaries, covering those who are poor or who become poor as they expend their resources to pay for needed services.[28] Because of their lower income and greater need for long-term care, female beneficiaries are more likely to qualify for Medicaid coverage. Nevertheless, Medicaid covers just one-half of all poor Medicare beneficiaries.[29] Although full Medicaid benefits are often restricted to the poorest Medicare beneficiaries, more limited benefits are available through the Qualified Medicare Beneficiary (QMB) program, which set eligibility levels at 100% of the FPL, and the Specified Low-Income Medicare Beneficiary (SLMB) program, which set eligibility levels at 120% to 135% of the FPL.[28] Unfortunately, participation in the SLMB is low. Some estimates indicate that only 16% of those eligible are enrolled.[30]

Out-of-Pocket Costs. Because of the gaps in Medicare coverage, beneficiaries can incur considerable out-of-pocket costs. Women on

Medicare spend a greater portion of their incomes on health care than men do (22% versus 17%, respectively).[22] Among women, those who are the most vulnerable spend considerably more (Figure 8-5). For example, women with activity limitations spend on average one-third of their income on health care costs. Poor women who do not have Medicaid to augment Medicare pay one-half (53%) of their incomes on their health care.[22] Most women on Medicare (78% of female beneficiaries of all ages) use prescription medicine, and, of those, nearly one-half spend $26 or more per month to cover the costs.[25]

Managed Care Access Issues

Managed care has been one of the most significant changes in health care delivery, serving an ever-larger proportion of the population. According to a recent survey, approximately three-quarters of insured women participate in some form of managed care, broadly defined as an HMO, a PPO, or a plan requiring referral for specialist care.[2] In 1999, more than one-half of the Medicaid population, mainly low-income women and their children, were enrolled in managed care primarily through mandatory enrollment policies at the state level.[7]

Part of the difficulty in examining managed care is the variety of forms that managed care takes. Managed care types range from staff models to POS models in which enrollees can receive services outside the plan but usually for a higher fee. To date, the findings on managed care's effects on access and quality of care have been generally inconclusive, although some trends have emerged. According to an analysis of the 1998 Commonwealth Fund Survey of Women's Health, women in managed care plans have similar or better access to care than women in traditional fee-for-service plans, and they receive significantly more gender-specific clinical preventive services compared with women in other plans. Across types of plans, the receipt of counseling services does not vary significantly. Nevertheless, women in managed care plans are less satisfied with their care, a finding that is reflected in lower ratings of their physicians and of quality of communication with their physicians.[31]

The shift to managed care has occurred rapidly in Medicaid, with low-income women and their children disproportionately affected by the shift. In 1991, 2.7 million Medicaid recipients were enrolled in managed care, increasing to 17.8 million by 1999,[32] most of whom were low-income women and their children. Issues of access to care are particularly important for Medicaid recipients, because they face several challenges in obtaining care. They have limited financial resources, often live in areas that are medically underserved, and frequently have poorer health status than those with higher incomes. In a study of low-income women in five states on several measures of access and satisfaction with care, women in Medicaid managed care generally did worse than women with either fee-for-service Medicaid or with private managed care. However, women in Medicaid managed care did have similar access to a regular provider and similar use rates as the other two groups.[33]

Managed care plans may present access barriers for low-income women. A 1997 study found that among managed care enrollees, compared to higher-income women, low-income women reported more difficulty obtaining care, were less likely to have a regular provider, and were more concerned about being denied a medical procedure.[34]

Concerns about limits on access to care in managed care plans have brought about legislative and regulatory action at both the federal and state levels. At the end of year 2000, 38 states and the District of Columbia had implemented policies that allow women enrolled in managed care greater access to obstetrician/gynecologists.[5] The 1998 Commonwealth Fund Survey of Women's Health found that less than 25% of nonelderly women enrolled in managed care plans needed a referral for an ob/gyn visit, compared to 75% who needed a referral for a specialist.[35] According to a national employer survey, 54% of employees and their dependents enrolled in their firm's largest HMO plan could have an ob/gyn serve as their primary care provider, a figure that is down somewhat from 1999.[3]

Access Issues for Subgroups of Women

Several subgroups of women, including racial and ethnic minorities, lesbians, disabled women, incarcerated women, and homeless women, experience major disparities in access to health care and health status.

Women of Color. Compared to white populations, women of color have a disproportionate share of morbidity and mortality across a wide range of health conditions.[36] They also are more likely to lack insurance coverage. A recent synthesis of the literature on racial and ethnic differences in access to medical care found that racial and ethnic subgroups generally have poorer access to care for several disease categories and service types.[37] Insurance status and socioeconomic status were identified as stronger predictors of access, but racial and ethnic differ ences often persisted even after controlling for these factors. Studies in progress are seeking to determine to what extent racial and ethnic differences in access are linked to systemic and financial barriers as opposed to cultural preferences.[37]

Lesbians. The lesbian population constitutes approximately 3% to 10% of the female population. A few studies indicate that lesbians face more and greater barriers to health care compared to heterosexual women and that these women may underuse needed health care services.[38] In 1999, the Institute of Medicine (IOM) Committee on Lesbian Health Research Priorities published a report, *Lesbian Health: Current Assessment and Directions for the Future*, which is the most recent and comprehensive study of lesbian health issues.[39] The committee did not find that lesbians are at greater risk for any particular health problem. However, the committee calls for greater research on lesbian health issues because the scant research on this population relies upon convenience samples rather than population–based samples, and most studies have been cross-sectional in design. The primary recommendation of the committee was to increase public and private funding to support research that focuses on risk, protective health factors, and access to health care services among lesbians to identify their specific health needs.[39]

Disabled Women. In 1999, 44 million adults aged 18 years and older (22%) reported having a disability.[40] The rate of disability was 24% among women and 20% among men. The two top health conditions associated with the disability for women were arthritis/rheumatism (22%) and back or spine problems (17%). These same two conditions were the main health conditions for men, but in different proportions, with back or spine problems affecting 17% and arthritis/rheumatism 11%.[40]

People with disabilities rank high among groups with elevated needs for short- and long-term

health services.[41] Medical expenditures for women with activity limitations are approximately three times higher than for women without activity limitations.[42] Women with disabilities were generally less likely to receive a Pap test or mammogram than were women without functional limitations.[43]

Considerable gaps exist in health care access for this population. A study of people (both women and men) with disabilities found that 21% did not get needed care in the past year, compared to 11% of adults without a disability.[44] One-fourth (28%) postponed getting needed care in the past year because they could not afford it. Although the vast majority of adults with disabilities were covered by insurance, one in three reported that they have special health care needs that were not covered by their health insurance.[44]

Incarcerated Women. The number of incarcerated women in the United States has increased dramatically over the last 10 years, growing by 92% since 1990. Illegal drug use by women accounts for nearly 40% of this increase.[45] Because the number of incarcerated men historically has been much greater than that of incarcerated women, little attention has been given to the unique and special health concerns of this population. Health concerns of incarcerated women include an already high risk for communicable disease, substance abuse, and mental health problems.[46,47] In one study of female prisoners, more than 50% reported having a medical condition requiring medical attention, yet only 28% received care.[48] The unique health issues female inmates face must be integrated into the development and implementation of health care standards and protocols.[49]

Homeless Women. Homeless women and men have extraordinary health care access barriers that can be overcome only through special outreach programs. It is difficult to determine the current number of homeless women, but it is estimated that 37% of the homeless population in 1999 were families with

Table 8-3

Use and access problems among women aged 18–64 years by insurance status, 1998

	Percent			
	All women	Continuously insured	Currently insured, but uninsured at some time in past year	Currently uninsured
In the past year did not:				
Get needed care	10	6	23	22
See specialist when needed	12	7	24	31
Fill prescription because of costs	15	10	27	31
One or more of the above	24	17	40	46
In the past year:				
No doctor visit	8	6	8	20
Had no regular doctor	22	14	29	51
Had difficulty getting needed care*	19	10	29	50

* Woman reported "extremely," "very," or "somewhat" difficult to get needed care.

Source: Collins K, Schoen C, Joseph S, Duchon L, Simantov E, Yellowitz M. Health concerns across a woman's lifespan: The Commonwealth Fund 1998 Survey of Women's Health. New York: The Commonwealth Fund; 1999.

children and 13% were single women.[50] Health care is often not a top priority for women who are homeless, and, consequently, homeless women suffer from common illness (e.g., colds, influenza) and chronic health problems (e.g., tuberculosis, arthritis) at disproportionate rates compared to women in the general population. These health problems are often exacerbated by increased stress, poor nutrition, and the lack of access to treatment, all of which are all too common in this population.[51] In addition to a lack of financial resources, homeless women tend to have little social support, earn little income, and are unemployed. Furthermore, there is a high rate of comorbidity of substance abuse and depression among homeless women.[51]

Utilization of Health Care Services

The types and amounts of health care services that women use are influenced by a wide range of factors including age, insurance coverage, and health needs. Considerable variation exists between women and men and among different subgroups of women.

Role of Insurance Coverage

Several studies have documented the relationship between insurance coverage and access to care among the nonelderly.[16,52] Uninsured women are much less likely than those with coverage to have had a doctor visit in the past year or a regular health care provider.[35] For example, the

1998 Commonwealth Fund Survey of Women's Health found that one-half of uninsured women have no regular doctor (compared to 14% of continuously insured women), and one-half report difficulties in getting needed care (compared to just 10% of insured women) (Table 8-3).[53] Continuity of coverage is an important component of access. Women who went without health insurance for part of the year face access difficulties at rates generally similar to those of women who are currently uninsured; thus, gaps in coverage increase the likelihood of going without care. Having coverage—either Medicaid or private—greatly improved access and use of health services for low-income women.[54] Even among elderly women there are differences in use by the presence and type of supplemental coverage.[55]

A usual source of care is also an important component in ensuring timely and consistent care. Having a usual source of care is associated with women's increased use of clinical preventive services and general medical checkups, even among insured women.[56, 57]

Health Care Visits

Women in the United States typically obtain health care services from many different sources. Women use the health care system more than men do, and their patterns of utilization are more complex than men's. Women use, on average, about two physicians at one time throughout their lifespan. There is considerable variation among women in the kinds of physicians used for regular care.[58]

According to the National Ambulatory Medical Care Survey, the number of visits made by women compared to men is higher in all age groups, except for the two oldest, (65–74 years, and 75 years and older). The visit rate increases for women with each successive age group, going from 2.4 visits per year for females aged 15–24 years to 6.5 for women aged 75 years and older (Table 8-4).[59] Differences in use rates between women and men appear to be medi-

Table 8-4

Number, percent distribution, and annual rate of office visits among men and women by age, 1997			
	Number of visits (in thousands)	**Percent distribution**	**Number of visits per person per year***
All visits	787,372	100.0	3.0
All men	315,891	40.1	2.4
All women	471,181	59.9	3.5
Under 15 years	63,042	8.0	2.2
15–24 years	43,042	5.5	2.4
25–44 years	137,486	17.5	3.3
45–64 years	113,756	14.4	4.0
65–74 years	57,918	7.4	5.8
75 + years	56,237	7.1	6.5

*Based on U.S. Bureau of Census monthly postcensus estimates of the civilian noninstitutionalized population as of July 1, 1997.

Source: Woodwell DA. National Ambulatory Medical Care Survey. 1997 summary. Advance data from Vital and Health Statistics; no. 305. Hyattsville (MD): National Center for Health Statistics; 1999.

ated by the type of service. According to a recent study of 509 new adult patients, women had more primary care visits (4 versus 3) and diagnostic services (10 versus 7) over a year period than men had.[60] Men and women had approximately the same mean number of specialty clinic visits (2.8 for women versus 2.3 for men), emergency department visits (0.31 for women versus 0.25 for men) and hospitalizations (0.17 for women versus 0.19 for men). However, women did have higher annual charges than men for all types of care including primary, specialty, emergency treatment, diagnostic services, and total annual charges (even after adjustments for health status, socioeconomic status, and clinic assignment).[60]

Inpatient Care

One important change in the U.S. health care system in recent years has been a decline in use of inpatient services and an increase in outpatient services, driven in large part by the movement to reduce health care costs. Between 1990 and 1996 the overall inpatient discharge rate in short-stay hospitals declined from 91.0 discharges per 1,000 population to 82.4 per 1,000. The average length of stay declined from 6.7 to 5.7 days.[61]

There is a recent increase in length of stay for childbirth. Length of stays for childbirth went from 3.8 days in 1980 to 2.1 days in 1995 and in 1997 increased to 2.4 days. State laws passed in 1995 were the precursor to federal legislation passed in 1996 that prohibited insurers from restricting hospital stays for vaginal deliveries to less than 2 days and 4 days for cesarean deliveries. Although the law became effective in 1998, its anticipated effects, as well as state legislation, may have resulted in the longer stays seen.[62]

Preventive Services

The use of preventive health care services has substantial and important positive effects on the long-term health status of women. Receipt of these services generally is a good indicator of overall access. Table 8-5 displays 1999 Behavioral Risk Factor Surveillance System (BRFSS) data on utilization of preventive care services for men and women. Nearly all women reported having their blood pressure taken by a health care professional in the past 2 years, and utilization is slightly better than for men. There is considerable room for improvement in other areas. Although colon cancer represents the third leading cause of cancer deaths among women and despite the recommendation for screening tests for both men and women 50 years of age and older (see chapter 4), rates of screening for this cancer are quite low. Based on the 1999 BRFSS data, approximately half of women 50 and older reported ever receiving the recommended screening (sigmoidoscopy), slightly less than the proportion of men screened.

Table 8-5

Preventive care service utilization by gender, 1999

	Percent	
	Women	**Men**
Cholesterol screening		
Blood cholesterol ever checked	76.0	81.9
Blood cholesterol checked within past 5 years	71.5	66.6
Hypertension screening		
Blood pressure taken by health professional within past 2 years	98.6	92.5
Colorectal cancer screening (≥50 years of age)		
Home blood stool test kit in past 2 years	23.3	16.4
Sigmoidoscopy ever	49.1	55.0
Breast cancer screening		
Clinical breast exam ever (≥18 years of age)	89.2	—
Clinical breast exam in past 2 years (≥50 years of age)	76.8	—
Mammogram in past 2 years (≥50 years of age)	75.5	—
Cervical cancer screening		
Pap smear in past 3 years (≥18 years of age, intact cervix)	85.4	—

Source: National Center for Chronic Disease Prevention and Health Promotion. 1999 Behavioral Risk Factor Surveillance System (BRFSS) prevalence report. Atlanta: U.S. Department of Health and Human Services, Centers for Disease Control and Prevention; 2000. Available from: URL: www.cdc.gov/nccdphp/brfss/pubrfdat.htm.

The 1999 BRFSS data suggest that screening for breast and cervical cancer still does not reach all women, even when focusing on a 2- to 3-year screening interval, rather than 12 months prior to interview only.[63] The 1998 Commonwealth Fund

Figure 8-6

Women receiving preventive care in the past year by income, 1998

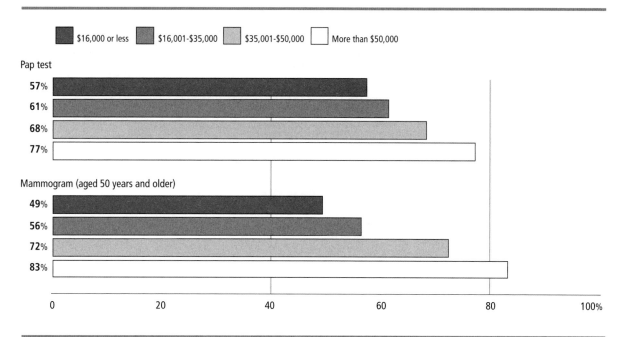

Source: Collins K. Schoen C, Joseph S, Duchon L, Simantov E, Yellowitz M. Health concerns across a woman's lifespan: The Commonwealth Fund 1998 Survey of Women's Health. New York: The Commonwealth Fund; 1999.

Survey of Women's Health found that the proportion of women who received a clinical breast examination (66%) or a Pap test (64%) to detect cervical cancer did not improve between 1993 and 1998.[35] Mammography rates for women 50 and older did increase, however, going from 55% to 61%. A further positive sign was the increase in mammography screening rates for both African American women and Hispanics between 1993 and 1998.

Uninsured women are at highest risk for not receiving preventive services.[35] And, as is seen for health care use overall, low-income women are much less likely to be screened than those with higher incomes (Figure 8-6).[35] The main barrier cited by women in the 1993 Commonwealth Fund Survey who did not receive a preventive screening was the cost.[56] Medicaid and private coverage make an important difference for low-income women, improving their low screening rates.[54]

Another component of prevention is counseling about health and risky behaviors. Studies generally find low levels of physician counseling on important health issues. Less than half of women report being counseled by physicians on health issues during the past year (Figure 8-7), suggesting that new strategies are needed to improve communication and to focus care and education on underlying health concerns.[35] Physicians can increase knowledge and potentially influence patients' behavior through counseling. Physicians are most likely to discuss issues of exercise, diet, and weight management; these topics are more likely to be discussed with African American women. Counseling rates for socially sensitive issues (e.g., HIV, violence) remain low across income and racial/ethnic groups.[35] In general low-income and less well-educated women are more likely to be counseled about smoking, sexually transmitted diseases, and safety and violence issues.[35]

Figure 8-7

Women receiving physician counseling on selected health issues, 1998

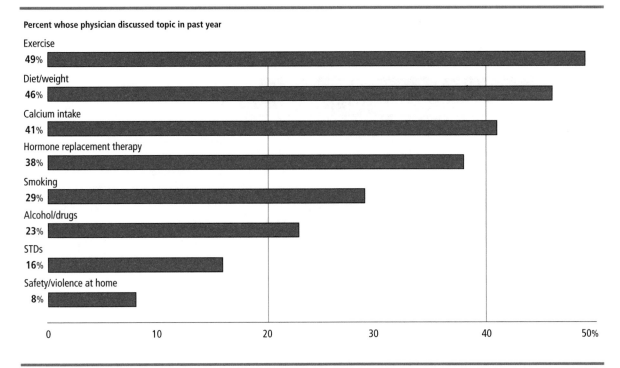

Percent whose physician discussed topic in past year

Exercise
49%

Diet/weight
46%

Calcium intake
41%

Hormone replacement therapy
38%

Smoking
29%

Alcohol/drugs
23%

STDs
16%

Safety/violence at home
8%

0   10   20   30   40   50%

Source: The Commonwealth Fund 1998 Survey of Women's Health. New York: The Commonwealth Fund; 1999.

Gynecologic Services

Women use the health care system differently than men do, often relying on a primary care provider, obstetrician/gynecologist, or both for their care. Nearly four out of 10 women see both an ob/gyn and a family practitioner or internist for their regular care, and 16% see only an ob/gyn as their regular source of care.[64] Access to ob/gyn providers is an important issue in meeting a woman's health needs. In a survey conducted by the Henry J. Kaiser Family Foundation, 84% of U.S. women aged 18–64 years reported having had a routine obstetric or gynecologic exam in the past 2 years, and 76% reported doing so within the last year. Uninsured women were the least likely to have had a recent routine ob/gyn examination (59%) by either an ob/gyn or other health provider. [65]

Women who use both a family practitioner or internist and an ob/gyn are more likely to receive recommended preventive services (e.g.,

pelvic exam, breast exam, Pap test).[58] Ob/gyns have also been found to counsel more frequently about family planning and STDs as compared to other primary care physicians.[66]

Obstetric Services

Infant mortality and low birth weight are strongly associated with time of entry into and continued use of prenatal care. The primary indicators of adequate prenatal care services are month of entry (or trimester of entry) into prenatal care and the total number of prenatal visits. These measures are available from standard U.S. birth certificates and are also compiled by the National Center for Health Statistics. The proportion of women beginning prenatal care in the first trimester of pregnancy has increased 10% since 1989 to a rate of 75% in 1998.[61] The largest increases in receipt of early prenatal care have occurred for racial and ethnic groups with the lowest levels of use, thereby reducing

Figure 8-8

Prenatal care begun during first trimester by race/ethnicity of mother, United States, 1997

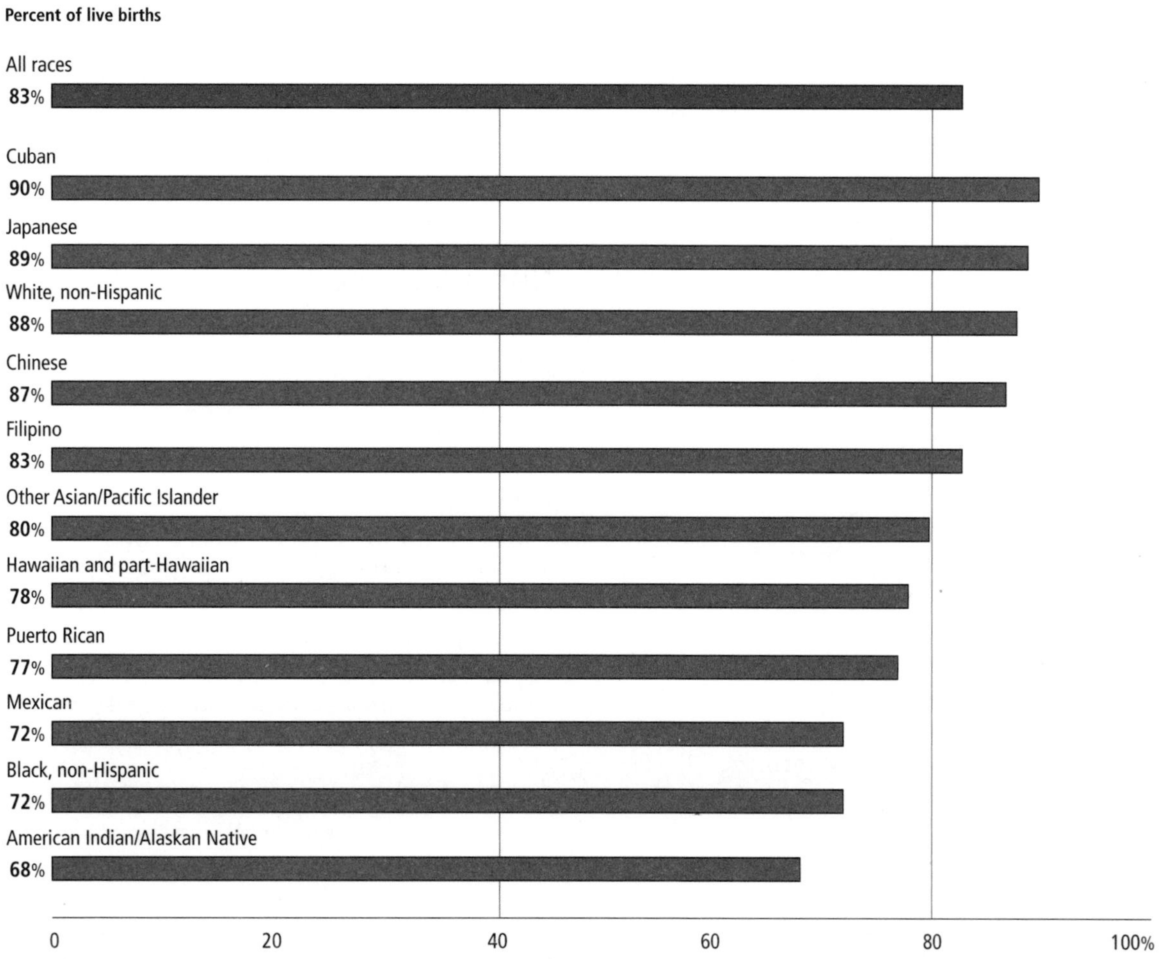

Percent of live births

All races
83%

Cuban
90%

Japanese
89%

White, non-Hispanic
88%

Chinese
87%

Filipino
83%

Other Asian/Pacific Islander
80%

Hawaiian and part-Hawaiian
78%

Puerto Rican
77%

Mexican
72%

Black, non-Hispanic
72%

American Indian/Alaskan Native
68%

0   20   40   60   80   100%

Source: National Center for Health Statistics. Health, United States, 1999. With health and aging chartbook. Table 6. (PHS)99–1232. Hyattsville (MD): U.S. Department of Health and Human Services; 1999.

disparities in use of early care. However, in 1997 the percent of mothers with early prenatal care still varied significantly among racial and ethnic groups, from 68% for American Indian mothers to 90% for Cuban mothers (Figure 8-8).[61]

Abortion Services

In 1996, 1.37 million abortions took place in the United States, a decrease from 1.61 million in 1990.[12] Several access issues are related to obtaining an abortion. The majority of U.S. abor-

tions (93%) are performed in clinics or physicians' offices. The number of abortion providers declined by 14% between 1992 and 1996, (from 2,380 to 2,042), leaving women in many areas of the country without access to these services unless they are able to travel significant distances.[12] Eighty-six percent of all U.S. counties lacked an abortion provider in 1996. Of abortion facilities, 43% provided services only through the 12th week of pregnancy in 1999. Almost half of women who have abortions beyond 15 weeks of gestation say they were delayed because of problems in affording, finding, or getting to abortion services.[12] Teens are more likely than older women to delay having an abortion until after 16 weeks of pregnancy, when medical risks increase.

The recent Food and Drug Administration (FDA) approval of mifepristone (RU486) provides a nonsurgical alternative to abortion. Obstacles remain to its use, however. Although many insurers will cover the drug, some may allow employers to exclude it from coverage. Other factors that may determine access to the drug are the availability of physicians trained in its use and variation in state laws on abortion.[67]

STD Management

According to the 1998 Commonwealth Fund Survey of Women's Health, STDs were one of the least discussed health prevention topics by physicians with their female patients. Sixteen percent of women report having been counseled regarding STDs during the past year.[35] Low-income women and those with less education were the most likely to be counseled. In another study, 67% of sexually active women aged 18–44 years who had a routine gynecological exam in the last 2 years reported that they were not counseled about or tested for HIV during their visit; 70% reported that they did not discuss nor were they tested for any other STD.[65] Insurance plans often do not reimburse health care providers for counseling and educational services provided to patients. Consequently, there is often little financial incentive to provide such services.

Mental Health

There are many barriers to treatment for mental health services. The Epidemiologic Catchment Area (ECA) study found that three-quarters of women who met diagnostic psychiatric criteria had not used mental health services in the previous 6 months even though women were more likely to seek mental health services than men were.[68] Several factors have been identified as barriers to seeking treatment. Among them

are financial barriers because of lack of or restrictive coverage for mental health services, lack of coordination of care or adequate referral sources, stigma attached to treatment, cultural and linguistic barriers, time constraints, and parenting responsibilities.[69] As of midyear 2000, 31 states had some form of mental health parity statute in insurance and managed care coverage to equalize benefits between physical and mental health.[70]

Nursing Home Care

In 1997, there were approximately 1.5 million nursing home residents 65 years of age and over,[61] representing 4% of the older population. As discussed in chapter 4, because women live longer than men, women are more likely to live with multiple chronic conditions, to have functional impairments, and to need long-term care. Women frequently outlive their spouses, leaving them more likely to live alone and live without a caregiver than are men. Living alone is a risk factor for nursing home admission. The U.S. female population has been and will increasingly be aging over the next 50 years (see chapter 1).

Women are the primary users of long-term care services; three quarters of all nursing home residents are females.[20] According to the National Center for Health Statistics (NCHS), half of current elderly residents of nursing homes are 85 years of age or older.[61] The rate of nursing home residence increases by age. In 1997, 12 in 1,000 women 65–74 years of age were nursing home residents, rising to 53 of 1,000 women 75-84 years of age and 222 per 1,000 for women 85 years of age and older.[61] Many elderly women live in the community, and 60% of women aged 85 years and older live alone.[61]

There are problems with access and quality in nursing homes. Medicaid's relatively low reimbursement rate deters nursing homes from making beds available to beneficiaries. The quality of care for nursing home residents, in particular Medicaid beneficiaries, has been an ongoing concern.[71]

Home Health Care

Women not only require more nursing home services than do older men, they also need more home health care services than men, again primarily due to their longer life spans and resulting effects of chronic illnesses. Medicare's coverage of home health services is limited to people who are homebound, in need of skilled nursing, physical therapy, or speech therapy, and under the care of a physician.[71] But, long-term care needs vary considerably. Some elderly or disabled need assistance only with shopping or paying bills, whereas others require full-time assistance. Because of limited insurance coverage, approximately two-thirds of the elderly depend upon family or friends as their only form of assistance.[71] These informal, unpaid caregivers are mainly women, who often feel the strain of balancing caregiving with other responsibilities.[72,73]

According to the NCHS, there were a total of 2.4 million home health care users in 1996, compared to 1.2 million in 1992. Females constitute 67% of those receiving home health care services.[61] Similarly, 66% of all Medicare beneficiaries who receive home health services are females.[20] Among women, use rates increase with age, with an average use of 130 users per 1,000 population for women aged 85 years and over. [61]

Many needs for assistance with daily living activities go unmet among the noninstitutionalized elderly. In 1995, among those aged 70 years and older who had difficulty and needed help with an activity of daily living (bathing, dressing) or a household activity (shopping, cleaning), 44% reported they had unmet needs.[61] That is, they either had no assistance or required additional assistance. In the majority of cases, those with unmet needs required hands-on help. Half of those who had an unmet need for assistance with activities of daily living reported a negative consequence.[61]

Quality of Health Care Services

Assessing the quality of health care services is important for consumers, purchasers, and providers. The Institute of Medicine defines quality of care as "the degree to which health services for individuals and populations increase the likelihood of desired health outcomes and are consistent with current professional knowledge."[74] This is an area of much activity in recent years, ranging from consumer-based report cards evaluating HMOs to federal policies requiring standardization of mammography equipment or those limiting the volume of Pap tests read per hour by laboratory technicians.

Framework to Evaluate Quality

The most commonly used framework to evaluate quality is based upon three dimensions of quality: structure, process, and outcomes.[75] Structure refers to the health care system characteristics (e.g., qualifications of providers, operating hours of the practice, infection control procedures), as well as the characteristics of the population needing services, which serve to either promote or impede access to care and the provision of services. Process refers to interactions between patients and providers and to what happens during assessment or treatment. It includes both technical and interpersonal aspects of care. Outcome measures are the short-term and long-term effects of health care and are viewed by many as the ultimate measure of the quality of the health care system.[76]

The availability and adequacy of health insurance is a structural factor that can affect entry into the health care system and provision of care when in the system. Other structural factors include such indicators as staffing patterns, organizational structure of the health care facility, and location of the facility.[76] Because of the way data are collected in managed care organizations, considerably more is known about the quality of care received by women enrolled in managed care

Table 8-6

Effectiveness of women's health care in managed care organizations: quality measures from HEDIS 2000* database/benchmarking project

Measure	Definition**	Percent		
		Plan performance		
		1999 average	10th percentile	90th percentile
Breast cancer screening	Percentage of women aged 52–69 years who had at least one mammogram in past 2 years	73	64	82
Cervical cancer screening	Percentage of women aged 21–64 years who had at least one Pap test in past 3 years	72	60	83
Prenatal care in first trimester	Percentage of pregnant women who began prenatal care in first 13 weeks of pregnancy	85	71	95
Check-ups after delivery	Percentage of women with live births who had postpartum visit 21–56 days after delivery	72	54	87
Chlamydia screening***	Percentage of sexually active women aged 16–26 years who had at least one test for chlamydia in past year			
	16–20 years	19	5	33
	21–26 years	16	5	28
Management of menopause***	Percentage of women aged 45–55 years who received sufficient/appropriate counseling about options for managing menopausal hormonal changes in past 2 years or ever			
	Exposure to counseling	73	66	79
	Breadth of counseling	50	41	58
	Personalization of counseling	47	38	56
	Composite score	57	49	64

*Data were collected in 1999 from HMO and POS health plans.

**For more information on the measures, see: National Committee for Quality Assurance. HEDIS 2000 technical specifications. Volume 2. Washington: National Committee for Quality Assurance; 1999.

***New measure in HEDIS 2000 database.

Source: National Committee for Quality Assurance. The state of managed care quality, 2000. Washington: National Committee on Quality Assurance; 2000.

organizations than those receiving care under a fee-for-service structure.[77]

Process of care measures relate to the appropriateness of care received, adherence to practice guidelines or standards, practice pattern profiling across communities, or consumer feedback on satisfaction with the care provided.[76] Studies examining differences in practice patterns across geographic areas are quite common. For example, differences in hormone replacement therapy (HRT) were seen between women in the West and those in the Northeast, with those in the West 3.5 times more likely to receive the therapy.[78] Variations by geographic area are also seen for mammography screening and surgical treatment among female Medicare recipients.[79]

Other studies focus on inappropriate use of services or differences in treatments across populations. For example, in a study comparing the appropriateness of hysterectomy across seven managed care organizations, 16% of women underwent hysterectomies for reasons judged to be clinically inappropriate by a panel of physicians.[80]

Quality of care received by women has been examined in comparison to that received by men for several conditions that they have in common, such as heart disease, kidney disease, and AIDS. For example, studies have demonstrated that African American women with coronary artery disease, compared with both white and African American men and white women, are significantly less likely to receive standard interventions, such as cardiac catheterization.[81]

Outcome measures, including clinical outcomes, functional status, and quality of life, are more challenging to investigate. These studies are often complex because of the difficulty in controlling several factors that might influence an outcome. The severity of illness needs to be controlled to eliminate the possibility that differences in outcome are really differences in health status. Also, because several factors affect outcomes, it is

sometimes difficult to attribute an outcome to a specific factor. In a study that examined outcome and process of care, it was found that women received less aggressive treatment after a heart attack than men and were more likely to die within the hospital. Both age and severity of illness were controlled for in this study.[82]

Measuring Quality

There are different ways to measure quality depending upon the intent of the assessment and the condition being examined. Until recently, the focus on quality assessment was on structural issues for accreditation. Now, more emphasis has been placed on process and outcome measures. One of the methods for capturing data on outcomes is the Health Plan and Employer Data and Information Set (HEDIS) database/benchmark project, developed by the National Committee for Quality Assurance in 1991.[83] The HEDIS project is used by commercial managed care plans and, now, public insurers, to measure quality. It is a set of standardized performance measures designed for use by both purchasers of insurance and consumers and is voluntary for reporting purposes.

Specific measures of interest to women's health include such items as breast and cervical cancer screening, chlamydia screening, rates of cesarean sections and vaginal births after cesarean delivery, prenatal care use in the first trimester, and counseling about women's options for management of menopuase.[83] Table 8-6 shows the average scores for these measures for health plans participating in the HEDIS 2000 project and scores for health plans performing at the tenth and 90th percentiles.[84]

Measures of controlling high blood pressure, beta blocker treatment after health attacks, and use of appropriate medications for people with asthma are also important for ensuring quality of care for chronic diseases, especially because recent research indicates that women's and men's rates of specific types of indicated procedures are dissimilar,[81] but these measures are not currently designed to be reported by gender. The HEDIS database can capture only a portion of quality issues, yet measurement of the quality of women's health care is an important area to develop.[85,86] The National Committee for Quality Assurance in 1997 appointed a Women's Health Measurement Advisory Panel to assist in the development of quality measures for possible inclusion in the HEDIS database. This panel developed the management of menopause measure, the first measure in the informed decision-making domain of the HEDIS database, and recommended development of measures related to osteoporosis screening and prevention of unintended pregnancy.[86]

The Institute of Medicine has recently released a report addressing quality issues in all aspects of the health care system.[87] The report is a call for action to dramatically improve the deficits in the current system and establishes several aims for the health care system. The health care system should be safe (avoid injuries to patients from care), effective (avoid overuse and underuse), patient-centered (care that is responsive to and respectful of patients and their preferences and values), timely (avoid waits and delays in care), efficient (avoid waste), and equitable (provide care that does not vary in quality based on a person's gender, ethnicity, geographic location, or income).[87] The report defines a vision of a health care system that provides care that is patient-centered, evidence-based, and systems-oriented.

Challenges in Ensuring High-Quality Care for Women

There are significant challenges in ensuring the delivery of high-quality health care for women. These challenges include information systems, privacy issues,[77] as well as fragmentation of care. Quality measurement relies on data and information systems that can track clinical care delivered to individuals, a consistent challenge for capitated systems where services are often bundled together for billing purposes. Also, automating clinical information requires significant investments of time and money from organizations. Even if all data system issues are solved, privacy and confidentiality concerns surround sensitive medical records—an issue that Congress has been grappling with for years and is of particular concern for women. Lastly, women often receive their health care from fragmented sources, using their regular doctors as well as other specialists and providers. No gold standard exists to ensure that women's health care is managed comprehensively across different providers and sites of care. Complicating matters, medical records are often fragmented and incomplete. The interface between seeing multiple doctors and ensuring quality for the whole woman, instead of body part by body part, remains a significant challenge.

References

1. Sandman D, Simantov E, An C. Out of touch: American men and the health care system. New York: The Commonwealth Fund; 2000.

2. Lewis-Idema D, Leiman J, Myers J, Collins, KS. Health care access and coverage for women: changing times, changing issues? New York: The Commonwealth Fund Commission on Women's Health; 1999.

3. Levitt L, Holve E, Wang J, Gabel J, Whitmore H, Pickreign J, et al. Employer health benefits, 2000 annual survey. Menlo Park (CA): Henry J. Kaiser Family Foundation and Health Research and Educational Trust; 2000.

4. Chollet D, Kirk AM. Understanding individual health insurance markets: structure, practices, and products in ten states. Menlo Park (CA): Henry J. Kaiser Family Foundation; 1998.

5. Henry J. Kaiser Family Foundation. State policies on access to gynecological care and contraception: an update on women's health policy. Menlo Park (CA): The Foundation; 2000.

6. Rowland D, Salganicoff A. The key to the door: Medicaid's role in improving health care for women and children. Annu Rev Public Health 1999;20:403–426.

7. Henry J. Kaiser Family Foundation. Medicaid's role for women. Women's health policy facts. Menlo Park (CA): The Foundation; 2000.

8. Henry J. Kaiser Family Foundation. Coverage of gynecological care and contraceptives. Women's health policy facts. Menlo Park (CA): The Foundation; 2000.

9. Schwalberg R, Zimmerman B, Mohamadi L, Giffin M, Mathis SA. Medicaid coverage of family planning services: results of a national survey. Menlo Park (CA): Henry J. Kaiser Family Foundation; 2001.

10. Henry J. Kaiser Family Foundation. Health coverage of contraceptive and other gynecological services. Women's health policy facts. Menlo Park (CA): The Foundation; 1999.

11. Breast and Cervical Cancer Prevention and Treatment Act of 2000. Public law #106-354, 106th U.S. Congress. Available from: URL: www.hcfa.gov/medicaid/bccpt/pl106.htm.

12. Alan Guttmacher Institute. Induced abortion (U.S.). Facts in brief. New York: The Institute, 2000. Available from: URL: www.agi-usa.org/pubs/fb_induced_abortion.html.

13. Thorpe KE. The distribution of health insurance coverage among pregnant women, 1990–1997. White Plains: March of Dimes; 1999.

14. U.S. Bureau of the Census. Current Population Survey. Washington: U.S. Department of Labor; March 2000.

15. Wyn R, Solis B, Ojeda V, Pourat N. Falling through the cracks: low-income women and their health insurance coverage. Menlo Park (CA): Henry J. Kaiser Family Foundation; 2001.

16. Schlobohm A, Hoffman C. Uninsured in America: a chart book. Washington: Kaiser Commission on Medicaid and the Uninsured; 2000.

17. Garrett B, Holahan J. Welfare leavers, Medicaid coverage, and private health insurance. Washington: The Urban Institute; 2000.

18. Personal Responsibility and Work Opportunity Act of 1996. 104th U.S. Congress; 1996.

19. Families USA. Losing health insurance: the unintended consequences of welfare reform. Washington: Families USA; 1999. Available from: URL: www.familiesusa.org/uninten.htm.

20. Henry J. Kaiser Family Foundation. Medicare and women. Fact sheet. Menlo Park (CA): The Foundation; 1998.

21. Population Reference Bureau. What the 1990 Census tells us about women: a state fact book. Washington: Population Reference Bureau; 1993.

22. Foley L, Gibson M. Older women's access to health care: potential impact of Medicare reform. Washington: AARP Public Policy Institute; 2000.

23. Anderson RN. United States life tables, 1998. Nat Vital Stat Rep. Centers for Disease Control; 2001.

24. Henry J. Kaiser Family Foundation. Medicare and women. Faces of Medicare. Menlo Park (CA): The Foundation; 1999.

25. Neuman P. Why Medicare is a woman's issue. Chart pack. Menlo Park (CA): Henry J. Kaiser Family Foundation; 1999.

26. Henry J. Kaiser Family Foundation. Analyses of the 1997 Medicare Consumer Beneficiary Survey. Menlo Park (CA): The Foundation; 1997.

27. Kasten J, Moon M, Segal M. What do Medicare HMO enrollees spend out-of-pocket? Washington: The Urban Institute; 2000.

28. O'Brien E, Rowland D. Medicare and Medicaid for the elderly and disabled poor. Washington: Kaiser Commission on Medicaid and the Uninsured; 1999.

29. Kaiser Commission on Medicaid and the Uninsured. Medicare and Medicaid for the elderly and disabled poor: Fact sheet. Washington: The Commission; 1999.

30.	Barents Group. A profile of QMB-eligible and SLMB-eligible Medicare beneficiaries. Washington: The Barents Group; 1999.

31.	Weisman CS, Henderson JT. Managed care and women's health: access, preventive services, and satisfaction. Women's Health Issues 2001; 11(3):201–215.

32.	Kaiser Commission on Medicaid and the Uninsured. Medicaid and managed care. Fact sheet. Washington: The Commission; 2001.

33.	Salganicoff A, Wyn R, Solis B. Medicaid managed care and low-income women: implications for access and satisfaction. Women's Health Issues 1998;8:339–349.

34.	Schoen C. The Kaiser/Commonwealth 1997 National Survey of Health Insurance: women's health insurance and managed care experiences. Presentation to The Commonwealth Fund Commission on Women's Health symposium entitled Access, Coverage, and Quality in Health Care for Women.

35.	Collins K, Schoen C, Joseph S, Duchon L, Simantov E, Yellowitz M. Health concerns across a woman's lifespan: The Commonwealth Fund 1998 Survey of Women's Health. New York: The Commonwealth Fund; 1999.

36.	Collins KS, Hall A, Neuhaus C. U.S. minority health: a chart book. New York: The Commonwealth Fund; 1999.

37.	Morehouse Medical Treatment Effectiveness Center. A synthesis of the literature: racial and ethnic differences in access to medical care. Menlo Park (CA): Henry J. Kaiser Family Foundation; 1999.

38.	Stevens PE. Lesbian health care research: a review of the literature from 1970 to 1990. Health Care Women Int 1992;13:91–120.

39.	Solarz AL. Lesbian health: current assessment and directions for the future. Washington: National Academy Press; 1999.

40.	Centers for Disease Control and Prevention. Prevalence of disabilities and associated health conditions among adults—United States, 1999. MMWR Morb Mortal Wkly Rep 2001;50(7):120–125.

41.	LaPlante MP. Disability, health insurance coverage, and utilization of acute health services in the United States. Washington: U.S. Department of Health and Human Services; 1993.

42.	Jans L, Stoddard S. Chart book on women and disability in the United States. Washington: U.S. Department of Education, National Institute on Disability and Rehabilitation Research; 1996.

43.	Centers for Disease Control and Prevention. Use of cervical and breast cancer screening among women with and without functional limitations—United States, 1994–1995. MMWR Morb Mortal Wkly Rep 1998; 47(RR-19): 1–33.

44.	1998 National Organization on Disability/Harris Survey of Americans with Disabilities. New York: Harris Interactive; 1998. Available from: URL: www.nod.org/presssurvey.html.

45.	Bureau of Justice Statistics. Prisoners in 1998. Washington: U.S. Department of Justice; 1999. Available from: URL: www.ojp.usdoj.gov/bjs/abstract/p98.htm.

46.	Hammett TM, Gaiter JL, Crawford C. Reaching seriously at-risk populations: health interventions in criminal justice settings. Health Education and Behavior 1998;25:99–120.

47.	Smith BV, Dailard C. Incarceration. In: Allen KM, Phillips JM, editors. Women's health across the lifespan: a comprehensive perspective. Philadelphia: Lippincott-Raven; 1997. p. 19, 464–478.

48.	Bureau of Justice Statistics. Profile of jail inmates, 1996. Washington: U.S. Department of Justice; 1998.

49.	Baldwin KM, Jones J. Health issues specific to incarcerated women: information for state maternal and child health programs. (research brief). Baltimore: Women's and Children's Health Policy Center, Johns Hopkins University; 2000.

50.	Lowe E, Slater A, Welfley J, Hardie D. A status report on hunger and homelessness in America's cities. Washington: United States Conference of Mayors; 1999. Available from: URL: www.usmayors.org.htm.

51.	Silver G, Panares R. The health of homeless women: information for state maternal and child health programs. Baltimore: Women's and Children's Health Policy Center, Johns Hopkins University; 2000.

52.	Weisman JS, Epstein AM. Falling through the safety net: insurance status and access to health care. Baltimore: Johns Hopkins University; 1994.

53.	The Commonwealth Fund. Health insurance coverage and access to care for working-age women. New York: The Commonwealth Fund; 1999.

54.	Salganicoff A, Wyn R. Access to care for low-income women: the impact of Medicaid. J Health Care Poor Underserved 1999;10:453–467.

55.	Blustein, J. Medicare coverage, supplemental insurance, and the use of mammography by older women. New Engl J Med 1995;332:1138–1143.

56. Wyn R, Brown ER, Yu H. Women's use of preventive health services. In: Falik M, Collins, KS, editors. Women's health: The Commonwealth Fund Survey. Baltimore: Johns Hopkins University; 1996.

57. Brown ER, Wyn R, Cumberland WG, Yu H, Abel E, Gelberg L, et al. Women's health-related behaviors and use of preventive services. New York: The Commonwealth Fund Commission on Women's Health; 1995.

58. Weisman C. Women's use of health care. In: Falik M, Collins, KS, editors. Women's Health: The Commonwealth Fund Survey. Baltimore: Johns Hopkins University Press; 1996.

59. Woodwell DA. National Ambulatory Medical Care Survey. 1997 summary. Advance data from Vital Health Stat; no. 305. Hyattsville (MD): National Center for Health Statistics; 1999.

60. Bertakis KD, Azari R, Helms LJ, Callahan EJ, Robbins JA. Gender differences in the utiliztion of health services. J Fam Pract 2000; 49:147–152.

61. National Center for Health Statistics. Health, United States, 1999. With health and aging chartbook. (PHS)99–1292. Hyattsville (MD): U.S. Department of Health and Human Services; 1999.

62. National Center for Health Statistics. Health E-Stats: longer hospital stays for childbirth. Hyattsville (MD): U.S. Department of Health and Human Services; 1997. Available from: URL: www.cdc.gov/nchs/products/pubs/pubd/hestats/hospbirth.htm.

63. National Center for Chronic Disease Prevention and Health Promotion. 1999 Behavioral Risk Factor Surveillance System (BRFSS) prevalence report. Atlanta: U.S. Department of Health and Human Services, Centers for Disease Control and Prevention; 2000. Available from: URL: www.cdc.gov/nccdphp/brfss/pubrfdat.htm.

64. Henderson JT, Weisman CS. Women's patterns of physician use: a life stage perspective. Paper presented at the annual meeting of the Population Association of America. Washington: 2001 Mar 29.

65. Henry J. Kaiser Family Foundation with Essence, Latina, and the Los Angeles Times. A national survey of women about their reproductive health care. Menlo Park (CA): The Foundation; 1999.

66. Horton JA, Murphy P, Hale RW. Obstetrician-gynecologists as primary care providers: a national survey of women. Prim Care Update Ob/Gyns 1994; 1(5): 212–215.

67. Kaiser Daily Reproductive Health Report. Mifepristone II: while most insurers will cover drug, obstacles still remain. Menlo Park (CA): The Henry J. Kaiser Family Foundation; Thursday October 5, 2000. Available from: URL: www.kaisernetwork.org/frame/index.cfm?goto=http://www.kaiser-network.org/reports/2000/10/kr001005.4.htm.

68. Robins LN, Locke BZ, Regier DA. An overview of psychiatric disorders in America. In: Robins L, Regier DA, editors. Psychiatric disorders in America. New York: The Free Press; 1991.

69. Glied S, Kofman S. Women and mental health: issues for health reform. New York: The Commonwealth Fund Commission on Women's Health; 1995.

70. Kirschstein ML. Insurance parity for mental health: cost, access, and quality. Appendix E: states with mental health parity statutes. Bethesda (MD): National Institute of Mental Health; 2000. Available from: URL: www.nimh.nih.gov/parity/appende.cfm.

71. Kaiser Commission on Medicaid and the Uninsured. Long-term care: Medicaid's role and challenges. Washington: The Commission; 1999.

72. Family Circle and Henry J. Kaiser Family Foundation. National survey on health care and other elder care issues. Menlo Park (CA): Henry J. Kaiser Family Foundation; 2000.

73. Donelan K, Falik M, DesRoches CM. Caregiving: challenges and implications for women's health. Women's Health Issues 2001; 11(3)185–200.

74. California HealthCare Foundation. Health care quality in California: a primer. Oakland (CA): California HealthCare Foundation; 2000.

75. Donabedian A. The definition of quality and approaches to its assessment. Chicago: Health Administration Press; 1980.

76. McGlynn E, Brook R. Ensuring quality of care. In: Andersen R, Rice T, Kominski G, editors. Changing the U.S. health care system: key issues in health services, policy, and management. San Francisco: Jossey-Bass; 1996.

77. McGlynn E. Quality of care for women: where are we and where are we headed? Women's Health Issues 1999;9(2):65–80.

78. Stafford R, Demet S Calusino N, Blumenthal D. Low rates of hormone replacement in visits to United States primary care physicians. Am J Obstet Gynecol 1997; 177(2):381–387.

79. California HealthCare Foundation. Geography is destiny: California variations in medical practice. In: Wennberg JE, Cooper MM, editors. The Dartmouth atlas of health care 1999. Chicago: American Hospital Association Press; 2000.

80. Bernstein S, McGlynn E, Siu A, Roth CP, Sherwood MJ, Keesey JW, et al. The appropriateness of hysterectomy: a comparison of care in seven health plans. JAMA 1993; 269:2398–402.

81. Sheifer SE, Escarce JJ, Schulman KA. Race and sex differences in the management of coronary artery disease. Am Heart J 2000; 139:848-857.

82. Iezzoni L, Ash A, Schwartz M, Mackiernan Y. Differences in procedure use, in-hospital mortality, and illness severity by gender for acute myocardial infarction patients: are answers affected by data source and severity measure? Med Care 1997;35(2):158–71.

83. National Committee for Quality Assurance. The health plan employer data and information set (HEDIS). Washington: National Committee for Quality Assurance. Available from: URL: www.ncqa.org.

84. National Committee for Quality Assurance. The state of managed care quality, 2000. Washington: The Committee; 2000.

85. Salganicoff A, Delbanco SF. Medicaid and managed care: meeting the reproductive needs of low-income women. J Public Health Manag Pract 1998;4(6):13–22.

86. Weisman C. Measuring quality in women's health care: issues and recent developments. Qual Manag Health Care 2000; 8(4): 14–20.

87. Committee on Quality of Health Care in America, Institute of Medicine. Crossing the quality chasm: a new health care system for the 21st century. Washington: National Academy Press; 2001.

Glossary

Age-adjusted rate

An age-adjusted rate is calculated to eliminate the effects of changes in the age composition of the population. Although these rates are not direct measures of mortality or morbidity, they are more useful than crude rates for assessing changes in risk over time and for comparing rates by sex or race because they take into account changes in the population size and age distribution. The National Center for Health Statistics calculates age-adjusted rates by applying age-specific rates to the U.S. standard million population, which is based on the relative age distribution of the 1940 population. Other age-adjusted rates may use different standard populations for adjustment.

Bacterial vaginosis (BV)

A vaginal infection in which there is an imbalance in the vaginal flora resulting in a predominance of gram-negative bacteria.

Birth cohort

A birth cohort consists of all persons born within a given time period.

Birth rate

The birth rate is calculated by dividing the number of live births in a population in a given year by the mid-year population. The rate can be restricted to births to women of specific age, race, marital status, or geographic location (birth-specific rates), or it can be related to the entire population (crude birth rate). It is expressed as the number of live births per 1,000 population.

Body mass index (BMI)

The BMI is calculated by dividing body weight measured in kilograms by the square of height measured in meters. This index is used to determine obesity and overweight categorizations.

Congenital

A congenital condition is one that is present at the time of birth.

Death rate

The death rate is calculated by dividing the number of deaths in a population in a given year by the mid-year population. The rate can be restricted to deaths in a specific age, race, sex, or geographic group or to deaths from specific causes, or it can be related to the entire population (crude death rate).

Discharge

The National Health Interview Survey defines a hospital discharge as the completion of any continuous period of stay of one night or more in a hospital as an inpatient, not including the period of stay of a well newborn infant. According to the National Hospital Discharge Survey and the American Hospital Association, discharge is the formal release of an inpatient by a hospital (excluding newborn infants), that is, the termination of a period of hospitalization (including stays of 0 nights) by death or by disposition to a place of residence, nursing home, or another hospital.

Endometrial ablation

Endometrial ablation is the removal of endometrial tissue, usually in women with abnormal bleeding. This can be done by hysterectomy, surgical removal of the endometrial tissue without removal of the uterus, or, more recently by thermal balloon methods (melting).

Endometriosis

Endometriosis is a disease of the reproductive system. Tiny cells of the endometrium, the lining of the uterus, move outside of the uterus and may implant on pelvic organs, pelvic walls, and the outside of ovaries or fallopian tubes. The condition is influenced by a woman's hormones. At the time of menstruation, these cells bleed in their new location, acting as if they are still in the uterus. This blood is absorbed by the organs nearby and causes inflammation. Over time, this disease can cause scarring and adhesions.

Episiotomy

An episiotomy is an incision into the perinatal body made before delivery to enlarge the area of the outlet and thereby facilitate delivery.

Estrogen

Estrogen is an ovarian hormone that is responsible for the sex characteristics of women and acts to regulate certain reproductive functions. A lack of estrogen has a significant effect on the health of postmenopausal women. Unopposed estrogen is estrogen given without progestin in hormone replacement therapy.

Fecund

A woman who is fecund is capable of having children.

Federal poverty level (FPL)

The U.S. Census Bureau defines poverty by using set of money income thresholds that vary by family size and composition. If a family's total income is less than that family's threshold, then that family, and every individual in it, is considered poor. The poverty thresholds do not vary geographically and are updated annually for inflation using the Consumer Price Index. The official poverty definition counts money income before taxes and does not include capital gains and noncash benefits (such as public housing, Medicaid, and food stamps). Poverty is not defined for people in military barracks, institutional group quarters, or for unrelated individuals under age 15 years (such as foster children).

Fee-for-service

A conventional indemnity system of payment that allows patients to choose any provider or location for health services. These doctors, hospitals, and other providers are paid a specific amount for each service performed, as identified by a claim for payment.

Fertility rate

The fertility rate is the number of live births per 1,000 women of reproductive age (15–44 years). It is calculated by dividing the number of reported live births in a population in a given year by the mid-year population of women 15–44 years of age.

Fetal death

The World Health Organization defines a fetal death as death before the complete expulsion or extraction from its mother of a product of conception, irrespective of the duration of pregnancy. The death is indicated by the fact that after such separation, the fetus does not breathe or show any other evidence of life, such as the beating of the heart, pulsation of the umbilical cord, or definite movement of voluntary muscles.

Fetal death rate

The fetal death rate is the number of fetal deaths with a stated or presumed gestation of 20 weeks or more divided by the sum of live births plus fetal deaths, stated per 1,000 live births plus fetal deaths. The late fetal death rate is the number of fetal deaths with a stated or presumed gestation of 28 weeks or more divided by the sum of live births plus late fetal deaths, stated per 1,000 live births plus late fetal deaths.

Five-year relative survival rate

The five-year relative survival rate is used as a measure of progress in detecting and treating cancer in its early stages. It takes normal life expectancy into account and provides an estimate of the proportion of persons with cancer that is potentially curable.

Gender

Gender refers to a person's self-representation as male or female, or how that person is responded to by social institutions based on the individual's gender presentation. Gender is rooted in biology and shaped by environment and experience.

Genital warts

Genital warts are cauliflower-like growths that are caused by the human papillomavirus (HPV).

Gestation

The National Vital Statistics System and the Centers for Disease Control and Prevention's Abortion Surveillance define the period of gestation as beginning with the first day of the last normal menstrual period and ending with the day of birth or day of termination of pregnancy.

Health maintenance organization (HMO)

A type of managed care plan that typically offers comprehensive health coverage for hospital, physician, and other health care services for a prepaid, fixed fee. HMOs contract with or directly employ health care providers. HMO enrollees are required to select their health care providers from a defined network of doctors and hospitals for all covered health care services.

Hispanic origin

Hispanic ethnicity includes persons of Mexican, Puerto Rican, Cuban, Central and South American, and other, unknown Spanish origins.

Hypertension

Hypertension is high blood pressure defined as a blood pressure of over 140 mmHg systolic and/or 90 mmHg diastolic.

Hysterectomy

A hysterectomy is a surgical procedure whereby a woman's uterus is removed. This procedure may be done via the abdomen or vagina.

Incidence

Incidence is a measure of morbidity or other events, expressed as the number of cases of disease having their onset during a prescribed period of time. It is often expressed as a rate.

Infant death

An infant death is the death of a live-born child before his or her first birthday. Deaths during the first year of life may be further classified according to age as neonatal and postneonatal. Neonatal deaths are those that occur before the 28th day of life; postneonatal deaths are those that occur between 28 and 365 days of age.

Infant mortality rate

The infant mortality rate is calculated by dividing the number of infant deaths during a calendar year by the number of live births reported in the same year. It is expressed as the number of infant deaths per 1,000 live births. The neonatal mortality rate is the number of deaths of children under 28 days of age per 1,000 live births. The postneonatal mortality rate is the number of deaths of children that occur between 28 days and 365 days after birth, per 1,000 live births.

Infecundity

Infecundity is the failure to achieve a live birth.

Infertility

Infertility is the inability of an individual or couple to achieve a recognized pregnancy after trying to conceive for more than 1 year (United States) or 2 years (World Health Organization).

Infertility, primary

Primary infertility is the absence of any prior pregnancy.

Infertility, secondary

Secondary infertility is when a woman or couple has achieved a prior pregnancy but fail to achieve additional pregnancies.

International Classification of Diseases, ninth edition (ICD-9)

The ICD codes mortality information for statistical purposes and is revised every 10 years.

Iron deficiency

According to the National Health and Nutrition Examination Survey III (NHANES III), iron deficiency is based on three laboratory tests of iron status: free erythrocyte protoporphyrin, transferrin, and serum ferritin, a similar approach as taken in NHANES II. To be considered iron deficient, an individual must have abnormal values for two or more indicators.

Iron deficiency anemia

Iron deficiency anemia is characterized by iron deficiency plus low hemoglobin.

Laparoscopy

A laparoscope is a device that allows doctors to view both the pelvic and upper abdominal regions. A laparoscopy is frequently used for tubal sterilizations and for diagnostic procedures to investigate infertility and pelvic pain.

Life expectancy

Life expectancy is the average number of years of life remaining to a person at a particular age and is based upon a given set of age-specific death rates, generally the mortality conditions existing in the period mentioned. Life expectancy can be determined by race, sex, or other characteristics using age-specific death rates for the population with that characteristic.

Live birth

The World Health Organization, the United Nations, and the National Center for Health Statistics define a live birth as the complete expulsion or extraction from its mother of a product of conception, irrespective of the duration of the pregnancy, which, after such separation, breathes or shows any other evidence of life such as heartbeat, umbilical cord pulsation, or definite movement of voluntary muscles, whether the umbilical cord has been cut or the placenta is attached. Each product of such a birth is considered liveborn.

Managed care

A broad term encompassing many different types of health care organizations, payment mechanisms, review mechanisms, and collaborations that link the financing and delivery of health care services. Managed care is sometimes used as a general term for the activity of organizing doctors, hospitals, and other providers into groups to enhance the quality and cost-effectiveness of health care. Managed care health plans typically include a review of medical necessity, incentives to use certain providers, and case management. While there are many types of managed care plans, the most common models are: health maintenance organizations (HMO), which are more heavily managed; point-of-service (POS) plans; and preferred provider organizations (PPOs), which are more loosely managed.

Marital status

Marital status is classified through self-reporting into the categories *married* and *unmarried*. The term *married* encompasses all married people including those separated from their spouses. *Unmarried* includes those who are single (never married), divorced, or widowed.

Maternal death

For a death to be classified as a maternal death, the certifying physician has to designate a maternal condition as the underlying cause of death.

Maternal mortality rate

The maternal mortality rate is defined as the number of maternal deaths per 100,000 live births. It is a measure of the likelihood that a pregnant woman will die from maternal causes. The number of live births used in the denominator is a proxy for the population of pregnant women who are at risk for maternal death.

Mean age

The mean age is the same as the average age.

Mistimed pregnancy

A mistimed pregnancy is one in which the woman expected to become pregnant but the pregnancy occurred earlier than anticipated.

Morbidity

Morbidity means illness or disease.

Myomectomy

Myomectomy is an alternative procedure to a hysterectomy. It is a way of removing fibroids either abdominally or vaginally without removing the uterus.

Nulliparity

Nulliparity means having had no prior live births.

Obesity

Current federal guidelines define moderate obesity as a body mass index (BMI) of 30.00 to 34.99 and severe obesity as a BMI greater than or equal to 35.00.

Oophorectomy

An oophorectomy is the surgical removal of the ovaries.

Outpatient visit

The American Hospital Association defines outpatient visits as visits for receipt of medical, dental, or other services by patients who are not lodged in the hospital. Each appearance by an outpatient to each unit of the hospital is counted individually as an outpatient visit.

Overweight

Current federal guidelines define overweight as a BMI of 25.00 to 29.99 (above normal weight but not obese).

Oxytocin

A hormone that stimulates uterine contractions.

Parity

Parity refers to the number of prior live births.

Pelvic inflammatory disease (PID)

A clinical syndrome resulting from the ascending spread of microorganisms from the vagina and endocervix to the endometrium, fallopian tubes, and/or contiguous structures. The Centers for Disease Control and Prevention (CDC) case definition can be found at www.cdc.gov/epo/mmwr/other/case_def/pelv_i97.html.

Point-of-service (POS) plan

A type of managed care arrangement that offers its enrollees the option to choose to receive a service from participating or nonparticipating providers, combining HMO features and out-of-network coverage. Enrollees can use health care providers outside of the plan's network, but the level of coverage generally decreases (or cost-sharing is increased) when services are received from nonparticipating providers.

Polychlorinated biphenyls (PCBs)

These chemical compounds are used in many products, including electrical transformers and paints. The Environmental Protection Agency banned the manufacture of PCBs, but they remain in the environment and may adversely affect individuals as an environmental toxin.

Perinatal mortality rate

The perinatal mortality rate is the sum of late fetal deaths plus infant deaths within 7 days of birth divided by the sum of live births plus late fetal deaths.

Preferred provider organization (PPO)

A type of managed care plan that contracts with independent providers to provide services at discounted fees for members. Members may also seek care from nonparticipating providers but generally are penalized financially for doing so by the loss of the discount and can be subject to higher copayments and/or deductibles.

Prevalence

Prevalence is the number of cases of a disease, infected persons, or persons with some other attribute present during a particular interval of time. It is often expressed as a rate.

Prevention, primary

Primary prevention is an action to prevent the development of disease.

Prevention, secondary

Secondary prevention is the early identification of people who have developed a particular disease at an early stage in the disease's natural history by effective screening or early intervention.

Prevention, tertiary

Tertiary prevention is the treatment of disease.

Preterm birth

A preterm birth occurs through the end of the last day of the 37th week after the onset of the last menstrual period.

Progestin

Progestin is any natural or synthetic form of progesterone, an ovarian hormone.

Sensitivity

The sensitivity of a test is the ability for that test to correctly identify those individuals who have the disease.

Sequelae

Complications or adverse effects following an attack of disease.

Sex

Sex refers to the classification of living things as male or female according to their reproductive organs and functions assigned by chromosomal complement.

Specificity

The specificity of a test is the ability for that test to correctly identify those individuals who do not have the disease.

Unwanted pregnancy

An unwanted pregnancy is one in which the woman does not anticipate pregnancy at that time or any time in the future.

Uterine artery embolization

Uterine artery embolization is a procedure that occludes blood flow into uterine arteries with the intent of cutting off the hormonal supply to the fibroid.

Uterine fibroids

Uterine fibroids or leiomyomas are noncancerous masses of muscle and connective tissue in the walls of the uterus and one of the most common conditions affecting premenopausal women.

Women, Infants and Children (WIC) program

The WIC program provides nutritional assessment, counseling, and education to poor pregnant or lactating women and their children up to age 5 years.

Frequently Cited Data Sources

The Commonwealth Fund Survey of Women's Health

The Commonwealth Fund Survey of Women's Health was a telephone interview survey conducted in 1995 and 1998 among a cross-sectional national sample of women 18 years of age and older in the United States. The goal of the survey was to collect information regarding significant health concerns such as access to health care, employment and marital status, mental health, and violence and abuse. The 1998 survey included 2,011 women, with an oversampling of minorities, blacks, Hispanics, and Asian Americans. Further information on the Commonwealth Fund and updated facts and figures may be obtained at the Fund's Website located at www.cmwf.org.

Continuing Survey of Food Intake by Individuals (CSFII)

During 1994–96, 16,103 people nationwide participated in the CSFII, popularly known as the "What We Eat in America" survey. Two nonconsecutive days of food intake data for individuals of all ages were collected 3–10 days apart during in-person interviews between January 1994 and January 1997, using the 24-hour recall method. The data are used to provide national probability estimates for the U.S. population. Estimates are based on combined data from all 3 years of the U.S. Department of Agriculture's (USDA) 10th nationwide food consumption survey. In future years, this survey will be integrated with the National Health and Nutrition Examination Survey (NHANES) to form the National Food and Nutrition Survey (NFNS). Further information is available at the Website supported by the USDA located at www.barc.usda.gov/bhnrc/foodsurvey/home.htm.

Epidemiologic Catchment Area (ECA) Program

The Epidemiologic Catchment Area (ECA) program of the National Institute of Mental Health (NIMH) was the first community-based study to provide prevalence rates of mental disorders in the United States. Although the ECA was not based on a national probability sample, data from five "catchment areas" (portions of New Haven, Connecticut; Baltimore, Maryland; Durham, North Carolina; St. Louis, Missouri; and Los Angeles, California) were expected to provide more reliable estimates than had been previously available.[1] Between 1980 and 1984, adults aged 18 years and older in each catchment area were selected to be interviewed.[1] Elderly, African American, and/or Hispanic residents were oversampled to allow for more precise estimates in these subgroups of the population. Subjects were interviewed using the NIMH Diagnostic Interview Scale, an instrument that uses DSM-III diagnostic criteria. Interview completion rates in each of the catchment areas ranged from 68% to 79%.[1]

National Center for Health Statistics (NCHS)

The National Center for Health Statistics (NCHS) is the federal government's principal vital and health statistics agency. Since 1960, when the National Office of Vital Statistics and the National Health Survey merged to form NCHS, the agency has provided a wide variety of data with which to monitor the nation's health. The data systems for NCHS include data on vital events as well as information on health status, lifestyle, exposure to unhealthy influences, the onset and diagnosis of illness and disability, and the use of health care services. Vital statistics are provided through state-operated registration systems of vital events such as births, deaths, marriages, divorces, and fetal deaths. Further information on the activities of the NCHS may be obtained through the CDC-maintained Website located at www.cdc.gov/nchs/.

National Center for HIV, STD, and TB Prevention (NCHSTP), Division of Sexually Transmitted Diseases

The NCHSTP is responsible for public health surveillance, prevention research, and programs to prevent and control HIV infection, AIDS, other STDs, and tuberculosis (TB). Center staff work in collaboration with governmental and nongovernmental partners at community, state, and national levels in the estimation of the incidence and prevalence of HIV, STD, and TB and the tracking of trends at all levels of government. Further information on current NCHSTP activities and updated fact and figures on HIV and STD incidence and prevalence may be obtained at the CDC-maintained Website located at www.cdc.gov/nchstp/od/nchstp.html.

National Comorbidity Survey (NCS)

The National Comorbidity Survey (NCS) was a nationally representative sample survey that was designed to study the comorbidity of psychiatric disorders and substance use disorders in the United States.[2] The survey was based on a stratified probability sample of the civilian noninstitutionalized population ages 15 to 54 years.[2] Subjects were interviewed in person by staff from the University of Michigan Survey Research Center, using a modified version of the Composite International Diagnostic Interview (CIDI) between September 14, 1990, and February 6, 1992.[2] The CIDI utilized the DSM-III-R diagnostic criteria and the response rate was 82.6%.

National Crime Victimization Survey (NCVS)

The U.S. Department of Justice's National Crime Victimization Survey gathers data on criminal victimization though a national sample of approximately 49,000 households. Respondents are included in the sample for 3 years and are interviewed at 6-month intervals. Unlike the FBI's Uniform Crime Reporting Program, the NCVS provides annual estimates of crimes, regardless of whether a law enforcement agency was contacted about the incident. The NCVS was extensively redesigned in the early 1990s to produce more accurate reporting of incidents of rape, sexual assault, and intimate and family violence. Questions were added to ensure respondents know that the survey is interested in a broad spectrum of crimes, not just those involving weapons, severe violence, or violence perpetrated by strangers. New methods of cueing respondents about experiences with victimizations increased the range of incident types reported. Criminal justice terminology was replaced with behavior-specific wording to make the questions more understandable.

National Health and Nutrition Examination Survey (NHANES)

The National Health and Nutrition Examination Survey (NHANES) is conducted by the National Center for Health Statistics (NCHS) and is designed to collect information about the health and diet of people in the United States. Among the various surveys, NHANES is unique in that it combines a home interview with direct measures of health via physical examination and blood tests conducted on participants. The first program, the National Health Examination Survey (NHES 1960–1962), focused on estimating the total prevalence of chronic disease and the distributions of various physical and physiologic measures, including blood pressure and serum cholesterol levels, among the sample of adults aged 18–79 years surveyed. NHES II (1963–1965) and NHES III (1966–1970) focused on the growth and development of children.

The first cycle of NHANES, or NHANES I (1971-1974), focused on chronic disease, specifically cardiovascular, respiratory, arthritic, and hearing conditions among adults, with the addition of the measurement of the nutritional status of the participants. In NHANES II (1976–1980), the nutritional component was expanded and focus was directed toward the measurement of diabetes, kidney and liver function, allergy, and speech pathology among the participants. The NHANES I and NHANES II focused on the general U.S. population between 1982 and 1984, and the Hispanic Health and Nutrition Examination Survey (HHANES) focused on specific ethnic groups, namely Mexican Americans, Cuban Americans, and Puerto Ricans. Recognizing the increasing burden of chronic disease among minority groups, the most recent

survey, NHANES III (1988–1994), included an oversampling of both black and Mexican Americans. NHANES III included participants as young as 2 months of age and adults with no upper age limit and focused on the effects of the environment upon health.

The current NHANES is the eighth in the series of national examination studies conducted in the United States since 1960. Approximately 5,000 national participants are screened using sample selection, followed by detailed household interviews. Sample individuals are invited to receive physical examinations and health and dietary interviews in mobile examination centers. Various medical tests and procedures are conducted to enable analysis of the relationship between health and nutrition status and disease risk factors, to measure the prevalence and co-morbidity of diseases and disorders, to establish reference standards, and to monitor secular trends in health and nutrition status. Beginning in 1999, NHANES became a continuous, annual survey that can be linked to related federal government surveys of the general U.S. population, specifically the National Health Interview Survey (NHIS) and, in the future, the U.S. Department of Agriculture's (USDA) Continuing Survey of Food Intakes by Individuals (CSFII). In January 2001, the USDA CSFII study will merge with NHANES to form the National Food and Nutrition Survey (NFNS). Further information on current NHANES activities and updated fact and figures may be obtained at the CDC-maintained Website located at www.cdc.gov/nchs/nhanes.htm.

National Health Interview Survey

The National Health Interview Survey (NHIS) is the principal source of information on the health of the civilian, noninstitutionalized population of the United States and is one of the major data collection programs of the National Center for Health Statistics (NCHS). The NHIS, initiated in July 1957, is a cross-sectional household interview survey conducted throughout each year among a sample of the population selected from each state. The NHIS data are collected annually through a personal household interview currently including approximately 43,000 households including about 106,000 persons. The annual response rate of NHIS is greater than 90 percent of the eligible households in the sample. Patients in long-term care facilities, persons on active duty with the armed forces (though their dependents are included), and U.S. nationals living in foreign countries are excluded from the survey. Because it is an annual survey, the NHIS allows public health researchers and policy makers to monitor trends in illness and disability and track progress toward achieving national health objectives. Further information on current NHIS activities and updated fact and figures may be obtained at the CDC-maintained Website located at www.cdc.gov/nchs/nhis.htm.

National Household Survey on Drug Abuse (NHSDA)

National Household Survey on Drug Abuse is the primary source of information on the prevalence, patterns, and consequences of drug and alcohol use and abuse in the general U.S. civilian, noninstitutionalized population, aged 12 years and older. Conducted each year by the federal government since 1971, the survey collects data by administering questionnaires to representative samples of the population at their place of residence. The survey covers residents of households, noninstitutional group quarters (e.g., shelters, rooming houses, dormitories), and civilians living on military bases. Persons excluded from the survey include homeless people who do not use shelters, active military personnel, and residents of institutional group quarters, such as jails and hospitals. Since October 1, 1992, the survey has been sponsored by the Substance Abuse and Mental Health Services Administration (SAMHSA). Further information on current NHSDA activities and updated fact and figures on substance abuse may be obtained at the SAMHSA Website located at www.samhsa.gov/.

National Maternal and Infant Health Survey (NMIHS)

The goal of the National Maternal and Infant Health Survey (NMIHS) is to collect data on factors related to poor pregnancy outcomes, including low birth weight, stillbirth, infant illness, and infant death. The NMIHS provides data on socioeconomic and demographic characteristics of mothers, prenatal care, pregnancy history, occupational background, health status of mother and infant, and types and sources of medical care received. The NMIHS is a "follow-back survey" meaning that it follows back informants named on vital records, such as birth and death certificates. The 1988 survey expanded on information available for birth, fetal death, and infant death vital records and is the first national survey that included data on those three pregnancy outcomes simultaneously. The latest NMIHS is based on questionnaires administered to nationally representative samples of mothers with live births, stillbirths, and infant deaths during 1988 and to physicians, hospitals, and other medical care providers associated with those outcomes. The survey is based on 10,000 live births, 4,000 fetal deaths, and 6,000 infant deaths. In 2000, a birth cohort study was planned in conjunction with the National Center for Education Statistics. Further information on current activities of the NMIHS and updated facts and figures on trends in maternal and infant health outcomes may be obtained through the CDC–maintained Website located at www.cdc.gov/nchs/about/major/nmihs/abnmihs.htm.

National Survey of Family Growth (NSFG)

The National Survey of Family Growth (NSFG) is a multipurpose survey based on personal interviews with a national sample of women 15–44 years of age in the civilian, noninstitutionalized population of the United States. The goal of the survey is to collect data on factors affecting pregnancy and women's health in the United States, such as the number of children women have had, intended and mistimed pregnancies, contracep tive use, infertility, impaired fecundity, and sterilization operations. Previous NSFG surveys were conducted in 1973, 1976, 1982, 1988, and 1990. The latest survey was conducted in 1995. Further information on current NSFG activities and updated facts and figures may be obtained at the CDC-maintained Website located at www.cdc.gov/nchs/nsfg.htm.

National Violence Against Women Survey (NVAW)

The National Violence Against Women Survey is a joint effort by the National Institute of Justice of the U.S. Department of Justice and the CDC of the U.S. Department of Health and Human Services. The survey, conducted from November 1995 to May 1996, involved interviewing a national sample of 8,000 women and 8,000 men aged 18 years and older. The survey screening questions gathered data on rape, physical assault, and stalking. The NVAW survey data are designed to be compared with the National Crime Victimization Survey (NCVS) to determine whether a dedicated ongoing survey, such as the NVAW, is needed on incidence and prevalence of violence against women.

Pregnancy-Related Mortality Surveillance System (PRMSS)

In 1987, the CDC's Division of Reproductive Health began to collect data on all deaths related to pregnancy through the PRMSS. A death is considered to be pregnancy related, and thus a maternal death, if it occurs during pregnancy or within 1 year of pregnancy termination and results from one of the following: (1) complications of the pregnancy itself, (2) a chain of events initiated by pregnancy, or (3) aggravation of an unrelated event by the physiologic effects of pregnancy. The number of maternal deaths identified through PRMSS classification is over 50% greater than the number classified using standard death certificate data.[3] Nevertheless, the PRMSS still cannot identify all pregnancy-related deaths, particularly those for which a record of the preg

nancy outcome is not generated, for example, in the case of an ectopic pregnancy.

Surveillance, Epidemiology, and End Results (SEER)

The Surveillance, Epidemiology, and End Results (SEER) program is a population-based system of registries funded by the National Cancer Institute (NCI). It is an outgrowth of the National Cancer Act of 1971, which included a mandate to collect, analyze, and disseminate data that would aid in the prevention, diagnosis, and treatment of cancer. The SEER program is composed of 11 registries in five states (Connecticut, Hawaii, Iowa, New Mexico, and Utah) and six metropolitan areas (Atlanta, Detroit, Los Angeles, San Francisco/Oakland, San Jose/Monterey, and Seattle/Puget Sound) covering about 14% of the U.S. population. The SEER program generates national estimates of cancer incidence for most cancer sites twice a year from a nonrandom, national sample for blacks, whites, and all races combined, and also by gender (with special monographs for other ethnic/racial groups). The registries provide data on all newly diagnosed cancer patients and give current follow-up information on previously diagnosed patients who were residents of the covered geographic areas at the time of initial diagnosis. Cases are followed annually to determine survival. The NCI processes, aggregates, and analyzes data from these 11 registries, along with cancer-related death records from the National Center for Health Statistics (NCHS). Further information on current SEER activities and updated facts and figures on trends in cancer incidence, prevalence and survival may be obtained at the Website maintained by the NCI located at www.seer.ims.nci.nih.gov/.

Uniform Crime Reporting Program (UCR)

The FBI's Uniform Crime Reporting Program annually compiles data on eight categories of crime (including homicide, rape, and aggravated assault) brought to the attention of law enforcement agencies nationwide. Over 16,000 city, county, and state agencies voluntarily submit summary reports on crimes within their jurisdictions on a monthly basis. Two additional components of the UCR—the National Incident-Based Reporting Program and the Supplementary Homicide Reports—provide further detail on the victim-perpetrator relationship in violent crimes. Because many crimes go unreported, UCR estimates are not considered comprehensive. For further information, see the Website at www.fbi.gov/ucr/ucr.htm.

Youth Risk Behavior Surveillance System (YRBSS)

The Youth Risk Behavior Surveillance System (YRBSS) monitors six categories of priority health-risk behaviors among youth and young adults—behaviors that contribute to unintentional and intentional injuries; tobacco use; alcohol and other drug use; sexual behaviors that contribute to unintended pregnancy and STDs (including HIV infection); unhealthy dietary behaviors; and physical inactivity. The YRBSS includes a national, school-based survey, the Youth Risk Behavior Survey (YRBS) conducted by CDC, as well as state, territorial, and local, school-based surveys conducted by education and health agencies. The first national, school-based YRBS was completed in 1990, and repeat surveys have been conducted every other year since 1991. The national YRBS is based on a national probability sample, and the data are representative of students in grades nine to 12 in public and private schools in the 50 states and the District of Columbia. In the 1999 YRBS, 15,349 surveys were completed by students in 144 schools across the nation, and the overall response rate was 66%. Further information on current YRBS activities and updated fact and figures may be obtained at the CDC-maintained Website located at www.cdc.gov/nccdphp/dash/yrbs/index.htm.

References

1. Regier DA, Boyd JH, Burke JD Jr, Rae DS, Myers JK, Kramer M, et al. One-month prevalence of mental disorders in the United States: based on five epidemiologic catchment area sites. Arch Gen Psychiatry 1988;45:977–986.

2. Kessler RC, McGonagle KA, Zhao S, Nelson CB, Hughes M, Eshleman S, et al. Lifetime and 12-month prevalence of DSM-III-R psychiatric disorders in the United States. Results from the National Comorbidity Survey. Arch Gen Psychiatry 1994;51:8–19.

3. Berg CJ, Atrash HK, Koonin LM, Tucker M. Pregnancy-related mortality in the United States 1987–1990. Obstet Gynecol 1996;88:161–167.

Index

and calcium, 135

and cancers, 75, 76, 83, 84, 85, 86, 87-88

and chronic conditions, 64, 65, 69

and diabetes, 73, 74

and eating disorders, 112, 113

and health care utilization, 177

and health conditions related to reproduction, 37, 39, 40

and heart/cardiovascular disease, 69-70

and hormone replacement therapy, 138

and illicit drugs, 127-28, 129

impact on women's health of, 2-3, 7

and infections, 47

and influenza and pneumonia, 59, 60

and iron, 136

and labor force participation, 7

mean, 196

and mental disorders, 105-6, 109-10, 111

and physical activity, 131, 132

and pregnancy and childbirth, 14-15, 17, 19-20, 22, 27, 30, 33, 35

and reproductive tract infections, 47-48, 49, 50, 53, 56, 57, 59

and smoking, 118, 119, 121, 123

and social and economic impacts on women's health, 2-3, 7

and vaginal douching, 141

and violence against women, 150, 153, 154-55, 159

women of childbearing, 14-15

Age-adjusted rate, 192

Agency for Health Care Policy and Research, 88

Agency for Healthcare Research and Quality, 164

Agoraphobia, 111

Agriculture, U.S. Department of, 133, 136, 202

AIDS. See Acquired immunodeficiency syndrome

Alan Guttmacher Institute, 15, 27

Alaskan Natives, 35, 47, 49, 53, 74, 131, 132, 159

Alcohol, 69, 79, 84, 110, 120-21, 124-26, 129, 130, 136, 205

Alzheimer's disease, 93

Amenorrhea, 112

American Academy of Pediatrics, 35

American Cancer Society, 85, 87

American College of Obstetricians and Gynecologists, 35

American Hospital Association, 193, 197

American Indians

and alcohol, 125, 126

and cervical cancer, 81

and diabetes, 74

and health care utilization, 182

and illicit drugs, 129

and physical activity, 131, 132

and pregnancy and childbirth, 35

and reproductive tract infections, 47, 49, 53

and smoking, 119

and violence against women, 159

Anemia, 136, 195

Anorexia nervosa, 112

Antenatal maternal health, 30-32

Antibiotics, 51, 59

Antidepressants, 108, 112

Anti-inflammatory drugs, 92

Antiretroviral therapy, 57

Antisocial personality disorder, 104

Antiviral therapy, 54

Anxiety, 104, 105, 110-11, 151, 154

Apolipoprotein E (APOE), 93

Arthritis, 65, 88-90, 175, 176

Arthritis Foundation, 89

Asbestos, 86, 87

Asian Americans, 3-4, 8, 90, 119, 120, 125, 126, 131

Asian/Pacific Islanders, 48, 49, 53, 69, 74, 81, 87 129, 159

Assault, 150, 153-56, 160, 204

Assisted reproductive technologies (ART), 24

Asthma, 31, 64, 65, 185

Atherosclerotic peripheral vascular disease, 123

Autoimmune diseases, 89, 92. See also specific disease

Azithromycin, 49, 50-51

B

Bacterial infections, 156

Bacterial vaginosis (BV), 36, 46, 58-59, 141, 192

Balanced Budget Act (1997), 172

Behavioral problems, 126, 129

Behavioral Risk Factor Surveillance System (BRFSS), 88, 120, 125, 130, 132, 133, 134, 178-79

Behavioral therapy, 112

Benzathine penicilin G, 53

Benzodiazepines, 126

Birth centers, 34

Birth certificates, 32, 180

Birth cohort, 192

Birth rate, 192

Birth. See Childbirth